Learning Disabilities Sourcebook, 3rd Edition

Leukemia Sourcebook

Liver Disorders Sourcebook

Lung Disorders Sourcebook

Medical Tests Sourcebook, 3rd Edition

Men's Health Concerns Sourcebook, 2nd Edition

Mental Health Disorders Sourcebook, 4th Edition

Mental Retardation Sourcebook

Movement Disorders Sourcebook, 2nd Edition

Multiple Sclerosis Sourcebook

Muscular Dystrophy Sourcebook

Obesity Sourcebook

Osteoporosis Sourcebook

Pain Sourcebook, 3rd Edition

Pediatric Cancer Sourcebook

Physical & Mental Issues in Aging Sourcebook

Podiatry Sourcebook, 2nd Edition

Pregnancy & Birth Sourcebook, 2nd Edition

Prostate & Urological Disorders Sourcebook

Prostate Cancer Sourcebook

Reconstructive & Cosmetic Surgery Sourcebook

Rehabilitation Sourcebook

Respiratory Disorders Sourcebook, 2nd Edition

Sexually Transmitted Diseases Sourcebook, 3rd Edition

Sleep Disorders Sourcebook, 3rd Edition

Smoking Concerns Sourcebook

Sports Injuries Sourcebook, 3rd Edition

Stress-Related Disorders Sourcebook, 2nd Edition

Stroke Sourcebook, 2nd Edition

Surgery Sourcebook, 2nd Edition

Thyroid Disorders Sourcebook

Transplantation Sourcebook

Traveler's Health Sourcebook

Urinary Tract & Kidney Diseases & Disorders Sourcebook, 2nd Edition

Vegetarian Sourcebook

Women's Health Concerns Sourcebook, 3rd Edition

Workplace Health & Safety Sourcebook

Worldwide Health Sourcebook

Teen Health Series

Abuse & Violence Information for Teens

Accident & Safety Information for Teens

Alcohol Information for Teens, 2nd Edition

Allergy Information for Teens

Asthma Information for Teens, 2nd Edition

Body Information for Teens

Cancer Information for Teens

Complementary & Alternative Medicine Information for Teens

Diabetes Information for Teens

Diet Information for Teens, 2nd Edition

Drug Information for Teens, 3rd Edition

Eating Disorders Information for Teens, 2nd Edition

Fitness Information for Teens, 2nd Edition

Learning Disabilities Information for Teens

Mental Health Information for Teens, 3rd Edition

Pregnancy Information for Teens

Sexual Health Information for Teens, 2nd Edition

Skin Health Information for Teens, 2nd Edition

Sleep Information for Teens

Sports Injuries Information for Teens, 2nd Edition

Stress Information for Teens

Suicide Information for Teens, 2nd Edition

Tobacco Information for Teens, 2nd Edition

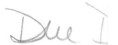

DATE DUE

JUN 03 2013	
MAY 24 2016	
NOV 03 2016	

GAYLORD   PRINTED IN U.S.A.

Complementary and Alternative Medicine
SOURCEBOOK

Fourth Edition

Health Reference Series

Fourth Edition

Complementary and Alternative Medicine SOURCEBOOK

Basic Consumer Health Information about Ayurveda, Acupuncture, Aromatherapy, Chiropractic Care, Diet-Based Therapies, Guided Imagery, Herbal and Vitamin Supplements, Homeopathy, Hypnosis, Massage, Meditation, Naturopathy, Pilates, Reflexology, Reiki, Shiatsu, Tai Chi, Traditional Chinese Medicine, Yoga, and Other Complementary and Alternative Medical Therapies

Along with Statistics, Tips for Selecting a Practitioner, Treatments for Specific Health Conditions, a Glossary of Related Terms, and a Directory of Resources for Additional Help and Information

Edited by
Amy L . Sutton

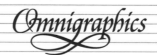

Omnigraphics

P.O. Box 31-1640, Detroit, MI 48231

Bibliographic Note
Because this page cannot legibly accommodate all the copyright notices, the Bibliographic Note portion of the Preface constitutes an extension of the copyright notice.

Edited by Amy L. Sutton

Health Reference Series

Karen Bellenir, *Managing Editor*
David A. Cooke, MD, FACP, *Medical Consultant*
Elizabeth Collins, *Research and Permissions Coordinator*
Cherry Edwards, *Permissions Assistant*
EdIndex, Services for Publishers, *Indexers*

* * *

Omnigraphics, Inc.
Matthew P. Barbour, *Senior Vice President*
Kevin M. Hayes, *Operations Manager*

* * *

Peter E. Ruffner, *Publisher*

Copyright © 2010 Omnigraphics, Inc.
ISBN 978-0-7808-1082-2

Library of Congress Cataloging-in-Publication Data

Complementary and alternative medicine sourcebook : basic consumer health information about ayurveda, acupuncture, aromatherapy, chiropractic care, diet-based therapies, guided imagery, herbal and vitamin supplements, homeopathy, hypnosis, massage, meditation, naturopathy, pilates, reflexology, reiki, shiatsu, tai chi, traditional chinese medicine, yoga, and other complementary and alternative medical therapies ; along with statistics, tips for selecting a practitioner, treatments for specific health conditions, a glossary of related terms, and a directory of resources for additional help and information / edited by Amy L. Sutton. -- 4th ed.
   p. cm. -- (Health reference series)
  Includes bibliographical references and index.
  Summary: "Provides basic consumer health information about alternative and complementary medical therapies, including treatments for specific diseases and conditions. Includes index, glossary of related terms, and other resources"--Provided by publisher.
  ISBN 978-0-7808-1082-2 (hardcover : alk. paper) 1. Alternative medicine--Popular works. I. Sutton, Amy L.
  R735.C66 2010
  610--dc22
                              2010013183

The information in this publication was compiled from the sources cited and from other sources considered reliable. While every possible effort has been made to ensure reliability, the publisher will not assume liability for damages caused by inaccuracies in the data, and makes no warranty, express or implied, on the accuracy of the information contained herein.

This book is printed on acid-free paper meeting the ANSI Z39.48 Standard. The infinity symbol that appears above indicates that the paper in this book meets that standard.

Printed in the United States

Table of Contents

Visit www.healthreferenceseries.com to view *A Contents Guide to the Health Reference Series*, a listing of more than 15,000 topics and the volumes in which they are covered.

Preface xi

Part I: An Overview of Complementary and Alternative Medicine (CAM)

Chapter 1—What Is Complementary and Alternative
           Medicine (CAM)? 3

Chapter 2—Common Questions and Answers about CAM 7

Chapter 3—The Use of CAM in the United States 13

Chapter 4—CAM Use and Children 17

Chapter 5—CAM Use in Older Adults 21

Chapter 6—Health Care Providers and CAM 31
        Section 6.1—Selecting a CAM Practitioner 32
        Section 6.2—Tips for Talking with Your
                Health Care Providers
                about CAM 37

Chapter 7—Insurance Issues and Paying
           for CAM Treatment 39

Chapter 8—Health Fraud Awareness 45

Chapter 9—Use Caution Buying Medical Products Online 51

Part II: Alternative Medicine Systems

Chapter 10—What Are Whole Medical Systems? 59

Chapter 11—Ayurvedic Medicine 65

Chapter 12—Other Indigenous Medical Systems 73

    Section 12.1—Traditional Chinese
               Medicine...................................... 74

    Section 12.2—Native American Medicine 78

Chapter 13—Acupuncture.. 81

Chapter 14—Homeopathy 85

Chapter 15—Naturopathy... 91

Part III: Dietary Supplements

Chapter 16—Questions and Answers about
           Dietary Supplements............................ 101

Chapter 17—Botanical Dietary Supplements 107

Chapter 18—Using Dietary Supplements Wisely 111

Chapter 19—Adolescents and Supplement Use...................... 117

Chapter 20—Tips for Older Dietary Supplement Users........... 121

Chapter 21—Vitamin A and Carotenoids................................ 129

Chapter 22—Vitamin B_6 137

Chapter 23—Vitamin B_{12} 143

Chapter 24—Vitamin D... 147

Chapter 25—Vitamin E 153

Chapter 26—Folate (Folic Acid) 161

Chapter 27—Magnesium... 169

Chapter 28—Omega-3 Fatty Acid Supplements 175

    Section 28.1—Fish Oils.................................... 176

    Section 28.2—Flaxseed and Flaxseed Oils 190

Chapter 29—Selenium... 193

Chapter 30—Bone and Joint Health Supplements................... 197

    Section 30.1—Calcium Supplements
               and Bone Health....................... 198

Section 30.2—Glucosamine/Chondroitin Supplements and Joint Health 201

Chapter 31—Immune System Support Supplements 205

Section 31.1—Echinacea 206

Section 31.2—Zinc 208

Chapter 32—Mood and Brain Health Supplements 213

Section 32.1—Ginkgo Biloba 214

Section 32.2—St. John's Wort 216

Chapter 33—Probiotics: Supplements for Gastrointestinal Health 219

Chapter 34—Sports and Energy Supplements 225

Section 34.1—Sports Supplements 226

Section 34.2—Energy Drinks 231

Chapter 35—Supplements Used for Weight Loss 235

Section 35.1—Green Tea 236

Section 35.2—Hoodia 238

Part IV: Biologically Based Therapies

Chapter 36—Biologically Based Therapies: An Overview 243

Chapter 37—Apitherapy 253

Chapter 38—Aromatherapy and Essential Oils 257

Chapter 39—Diet-Based Therapies 263

Section 39.1—Detoxification Diets 264

Section 39.2—Fasting 267

Section 39.3—Gerson Therapy 269

Section 39.4—Macrobiotics 273

Section 39.5—Veganism 275

Section 39.6—Vegetarianism 279

Chapter 40—Oxygen Therapy 285

Part V: Mind-Body Medicine

Chapter 41—Mind-Body Medicine: An Overview 293

Chapter 42—Art Therapy 299

Chapter 43—Biofeedback 303

Chapter 44—Deep Breathing Exercises 311

Chapter 45—Feng Shui 317

Chapter 46—Guided Imagery and Hypnosis........................... 321

    Section 46.1—Guided Imagery........................ 322

    Section 46.2—Hypnosis 324

Chapter 47—Meditation 329

Chapter 48—Music Therapy 335

Chapter 49—Prayer and Spirituality 341

Chapter 50—Relaxation Training..................................... 345

Chapter 51—Tai Chi... 349

Chapter 52—Yoga 353

Chapter 53—Other Mind-Body Medicine
    Therapies.. 357

    Section 53.1—Color Therapy.......................... 358

    Section 53.2—Dance Therapy......................... 359

Part VI: Manipulative and Body-Based Therapies

Chapter 54—Manipulative and Body-Based Therapies:
    An Overview... 363

Chapter 55—Alexander Technique 371

Chapter 56—Aquatic Therapy (Hydrotherapy)....................... 383

Chapter 57—Chiropractic Care and Osteopathic
    Manipulation... 399

Chapter 58—Craniosacral Therapy 403

Chapter 59—Feldenkrais Method..................................... 407

Chapter 60—Massage Therapy 413

    Section 60.1—Massage Therapy Overview..... 414

    Section 60.2—Lymphatic Drainage
        Massage 419

    Section 60.3—Tui Na: Chinese Massage 421

Chapter 61—Pilates.. 423

Chapter 62—Qigong 427

Chapter 63—Reflexology 431

Chapter 64—Structural Integration Techniques 435

    Section 64.1—Hellerwork Structural
                 Integration............................... 436

    Section 64.2—Rolfing.. 438

Chapter 65—Other Manipulative and Body-Based
    Therapies... 447

    Section 65.1—Applied Kinesiology................. 448

    Section 65.2—Bowen Technique...................... 449

    Section 65.3—Trager Approach...................... 450

Part VII: Energy-Based Therapies

Chapter 66—Energy Medicine: An Overview............................ 455

Chapter 67—Magnet Therapy.. 463

Chapter 68—Polarity Therapy 467

Chapter 69—Reiki 471

Chapter 70—Shiatsu 475

Chapter 71—Therapeutic Touch 479

Chapter 72—Other Energy-Based Therapies........................... 483

    Section 72.1—Bioresonance Therapy.............. 484

    Section 72.2—Crystal and Gem Therapy........ 486

    Section 72.3—Zero Balancing......................... 487

Part VIII: Alternative Treatments for Specific Diseases and Conditions

Chapter 73—Arthritis and CAM.. 491

Chapter 74—Asthma, Allergies, and CAM 503

Chapter 75—Cancer and CAM... 507

Chapter 76—Cognitive Decline and CAM 517

Chapter 77—Diabetes and CAM.. 523

Chapter 78—Fibromyalgia and CAM 529

Chapter 79—Headache and CAM 533

Chapter 80—Heart Disease and Chelation Therapy 537

Chapter 81—Hepatitis C and CAM 541

Chapter 82—Hormones, CAM, and Aging 547

Chapter 83—Infertility and CAM 559

    Section 83.1—Herbal Remedies for
             Infertility 560

    Section 83.2—Infertility and CAM 561

Chapter 84—Low Back Pain and CAM 563

Chapter 85—Menopausal Symptoms and CAM 567

Chapter 86—Mental Health Care and CAM 573

    Section 86.1—Overview of CAM Used in
             Mental Health Care 574

    Section 86.2—Alcohol Addiction and
             Electroacupuncture 579

    Section 86.3—Attention Deficit
             Hyperactivity Disorder
             (ADHD) and CAM 580

    Section 86.4—Anxiety and Self-Hypnosis 582

    Section 86.5—Posttraumatic Stress Disorder
             and Acupuncture 583

Chapter 87—Sleep Disorders and CAM 585

Part IX: Additional Help and Information

Chapter 88—Glossary of Terms Related to Alternative
    and Complementary Medicine 593

Chapter 89—Directory of Organizations That Provide
    Information about Alternative and
    Complementary Medicine 599

Index... 615

Preface

About This Book

Complementary and alternative medicine (CAM) therapies play a key role in the health care of many Americans. The National Center for Complementary and Alternative Medicine reports that in the United States, about four in 10 adults and about one in nine children use some form of CAM, such as deep breathing, dietary supplements, massage, meditation, or yoga. CAM, alone or in conjunction with mainstream medicine, is often used to treat an increasing variety of diseases and conditions, such as arthritis, anxiety, back pain, cancer, diabetes, heart disease, and sleep problems.

Complementary and Alternative Medicine Sourcebook, Fourth Edition provides updated information for people considering these therapies for general well-being or specific health conditions. It discusses how to select a CAM practitioner, talk with a primary health care provider about using CAM, evaluate information on the internet, and pay for CAM therapies. It describes whole medical systems, such as Ayurveda, traditional Chinese medicine, Native American medicine, acupuncture, homeopathy, and naturopathy. It also talks about the safe use of dietary supplements, including vitamins, minerals, and herbs. Information on biologically based therapies, mind-body medicine, manipulative and body-based therapies, and energy-based therapies is also included. A glossary of related terms and a directory of additional resources provide additional help and information.

How to Use This Book

This book is divided into parts and chapters. Parts focus on broad areas of interest. Chapters are devoted to single topics within a part.

Part I: An Overview of Complementary and Alternative Medicine (CAM) defines CAM, identifies common therapies, and answers questions consumers often have about choosing a CAM practitioner and paying for treatments. Information and statistics on CAM use in specific populations, including children and the elderly, is also included, along with tips on avoiding health fraud and spotting internet scams.

Part II: Alternative Medicine Systems describes whole medical systems practiced in cultures throughout the world that evolved separately from conventional medicine as it is practiced in the United States. These include Ayurvedic medicine, traditional Chinese medicine, Native American medicine, acupuncture, homeopathy, and naturopathy.

Part III: Dietary Supplements identifies vitamins, minerals, herbs and botanicals, and other food and dietary substances taken to improve health or nutrition. Readers will also find tips on ensuring supplement safety and selecting specific products to support bone and joint health, immune system functioning, mood regulation, and weight loss efforts.

Part IV: Biologically Based Therapies discusses CAM practices that strive to enhance or improve health using substances found in nature. This part highlights biologically based techniques including apitherapy, aromatherapy and essential oils, and diet-based therapies such as detoxification diets, fasting, macrobiotics, and vegetarianism.

Part V: Mind-Body Medicine describes CAM techniques that focus on using the mind to improve health or reduce unwanted symptoms, such as biofeedback, deep breathing, guided imagery and hypnosis, meditation, prayer and spirituality, relaxation training, tai chi, and yoga. In addition, readers will find information about practices focused on healing via creative expression in art, music, and dance.

Part VI: Manipulative and Body-Based Therapies offers information about massage therapy, chiropractic care and osteopathic manipulation, hydrotherapy, Pilates, reflexology, qigong, and other CAM therapies that involve movement or manipulation of one or more parts of the body.

Part VII: Energy-Based Therapies discusses CAM therapies that encourage healing through the manipulation of energy fields. CAM practitioners of reiki, shiatsu, polarity therapy, and therapeutic touch use pressure and touch to manipulate the energy fields in and around a person's body. With magnet and bioresonance therapies, practitioners influence electromagnetic fields, which purports to increase energy and vitality in the patient.

Part VIII: Alternative Treatments for Specific Diseases and Conditions highlights scientific research of CAM therapies for treating arthritis, asthma and allergies, cancer, dementia, diabetes, fibromyalgia, headache, heart disease, hepatitis, and sleep disorders. The use of CAM for treating mental health problems, including anxiety and addiction, is also discussed.

Part IX: Additional Help and Information provides a glossary of important terms related to complementary and alternative medicine. A directory of organizations that provide information to consumers about complementary and alternative therapies is also included.

Bibliographic Note

This volume contains documents and excerpts from publications issued by the following U.S. government agencies: Agency for Healthcare Research and Quality (AHRQ); National Cancer Institute (NCI); National Center for Complementary and Alternative Medicine (NCCAM); National Institute of Arthritis and Musculoskeletal and Skin Diseases (NIAMS); National Institute of Neurological Disorders and Stroke (NINDS); National Institute on Aging (NIA); National Institutes of Health (NIH); Office of Dietary Supplements (ODS); Substance Abuse and Mental Health Services Administration (SAMHSA); and the U.S. Food and Drug Administration (FDA).

In addition, this volume contains copyrighted documents from the following organizations: A.D.A.M., Inc.; American Apitherapy Society; American Art Therapy Association; American Dance Therapy Association; American Music Therapy Association; American Polarity Therapy Association; American Pregnancy Association; American Psychological Association; American Reflexology Certification Board; American Society for the Alexander Technique; Association for Applied Psychophysiology and Biofeedback; Asthma and Allergy Foundation of America; Center for Integrative Health and Healing; ChiEnergy; Feldenkrais Educational Foundation of North America; Gannett Company, Inc.; Hellerwork International; National Center on Physical Activity and Disability; National Headache Foundation; National Qigong Association; Natural Medicines Comprehensive Database; Natural Standard;

The Nemours Foundation; Rolf Institute of Structural Integration; Trager International; University of California–San Diego; Vegetarian Resource Group; and the Zero Balancing Health Association.

Full citation information is provided on the first page of each chapter or section. Every effort has been made to secure all necessary rights to reprint the copyrighted material. If any omissions have been made, please contact Omnigraphics to make corrections for future editions.

Acknowledgements

Thanks go to the many organizations, agencies, and individuals who have contributed materials for this *Sourcebook* and to medical consultant Dr. David Cooke and document engineer Bruce Bellenir. Special thanks go to managing editor Karen Bellenir and research and permissions coordinator Liz Collins for their help and support.

About the Health Reference Series

The *Health Reference Series* is designed to provide basic medical information for patients, families, caregivers, and the general public. Each volume takes a particular topic and provides comprehensive coverage. This is especially important for people who may be dealing with a newly diagnosed disease or a chronic disorder in themselves or in a family member. People looking for preventive guidance, information about disease warning signs, medical statistics, and risk factors for health problems will also find answers to their questions in the *Health Reference Series*. The *Series*, however, is not intended to serve as a tool for diagnosing illness, in prescribing treatments, or as a substitute for the physician/patient relationship. All people concerned about medical symptoms or the possibility of disease are encouraged to seek professional care from an appropriate health care provider.

A Note about Spelling and Style

Health Reference Series editors use *Stedman's Medical Dictionary* as an authority for questions related to the spelling of medical terms and the *Chicago Manual of Style* for questions related to grammatical structures, punctuation, and other editorial concerns. Consistent adherence is not always possible, however, because the individual volumes within the *Series* include many documents from a wide variety of different producers and copyright holders, and the editor's primary goal is to present material from each source as accurately as is possible following the terms specified by each document's producer. This sometimes means that information in different chapters or sections may follow other guidelines and alternate spelling authorities. For example, occasionally a copyright holder may require that eponymous terms be shown in possessive forms (Crohn's disease *vs.* Crohn disease) or that British spelling norms be retained (leukaemia *vs.* leukemia).

Locating Information within the Health Reference Series

The *Health Reference Series* contains a wealth of information about a wide variety of medical topics. Ensuring easy access to all the fact sheets, research reports, in-depth discussions, and other material contained within the individual books of the *Series* remains one of our highest priorities. As the *Series* continues to grow in size and scope, however, locating the precise information needed by a reader may become more challenging.

A Contents Guide to the Health Reference Series was developed to direct readers to the specific volumes that address their concerns. It presents an extensive list of diseases, treatments, and other topics of general interest compiled from the Tables of Contents and major index headings. To access *A Contents Guide to the Health Reference Series*, visit www.healthreferenceseries.com.

Medical Consultant

Medical consultation services are provided to the *Health Reference Series* editors by David A. Cooke, MD, FACP. Dr. Cooke is a graduate of Brandeis University, and he received his M.D. degree from the University of Michigan. He completed residency training at the University of Wisconsin Hospital and Clinics. He is board-certified in Internal Medicine. Dr. Cooke currently works as part of the University of Michigan Health System and practices in Ann Arbor, MI. In his free time, he enjoys writing, science fiction, and spending time with his family.

Our Advisory Board

We would like to thank the following board members for providing guidance to the development of this *Series*:

- Dr. Lynda Baker, Associate Professor of Library and Information Science, Wayne State University, Detroit, MI

- Nancy Bulgarelli, William Beaumont Hospital Library, Royal Oak, MI

- Karen Imarisio, Bloomfield Township Public Library, Bloomfield Township, MI

- Karen Morgan, Mardigian Library, University of Michigan-Dearborn, Dearborn, MI

- Rosemary Orlando, St. Clair Shores Public Library, St. Clair Shores, MI

Health Reference Series *Update Policy*

The inaugural book in the *Health Reference Series* was the first edition of *Cancer Sourcebook* published in 1989. Since then, the *Series* has been enthusiastically received by librarians and in the medical community. In order to maintain the standard of providing high-quality health information for the layperson the editorial staff at Omnigraphics felt it was necessary to implement a policy of updating volumes when warranted.

Medical researchers have been making tremendous strides, and it is the purpose of the *Health Reference Series* to stay current with the most recent advances. Each decision to update a volume is made on an individual basis. Some of the considerations include how much new information is available and the feedback we receive from people who use the books. If there is a topic you would like to see added to the update list, or an area of medical concern you feel has not been adequately addressed, please write to:

Editor
Health Reference Series
Omnigraphics, Inc.
P.O. Box 31-1640
Detroit, MI 48231
E-mail: editorial@omnigraphics.com

Part One

An Overview of Complementary and Alternative Medicine (CAM)

Chapter 1

What Is Complementary and Alternative Medicine (CAM)?

There are many terms used to describe approaches to health care that are outside the realm of conventional medicine as practiced in the United States. This text explains how the National Center for Complementary and Alternative Medicine (NCCAM), a component of the National Institutes of Health, defines some of the key terms used in the field of complementary and alternative medicine (CAM). Complementary medicine is used together with conventional medicine, and alternative medicine is used in place of conventional medicine.

What is CAM?

CAM is a group of diverse medical and health care systems, practices, and products that are not generally considered to be part of conventional medicine. While scientific evidence exists regarding some CAM therapies, for most there are key questions that are yet to be answered through well-designed scientific studies—questions such as whether these therapies are safe and whether they work for the purposes for which they are used.

Are complementary medicine and alternative medicine different from each other?

Yes, they are different. **Complementary medicine** is used together with conventional medicine. An example of a complementary therapy

From "What is CAM?" by the National Center for Complementary and Alternative Medicine (NCCAM, nccam.nih.gov), part of the National Institutes of Health, February 2007.

is using aromatherapy to help lessen a patient's discomfort following surgery. **Alternative medicine** is used in place of conventional medicine. An example of an alternative therapy is using a special diet to treat cancer instead of undergoing surgery, radiation, or chemotherapy that has been recommended by a conventional doctor.

What is integrative medicine?

Integrative medicine combines treatments from conventional medicine and CAM for which there is evidence of safety and effectiveness. It is also called integrated medicine.

What are the major types of complementary and alternative medicine?

NCCAM groups CAM practices into four domains, recognizing there can be some overlap. In addition, NCCAM studies CAM whole medical systems, which cut across all domains.

Whole medical systems: Whole medical systems are built upon complete systems of theory and practice. Often, these systems have evolved apart from and earlier than the conventional medical approach used in the United States. Examples of whole medical systems that have developed in Western cultures include homeopathic medicine and naturopathic medicine. Examples of systems that have developed in non-Western cultures include traditional Chinese medicine and Ayurveda.

Mind-body medicine: Mind-body medicine uses a variety of techniques designed to enhance the mind's capacity to affect bodily function and symptoms. Some techniques that were considered CAM in the past have become mainstream (for example, patient support groups and cognitive-behavioral therapy). Other mind-body techniques are still considered CAM, including meditation, prayer, mental healing, and therapies that use creative outlets such as art, music, or dance.

Biologically based practices: Biologically based practices in CAM use substances found in nature, such as herbs, foods, and vitamins. Some examples include dietary supplements, herbal products, and the use of other so-called natural but as yet scientifically unproven therapies (for example, using shark cartilage to treat cancer).

Manipulative and body-based practices: Manipulative and body-based practices in CAM are based on manipulation and/or movement of one or more parts of the body. Some examples include chiropractic or osteopathic manipulation.

Energy medicine: Energy therapies involve the use of energy fields. They are of two types:

- Biofield therapies are intended to affect energy fields that purportedly surround and penetrate the human body. The existence of such fields has not yet been scientifically proven. Some forms of energy therapy manipulate biofields by applying pressure and/or manipulating the body by placing the hands in, or through, these fields. Examples include qi gong, Reiki, and therapeutic touch.

- Bioelectromagnetic-based therapies involve the unconventional use of electromagnetic fields, such as pulsed fields, magnetic fields, or alternating-current or direct-current fields.

What is NCCAM's role in the field of CAM?

NCCAM is the Federal Government's lead agency for scientific research on CAM. NCCAM's mission is to explore complementary and alternative healing practices in the context of rigorous science, train CAM researchers, and disseminate authoritative information to the public and professionals.

Chapter 2

Common Questions and Answers about CAM

For thousands of Americans, health care includes some form of complementary and alternative medicine (CAM). Like any decision concerning your health, decisions about whether to use CAM are important.

What is CAM?

CAM is a group of diverse medical and health care systems, practices, and products that are not generally considered part of conventional medicine. Conventional medicine is medicine as practiced by holders of MD (medical doctor) or DO (doctor of osteopathy) degrees and by their allied health professionals, such as physical therapists, psychologists, and registered nurses. Integrative medicine combines conventional and CAM treatments for which there is evidence of safety and effectiveness.

How can I get reliable information about a CAM therapy?

It is important to learn what scientific studies have discovered about the CAM therapy you are considering. Making a decision based on the facts is a better idea than using a therapy simply because of something you have seen in an advertisement or on a website or because someone has told you that it worked for them.

From "Are You Considering CAM?" by the National Center for Complementary and Alternative Medicine (NCCAM, nccam.nih.gov), part of the National Institutes of Health, April 2009.

Understanding a therapy's potential benefits, risks, and scientific evidence is critical to your health and safety. Scientific research on many CAM therapies is relatively new, so this kind of information may not be available for every therapy. However, many studies are under way, including those that NCCAM supports, and knowledge and understanding of CAM are increasing all the time.

Here are some ways to find reliable information:

- **Talk with your doctor or other health care providers.** Tell them about the therapy you are considering and ask any questions you may have about safety, effectiveness, or interactions with medications (prescription or nonprescription) or other dietary supplements. They may know about the therapy and be able to advise you on its safety and use.

- **Visit the NCCAM website (nccam.nih.gov).** The Health Information page has information on specific CAM therapies, and links to other online sources of information. It also has contact information for the NCCAM Clearinghouse, where information specialists are available to assist you in searching the peer-reviewed literature and to suggest useful NCCAM publications.

- **Visit your local library or a medical library.** Ask the reference librarian to help you find books and scientific journals with information on the therapy that interests you.

Are CAM therapies safe? How can I minimize risks in using CAM therapies?

As with any medical treatment, there can be risks with CAM therapies. These risks depend on the specific therapy. Each CAM therapy needs to be considered on its own. However, if you are considering a CAM therapy, the following general suggestions can help you think about safety and minimize risks.

- Take charge of your health by being an informed consumer. Find out what the scientific evidence is about any therapy's safety and whether it works.

- Be aware that individuals respond differently to treatments, whether conventional or CAM. How a person might respond to a CAM therapy depends on many things, including the person's state of health, how the therapy is used, or the person's belief in the therapy.

- Keep in mind that "natural" does not necessarily mean "safe." (Think of mushrooms that grow in the wild: some are safe to eat, while others are not.)

- Learn about factors that affect safety. For a CAM therapy that is administered by a practitioner, these factors include the training, skill, and experience of the practitioner. For a CAM product such as a dietary supplement, the specific ingredients and the quality of the manufacturing process are important factors.

- If you decide to use a CAM therapy that would be given by a practitioner, choose the practitioner carefully.

- If you decide to use a dietary supplement, such as an herbal product, be aware that some products may interact with medications (prescription or over-the-counter) or other dietary supplements, and some may have side effects on their own.

- Tell all your health care providers about any complementary and alternative practices you use. Give them a full picture of what you do to manage your health. This will help ensure coordinated and safe care.

How can I determine whether statements made about the effectiveness of a CAM therapy are true?

Statements that manufacturers and providers of CAM therapies may make about effectiveness and benefits can sound reasonable and promising. However, the statements may not be backed up by scientific evidence. Before you begin using a CAM therapy, it is a good idea to ask the following questions:

- Is there scientific evidence (not just personal stories) to back up the statements?

- Does the federal government have anything to report about the therapy?
  - Visit the NCCAM website or contact the NCCAM Clearinghouse to see if NCCAM has information about the therapy.
  - Visit the FDA [U.S. Food and Drug Administration, www.fda.gov] online to see if there is any information available about the product or practice. Information specifically about dietary supplements can be found on FDA's Center for Food Safety and Applied Nutrition website. Or visit the FDA's page on recalls and safety alerts.

- Check with the Federal Trade Commission (FTC, www.ftc .gov) to see if there are any enforcement actions for deceptive advertising regarding the therapy. Also, visit the site's Diet, Health, and Fitness Consumer Information section.

- How does the provider or manufacturer describe the therapy?

  - Question terms like "scientific breakthrough," "miracle cure," "secret ingredient," or "ancient remedy."

  - If you encounter claims of a "quick fix" that departs from previous research, keep in mind that science usually advances over time by small steps, slowly building toward an evidence base.

  - Remember: If it sounds too good to be true—for example, claims that a therapy can cure a disease or works for a wide variety of ailments—it usually is.

Are CAM therapies tested to see if they work?

While some scientific evidence exists regarding the effectiveness of some CAM therapies, for most there are key questions that are yet to be answered through well-designed scientific studies—questions such as how the therapies work, and whether they work for the diseases or medical conditions for which they are used. As the federal government's lead agency for scientific research on CAM, NCCAM supports studies to answer these questions and determine who might benefit most from the use of specific therapies.

I am interested in a CAM therapy that involves treatment from a practitioner. How do I go about selecting a practitioner?

Your health care provider or local hospital may be able to recommend a practitioner. The professional organization for the type of practitioner you are seeking may have helpful information, such as licensing and training requirements. Many states have regulatory agencies or licensing boards for certain types of practitioners; they may be able to help you locate practitioners in your area.

Can I receive treatment or a referral to a practitioner from NCCAM?

NCCAM does not provide CAM treatments or referrals to practitioners. NCCAM's mission is to explore CAM practices using rigorous scientific methods and build an evidence base for the safety and effectiveness of these practices.

Can I participate in a CAM clinical trial?

NCCAM supports clinical trials (research studies in people) on CAM therapies. Clinical trials on CAM are taking place in many locations worldwide, and study participants are needed. To find trials that are recruiting participants, go to the website nccam.nih.gov/research/clinicaltrials. You can search this site by type of therapy or by disease or condition.

Chapter 3

The Use of CAM in the United States

In December 2008, the National Center for Complementary and Alternative Medicine (NCCAM) and the National Center for Health Statistics (part of the Centers for Disease Control and Prevention) released new findings on Americans' use of complementary and alternative medicine (CAM). The findings are from the 2007 National Health Interview Survey (NHIS), an annual in-person survey of Americans regarding their health- and illness-related experiences. The CAM section gathered information on 23,393 adults aged 18 years or older and 9,417 children aged 17 years and under. A similar CAM section was included in the 2002 NHIS, providing the opportunity to examine trends in CAM use, too.

About CAM

CAM is a group of diverse medical and health care systems, practices, and products that are not generally considered part of conventional medicine. Complementary medicine is used together with conventional medicine, and alternative medicine is used in place of conventional medicine. Integrative medicine combines conventional and CAM treatments for which there is evidence of safety and effectiveness. While scientific evidence exists regarding some CAM therapies, for most there are key questions that are yet to be answered through well-designed

Excerpted from "The Use of Complementary and Alternative Medicine in the United States," by the National Center for Complementary and Alternative Medicine (NCCAM, nccam.nih.gov), December 2008.

scientific studies—questions such as whether these therapies are safe and whether they work for the purposes for which they are used. NC-CAM's mission is to explore CAM practices using rigorous scientific methods and build an evidence base for the safety and effectiveness of these practices.

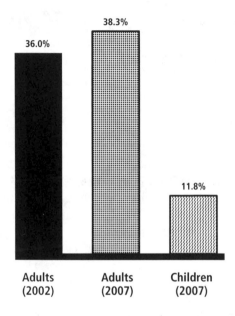

Figure 3.1. *CAM Use by U.S. Adults and Children*

How Many People Use CAM

In the United States, approximately 38 percent of adults (about 4 in 10) and approximately 12 percent of children (about 1 in 9) are using some form of CAM, shown in Figure 3.1.

Who Uses CAM Most

People of all backgrounds use CAM. However, CAM use among adults is greater among women and those with higher levels of education and higher incomes.

CAM Therapies Used the Most

Nonvitamin, nonmineral natural products are the most commonly used CAM therapy among adults. Use has increased for several therapies, including deep breathing exercises, meditation, massage therapy, and yoga.

CAM therapies included in the 2007 NHIS:

- Acupuncture*

- Ayurveda*

- Biofeedback*

- Chelation therapy*

- Chiropractic or osteopathic manipulation*

- Deep breathing exercises

- Diet-based therapies
    - Atkins diet
    - Macrobiotic diet
    - Ornish diet
    - Pritikin diet
    - South Beach diet
    - Vegetarian diet
    - Zone diet

- Energy healing therapy/Reiki*

- Guided imagery

- Homeopathic treatment

- Hypnosis*

- Massage*

- Meditation

- Movement therapies
    - Alexander technique
    - Feldenkrais
    - Pilates
    - Trager psychophysical integration

- Natural products (nonvitamin and nonmineral, such as herbs and other products from plants, enzymes, etc.)

- Naturopathy*

- Progressive relaxation

- Qi gong

- Tai chi

- Traditional healers*
  - Botanica
  - Hierbero or Yerbera
  - Shaman
  - Curandero
  - Native American healer/Medicine man
  - Sobador
  - Espiritista
- Yoga

Note: An asterisk (*) indicates a practitioner-based therapy.

Use of Natural Products

The most popular natural products are fish oil/omega-3 fatty acids, glucosamine, echinacea, and flaxseed.

Health Conditions Prompting CAM Use

People use CAM for an array of diseases and conditions. American adults are most likely to use CAM for musculoskeletal problems such as back, neck, or joint pain. The use of CAM therapies for head or chest colds showed a substantial decrease from 2002 to 2007.

CAM Use among Children

The 2007 NHIS asked selected adult respondents about CAM use by children in their households. Overall, approximately 12 percent of children use some form of CAM. Use is greater among the following groups:

- Children whose parents used CAM (23.9%)
- Adolescents aged 12–17 (16.4%), compared to younger children
- White children (12.8%), compared to Hispanic children (7.9%) and black children (5.9%)
- Children whose parents had higher education levels (more than high school: 14.7%)
- Children with six or more health conditions (23.8%)
- Children whose families delayed conventional care because of cost (16.9%)

Chapter 4

CAM Use and Children

A wide range of complementary and alternative medicine (CAM) therapies are used in children, including herbs and dietary supplements, massage, acupuncture, chiropractic care, naturopathy, and homeopathy. This text offers information for parents who are thinking about using a CAM therapy for their child.

Patterns of CAM Use in Children

The 2007 National Health Interview Survey gathered information on CAM use among more than 9,000 children aged 17 and under. Nearly 12 percent of the children had used some form of CAM during the past 12 months. CAM use was much more likely among children whose parents also used CAM. Adolescents aged 12–17, children with multiple health conditions, and those whose families delayed or did not use conventional medical care because of cost were also more likely to use CAM.

In addition, a 2001 survey of 745 members of the American Academy of Pediatrics found that 87 percent of pediatricians had been asked about CAM therapies by a patient or a parent in the 3 months prior to the survey. The pediatricians were asked most often about herbs and dietary supplements.

From "CAM Use and Children," by the National Center for Complementary and Alternative Medicine (NCCAM, nccam.nih.gov), part of the National Institutes of Health, February 2009.

Safety of Childhood CAM Use

Few high-quality studies have examined how CAM therapies may affect young people, and results from studies in adults do not necessarily apply to children. Children are not small adults. Their immune and central nervous systems are not fully developed, which can make them respond to treatments differently from adults. This is especially true for infants and young children.

Herbs and other dietary supplements may interact with medicines or other supplements, or they may cause problems during surgery, such as bleeding-related complications. In addition, "natural" does not necessarily mean "safe." CAM therapies can have side effects, and these may be different in children than in adults.

Parents should seek information from scientific studies about how safe and effective a specific CAM therapy is in children. However, since few, if any, rigorous studies in young people exist, additional scientific studies are needed. Anecdotes and testimonials (personal stories) about CAM therapies are common and can be compelling, but they are not evidence.

Discussing CAM with Your Pediatrician

Parents often do not tell pediatricians or other health care providers that their child is receiving CAM. It is important, however, that families speak with their child's health care provider about any CAM therapy being used or considered. Providing a full picture of what is being done to manage your child's health will help ensure coordinated and safe care.

When seeking care from a CAM practitioner, it is important to ask about the practitioner's qualifications, including the following:

- Education and training

- Experience in delivering care to children

- Experience working with other providers, including physicians, to ensure coordinated care

- Licensing (some states have licensing requirements for certain CAM practitioners, such as chiropractors, naturopathic doctors, massage therapists, and acupuncturists)

In addition to asking your child's physician what is known about whether a therapy works and is safe for children, consider these points when making decisions about using CAM in children:

- Ensure that your child has received an accurate diagnosis from a licensed health care provider and that CAM use does not replace or delay conventional medical care.

- If you decide to use CAM for your child, do not increase the dose or length of treatment beyond what is recommended. More is not necessarily better.

- If your child experiences an effect from a CAM therapy that concerns you, contact your child's health care provider.

- Store herbal and other dietary supplements out of the sight and reach of children.

- If you are a woman who is pregnant or breastfeeding, remember that some CAM therapies may affect your fetus or nursing infant.

Chapter 5

CAM Use in Older Adults

What is CAM?

Today, many people use complementary and alternative medicine, or CAM, for a wide variety of diseases or conditions, and use of CAM has increased in recent years. But what exactly is CAM, and how is it different from standard medical care?

Definition of CAM

Complementary medicine is used together with standard medical care. An example is using acupuncture to help with side effects of cancer treatment.

Alternative medicine is used in place of standard medical care. An example is treating heart disease with chelation therapy (which seeks to remove excess metals from the blood) instead of using a standard approach.

A related concept, "integrative medicine," is a total approach to care that involves the patient's mind, body, and spirit. It combines standard medical treatments with CAM practices that have shown the most promise. An example is taking an omega-3 fatty acid supplement in addition to a prescription statin medication to reduce cholesterol.

Experts group CAM practices into four major categories. These include the following:

Excerpted from "Complementary and Alternative Medicine (CAM)," by the National Institute on Aging (NIA, nihseniorhealth.gov), part of the National Institutes of Health, December 2008.

- Biologically based practices
- Energy medicine
- Manipulative and body-based practices
- Mind-body medicine

These four categories sometimes overlap.

Another term, "whole medical systems," refers to complete systems of care that have evolved over time in different cultures and parts of the world. Whole medical systems may include practices from the four major CAM categories.

CAM Practices

The four major categories of complementary and alternative medicine include biologically based practices, energy medicine, manipulative and body-based practices, and mind-body medicine. These categories sometimes overlap.

Biologically Based Practices

Biologically based practices involve adding dietary supplements, functional foods, and other products found in nature to one's diet. A dietary supplement is a product that contains vitamins, minerals, herbs or botanicals, amino acids, enzymes, probiotics, or other ingredients that supplement the diet. Examples of dietary supplements include vitamin B_{12}, St. John's wort (a botanical), and acidophilus (a probiotic).

Energy Medicine

Energy medicine uses energy fields with the intent to affect health. Some fields, such as magnetic fields, have been measured. Others, such as biofields, have not. Therapies involving biofields are based on the idea that people have a subtle form of energy; energy medicine practitioners believe that illness results from disturbances of these subtle energies.

Examples of energy medicine include magnet therapy, healing touch, and Reiki.

Magnet therapy uses magnets or magnetic devices to treat or ease the symptoms of various diseases and conditions, including pain.

Healing touch practitioners pass their hands over or gently touch a person's body to try to identify imbalances in the body's energy field.

Reiki is based on the idea that there is a universal (or source) energy that supports the body's innate healing abilities. Practitioners seek to access the energy and allow it to flow to the body to help with healing. In a Reiki session, the practitioner's hands are placed lightly on or just above the client's body.

Manipulative and Body-Based Practices

Manipulative and body-based practices focus mainly on the structures and systems of the body, including the bones and joints, the soft tissues, and the circulatory and lymphatic systems. Some practices come from traditional systems of medicine, such as those from China and India, while others, like spinal manipulation, were developed within the last 150 years.

Examples of manipulative and body-based practices are massage, spinal manipulation, and reflexology. Spinal manipulation is performed by chiropractors and other health professionals such as physical therapists and osteopaths.

There are over 80 types of massage therapy. In all of them, therapists press, rub, and otherwise manipulate the muscles and other soft tissues of the body, often varying pressure and movement. They most often use their hands and fingers, but may also use their forearms, elbows, or feet. The goal of the therapy is usually to relax the soft tissues, increase delivery of blood and oxygen to the massaged areas, warm them, and decrease pain.

The goal of chiropractic medicine is to help the body heal by correcting its alignment.

Doctors of chiropractic, who are also called chiropractors or chiropractic physicians, use a type of hands-on therapy called manipulation, or adjustment, as their main type of procedure. Adjustments are done to increase the range and quality of motion in the area being treated.

Conditions commonly treated by chiropractors include back pain, neck pain, headaches, sports injuries, and repetitive strains. Patients also seek treatment of pain associated with other conditions, such as arthritis.

In reflexology, pressure points on the feet or hands are used to help other parts of the body relax and heal.

Mind-Body Medicine

Mind-body medicine, which focuses on how the mind and body interact, uses a variety of techniques designed to enhance the mind's capacity to affect bodily function and symptoms.

Examples of mind-body medicine are meditation, yoga, tai chi, qi gong, imagery, and creative outlets.

The term meditation refers to a group of techniques, most of which started in Eastern religious or spiritual traditions. These techniques have been used by many different cultures throughout the world for thousands of years. Today, many people use meditation outside of its traditional religious or cultural settings for health and wellness purposes.

In meditation, people learn to focus their attention and suspend the stream of thoughts that normally occupy the mind. This practice is believed to result in a state of greater calmness, physical relaxation, and psychological balance. Practicing meditation can change how a person relates to the flow of emotions and thoughts in the mind.

Yoga is an ancient system of exercise, breathing, and relaxation that originated in India.

In yoga, people use stretches and poses and pay special attention to their breathing to balance the mind, body, and spirit.

Tai chi is a practice that uses a series of slow, gentle movements co-ordinated with breathing and meditation. The goal is to enhance physical functioning, improve balance and concentration, and reduce stress.

Qi gong is also a practice that combines movement, meditation, and controlled breathing.

In imagery, people imagine scenes, pictures, or experiences to achieve a desired physical response such as stress reduction.

Creative outlets such as art, music, or dance are also sometimes used for health purposes.

Whole Medical Systems

Whole medical systems are built upon complete systems of theory and practice. Often, these systems have evolved apart from, and earlier than, the standard medical approach used in the United States. Examples of whole medical systems that have developed in non-Western cultures include traditional Chinese medicine and Ayurvedic medicine. Examples of systems that have developed in Western cultures include homeopathic medicine and naturopathic medicine.

Traditional Chinese Medicine (TCM)

Traditional Chinese medicine, or TCM, is a healing system that dates back more than 2,000 years. It is based on the concept that disease results from disruption in the flow of vital energy, or qi in the body. The flow of qi is maintained by keeping a balance in the two forces known as yin and yang.

TCM uses three main therapeutic approaches: acupuncture and moxibustion, herbs and other natural products, and massage and manipulation.

Acupuncture is the stimulation of specific points on the body by a variety of techniques, including the insertion of thin metal needles through the skin. It is intended to remove blockages in the flow of qi and restore and maintain health.

Moxibustion is the application of heat from the burning of the herb moxa at the acupuncture point.

Herbs and botanicals used in TCM are usually used together in formulas, and the formulas are usually adjusted to fit a person's specific diagnosis. TCM is an example of personalized medicine.

Ayurvedic Medicine

Ayurveda, which means "the science of life" in Sanskrit, originated in India and evolved there over thousands of years. Its goal is to prevent and treat disease by bringing the body, mind, and spirit into balance. Ayurveda also proposes treatments for specific health problems.

Three qualities called doshas are believed to form important characteristics of each person's body constitution and to control bodily activities. Imbalances in the doshas, which can be caused by an unhealthy lifestyle, diet, stress, the weather, chemicals, or germs, can lead to illness.

Ayurvedic medicine relies on therapies such as diet, exercise, meditation, herbs, massage, exposure to sunlight, and controlled breathing. The goals of treatment are to eliminate impurities, reduce symptoms, reduce worry, increase harmony in a person's life, and help resolve both physical and psychological problems.

Homeopathy

Homeopathy originated in Europe and has been practiced in the United States since the early 19th century. Its goal is to help the body heal itself by using very small doses of highly diluted substances that in larger doses would produce illness or symptoms. Most homeopathic remedies are derived from natural substances that come from plants, minerals, or animals.

A homeopathic practitioner will select treatments based upon a total picture of a person's symptoms, not solely upon the symptoms of a disease. Homeopaths evaluate not only a person's physical symptoms but emotions, psychological state, lifestyle, nutrition, and other aspects. In homeopathy, different people with the same symptoms may receive different homeopathic remedies.

Naturopathy

Like homeopathy, naturopathy originated in Europe, but it also includes ancient and modern therapies from other traditions. Naturopathy attempts to help the body heal itself, and naturopaths consider a person's physical, emotional, genetic, environmental, and social circumstances when evaluating treatment. The emphasis is on supporting health rather than fighting disease.

Practitioners of naturopathy prefer to use treatment approaches that they consider to be the most natural and least invasive, relying on methods other than standard medications and surgery. They focus on changes in diet and lifestyle and on preventing disease, together with CAM therapies such as herbs and massage.

CAM Research and Diseases Affecting Older Adults

The National Institutes of Health (NIH) funds research into the safety and effectiveness of complementary and alternative medicine (CAM) therapies. Much of the research looks at CAM for medical conditions that are common in older people, such as heart disease, cancer, arthritis, and Alzheimer's disease.

NIH supports many studies of CAM and heart disease, including studies of chelation therapy, meditation, and garlic.

NIH is leading a large, nationwide study to find out whether chelation therapy is safe and effective for people with heart disease. Chelation uses a chemical called EDTA [ethylene-diamine-tetra-acetic acid] to remove heavy metals from the body.

Researchers are also conducting studies of how meditation and related practices affect heart disease. One study is looking at whether a technique called mindfulness-based stress reduction can help patients who have decreased blood flow to the heart.

In another study, researchers are focusing on ways that garlic might prevent blood clots, which can lead to a heart attack. Research shows that garlic can thin the blood in a manner similar to aspirin. An earlier study found that garlic does not seem to lower LDL (low-density lipoprotein), the "bad cholesterol" that increases heart disease risk.

NIH-supported research into CAM therapies for cancer includes studies of acupuncture, massage, and vitamin E and selenium.

Researchers have found evidence that acupuncture can reduce nausea and vomiting caused by cancer chemotherapy. Other researchers are currently studying whether acupuncture can improve quality of life in patients with advanced ovarian and colorectal cancers.

Acupuncture is one of many CAM therapies that people with cancer seek out—not as cures, but as complementary therapies that may help them feel better and recover faster.

Studies are evaluating whether massage can help people who have cancer cope with various physical and emotional challenges. Researchers are looking at whether massage can reduce pain and swelling related to cancer.

Vitamin E and selenium are dietary supplements that were tested in a large study for prostate cancer prevention. The study, known as SELECT (the Selenium and Vitamin E Cancer Prevention Trial) found that the supplements, taken either alone or together, did not prevent prostate cancer. Over 35,000 men age 50 and over participated in this study. The researchers will continue to monitor the volunteers' health for another 3 years to learn more about prostate cancer and other diseases faced by older men.

NIH-supported research into CAM therapies for osteoarthritis, the most common kind of arthritis, include studies of acupuncture and glucosamine and chondroitin.

A study of acupuncture in people with osteoarthritis of the knee recently found that the therapy can reduce pain and improve ability to function in people with this condition. The study was the largest, lengthiest acupuncture study of its kind.

In a study of the dietary supplements glucosamine and chondroitin in people with pain from osteoarthritis of the knee, the combination did not help the participants as a whole, but it did help a small group of people with moderate to severe pain. A follow-up study, showed that the supplements, together or alone, also appeared to fare no better than placebo in slowing the loss of cartilage in knee osteoarthritis.

NIH-supported research into CAM therapies for Alzheimer disease and other kinds of dementia (age-related changes in memory, thinking ability, and personality) includes studies of ginkgo biloba, antioxidants, B vitamins, and omega-3 fatty acids.

Although researchers had hoped that extracts from the leaves of the ginkgo biloba tree might be of some help in preventing dementia, a large study called the Ginkgo Evaluation in Memory study (GEM) recently found that the ginkgo product researched was not effective in delaying or preventing Alzheimer's disease or other types of dementia. This study, which recruited more than 3,000 volunteers age 75 and over, was the largest study ever to investigate ginkgo's effect on dementia.

Some studies are considering whether antioxidants—such as vitamin E and C—can slow Alzheimer disease. One clinical trial is examining whether vitamin E and/or selenium supplements can prevent

Alzheimer disease or stop mental decline. More studies on other anti-oxidants are ongoing or being planned.

Studies have shown that people with Alzheimer disease often have higher levels of an amino acid called homocysteine in their blood. High levels of homocysteine are known to increase the risk of heart disease. Folic acid and vitamins B6 and B12 can reduce levels of homocysteine in the blood, and scientists are conducting clinical trials to see whether these substances can also slow rates of mental decline.

Omega-3 fatty acids are found in the oil of certain fish. One study is looking at whether an omega-3 fatty acid called DHA [docosahexaenoic acid] can slow the progression of Alzheimer disease.

Be an Informed Consumer

Take charge of your health by being an informed consumer.

Talk with your health care providers when making any decisions about using complementary and alternative medicine (CAM). Your health care providers can give you advice based on your medical needs.

If you are thinking about using a CAM therapy, learn the facts. Is it safe? Does it work?

Find out what scientific studies have been done. It is not a good idea to use a CAM therapy simply because you have seen it in an advertisement or on a website or because people have told you that it worked for them.

Keep in mind that the number of websites offering health-related resources grows every day. Many sites provide valuable information, while others may have information that is unreliable or misleading. To evaluate the quality of a website, take a look at who runs the site, who pays for it, and the purpose of the site. Also, check out where the information comes from, how it is selected, and how current it is.

Scientific research on many CAM therapies is relatively new, so information about safety and effectiveness may not be available for every therapy. However, many studies of CAM treatments are under-way, and researchers are always learning more about CAM.

You can find reliable information on CAM through the National Institutes of Health's National Center for Complementary and Alternative Medicine (NCCAM). The NCCAM website (nccam.nih.gov) provides a variety of useful information as well as links to other trustworthy sources. You can also contact the NCCAM Clearinghouse staff [call toll-free at: 888-644-6226 or e-mail info@nccam.nih.gov] for help).

Your health care providers and pharmacist are also good resources for learning about CAM. If you are considering a new CAM therapy, ask them about its safety, effectiveness, and possible interactions with medications (both prescription and over-the-counter). Your health care team can find the latest scientific studies or help you to understand the results of studies you have found.

Dietary supplements—such as vitamins, minerals, and herbs and other botanicals—can be a form of CAM. Some dietary supplements can interact with your prescription medicines. Supplements may also have side effects if not used correctly, if taken in large amounts, or sometimes even if taken according to the instructions on the label.

While many supplements come from natural sources, "natural" does not always mean "safe." Natural supplements may have active ingredients that cause strong biological effects in the body. Some supplements will affect how your medicines work.

Also, if you are considering or using dietary supplements, it is important to know that they are not regulated in the same way as drugs. The federal government does not review supplements for safety and effectiveness before they are sold. However, in 2007 the U.S. Food and Drug Administration (FDA) established a rule requiring current good manufacturing practices for dietary supplements. The rule will help ensure that dietary supplements are produced in a quality manner, do not contain contaminants or impurities, and are accurately labeled.

For CAM therapies provided by a practitioner, such as acupuncture or chiropractic treatments, choose a practitioner with care.

Tell Your Health Care Providers

Almost two thirds of people aged 50 and older use some form of complementary and alternative medicine (CAM). But less than one third of those who use CAM talk with their doctors about it, according to a recent survey by AARP [American Association of Retired Persons] and the National Institutes of Health (NIH). If you use CAM, it is important to tell your health care providers.

Giving your health care providers a full picture of what you do to manage your health helps you stay in control. Some CAM approaches can have an effect on standard medicine. For example, certain supplements can interact with over-the-counter or prescription medicines. Also, some supplements—such as garlic or ginkgo—can increase the risk of bleeding problems during surgery. Talking with your health care providers about CAM use will help ensure coordinated and safe care. Your pharmacist may also have information on any dietary supplements you are considering or using.

Be proactive—don't wait for your health care providers to ask about your CAM use. Tell them about all of the therapies you use—standard and CAM. Talking to your providers about your CAM use helps them to be your fully informed partners in health care. Similarly, it is important to tell your CAM practitioners about the conventional medications you use.

When filling out the patient history form at a medical office or hospital, list all over-the-counter and prescription medicines, as well as dietary supplements. Tell your health care provider about other CAM therapies that you use, as well. It may help to make a list in advance and bring it with you.

If you are considering a new CAM therapy, ask your health care providers about its safety, effectiveness, and possible interactions with medicines (both prescription and over-the-counter).

It is especially important to talk with your health care providers if you are:

- thinking about replacing your regular medical care with one or more supplements;

- taking other medications for a chronic medical condition; or

- planning to have surgery.

Chapter 6

Health Care Providers and CAM

Chapter Contents

Section 6.1—Selecting a CAM Practitioner 32

Section 6.2—Tips for Talking with Your Health
Care Providers about CAM 37

Section 6.1

Selecting a CAM Practitioner

Excerpted from text by the National Center for Complementary and Alternative Medicine (NCCAM, nccam.nih.gov), part of the National Institutes of Health, February 2007.

Selecting a health care practitioner—of conventional or complementary and alternative medicine (CAM)—is an important decision and can be key to ensuring that you are receiving the best health care.

What is CAM?

CAM is a group of diverse medical and health care systems, practices, and products that are not presently considered to be part of conventional medicine. Complementary medicine is used together with conventional medicine, and alternative medicine is used in place of conventional medicine. Some health care providers practice both CAM and conventional medicine. The list of what is considered to be CAM changes continually as those therapies that are proven to be safe and effective become adopted into conventional health care and as new approaches to health care emerge.

I am interested in a CAM therapy that involves treatment from a practitioner. How do I go about finding a practitioner?

Before selecting a CAM therapy or practitioner, talk with your primary health care provider(s). Tell them about the therapy you are considering and ask any questions you may have. They may know about the therapy and be able to advise you on its safety, use, and effectiveness, or possible interactions with medications. Here are some suggestions for finding a practitioner:

- Ask your doctor or other health professionals whether they have recommendations or are willing to make a referral.

- Contact a nearby hospital or a medical school and ask if they maintain a list of area CAM practitioners or could make a recommendation. Some regional medical centers may have CAM centers or CAM practitioners on staff.

- Ask if your therapy will be covered by insurance; for example, some insurers cover visits to a chiropractor. If the therapy will be covered, ask for a list of CAM practitioners who accept your insurance.

- Contact a professional organization for the type of practitioner you are seeking. Often, professional organizations have standards of practice, provide referrals to practitioners, have publications explaining the therapy (or therapies) that their members provide, and may offer information on the type of training needed and whether practitioners of a therapy must be licensed or certified in your state. Professional organizations can be located by searching the internet or directories in libraries (ask the librarian). One directory is the Directory of Information Resources Online (DIRLINE) compiled by the National Library of Medicine (dirline.nlm.nih.gov). It contains locations and descriptive information about a variety of health organizations, including CAM associations and organizations. You may find more than one member organization for some CAM professions; this may be because there are different "schools" of practice within the profession or for other reasons.

- Many states have regulatory agencies or licensing boards for certain types of practitioners. They may be able to provide you with information regarding practitioners in your area. Your state, county, or city health department may be able to refer you to such agencies or boards. Licensing, accreditation, and regulatory laws for CAM practices are becoming more common to help ensure that practitioners are competent and provide quality services.

Will insurance cover the cost of a CAM practitioner?

Few CAM therapies are covered by insurance, and the amount of coverage offered varies depending on the insurer. Before agreeing to a treatment that a CAM practitioner suggests, you should check with your insurer to see if they will cover any portion of the therapy's cost. If insurance does cover a portion of the cost, you will want to ask if the practitioner accepts your insurance or participates in your insurer's network. Even with insurance, you may be responsible for a percentage of the cost of therapy.

I have located the names of several practitioners. How do I select one?

Begin by contacting the practitioners on your list and gathering information.

- Ask what training or other qualifications the practitioners have. Ask about their education, additional training, licenses, and certifications. If you have contacted a professional organization, see if the practitioners' qualifications meet the standards for training and licensing for that profession.

- Ask if it is possible to have a brief consultation in person or by phone with the practitioners. This will give you a chance to speak with them directly. The consultation may or may not involve a charge.

- Ask if there are diseases/health conditions in which the practitioners specialize and how frequently they treat patients with problems similar to yours.

- Ask if the practitioners believe the therapy can effectively address your complaint and if there is any scientific research supporting the treatment's use for your condition.

- Ask how many patients the practitioners typically see in a day and how much time they spend with each patient.

- Ask whether there is a brochure or website to tell you more about the practice.

- Ask about charges and payment options. How much do treatments cost? If you have insurance, do the practitioners accept your insurance or participate in your insurer's network? Even with insurance, you may be responsible for a percentage of the cost.

- Ask about the hours appointments are offered. How long is the wait for an appointment? Consider whether this will be convenient for your schedule.

- Ask about office location. If you need a building with an elevator or a wheelchair ramp, ask about it.

- Ask what will be involved in the first visit or assessment. Observe how comfortable you feel during these first interactions.

Once you have gathered the information, assess the answers and determine which practitioner was best able to respond to your questions and best suits your needs.

I have selected a practitioner. What questions should I ask at my first visit?

The first visit is very important. Come prepared to answer questions about your health history, such as surgeries, injuries, and major illnesses, as well as prescriptions, vitamins, and other supplements you take. Not only will the practitioner wish to gather information from you, but you will want to ask questions, too. Write down ahead of time the questions you want to ask, or take a family member or friend with you to help you remember the questions and answers. Some people bring a tape recorder to record the appointment. (Ask the practitioner for permission to do this in advance.) Here are some questions you may want to ask:

- What benefits can I expect from this therapy?
- What are the risks associated with this therapy?
- Do the benefits outweigh the risks for my disease or condition?
- What side effects can be expected?
- Will the therapy interfere with any of my daily activities?
- How long will I need to undergo treatment? How often will my progress or plan of treatment be assessed?
- Will I need to buy any equipment or supplies?
- Do you have scientific articles or references about using the treatment for my condition?
- Could the therapy interact with conventional treatments?
- Are there any conditions for which this treatment should not be used?

How do I know if the practitioner I have selected is right for me?

After your first visit with a practitioner, evaluate the visit. Ask yourself:

- Was the practitioner easy to talk to? Did the practitioner make me feel comfortable?
- Was I comfortable asking questions? Did the practitioner appear willing to answer them, and were they answered to my satisfaction?
- Was the practitioner open to how both CAM therapy and conventional medicine might work together for my benefit?
- Did the practitioner get to know me and ask me about my condition?
- Did the practitioner seem knowledgeable about my specific health condition?

- Does the treatment recommended seem reasonable and acceptable to me?

- Was the practitioner clear about the time and costs associated with treatment?

Can I change my mind about the treatment or the practitioner?

Yes, if you are not satisfied or comfortable, you can look for a different practitioner or stop treatment. However, as with any conventional treatment, talk with your practitioner before stopping to make sure that it is safe to simply stop treatment—it may not be advisable to stop some therapies midway through a course of treatment.

Discuss with your practitioner the reasons you are not satisfied or comfortable with treatment. If you decide to stop a therapy or seek another practitioner, make sure that you share this information with any other health care practitioners you may have, as this will help them make decisions about your care. Communicating with your practitioner(s) can be key to ensuring the best possible health care.

Can I receive treatment or a referral to a practitioner from NCCAM?

NCCAM is the federal government's lead agency for scientific research on CAM. NCCAM's mission is to explore CAM healing practices in the context of rigorous science, train CAM researchers, and disseminate authoritative information to the public and professionals. NCCAM does not provide CAM therapies or referrals to practitioners.

Can I receive CAM treatment through a clinical trial?

NCCAM supports clinical trials (research studies in people) on CAM therapies. Clinical trials on CAM are taking place in many locations worldwide, and study participants are needed. To find trials that are recruiting participants, go to the website nccam.nih.gov/clinicaltrials. You can search this site by the type of therapy being studied or by disease or condition.

Section 6.2

Tips for Talking with Your Health Care Providers about CAM

From text by the National Center for Complementary and Alternative Medicine (NCCAM, nccam.nih.gov), part of the National Institutes of Health, October 2008.

Like many Americans, you may be using or considering some form of complementary and alternative medicine (CAM). If so, it is a good idea to talk with your health care providers about your CAM use.

About CAM

CAM refers to health-related products and practices that are not presently considered part of conventional medicine. Examples include herbal supplements, acupuncture, chiropractic manipulation, and many others.

Reasons for Talking with Your Health Care Providers about CAM Use

Some CAM approaches can have an effect on conventional medicines. Talking with your health care providers about your CAM use will help ensure coordinated and safe care.

Doctors, nurses, pharmacists, and other health care providers can help you decide whether a particular CAM therapy is right for you. They can answer questions, suggest reliable sources of information, and point out potential benefits and risks.

You are an important part of a team that includes all of the health care providers you rely on to manage your health. Giving your team a complete picture of everything you do to take care of your health makes them your fully informed partners—and it helps you stay in control of your own health care.

Tips for Talking with Your Health Care Providers about CAM

- Don't wait for your health care providers to ask about your CAM use. Be proactive—start the conversation.

- Keep a current list of all of your therapies and treatments, including over-the-counter and prescription medicines as well as any CAM products such as herbal and dietary supplements. Also note any medical specialists or CAM practitioners you see. Take the list with you whenever you visit a health care provider. Be sure to tell your health care providers about all of your therapies and treatments. Also include all therapies and treatments on any patient history forms you fill out.

- Gather information on the CAM therapy you're interested in. You may want to take copies with you; that way, you and your health care provider can refer to them as you talk, and your health care provider can help you evaluate the information.

- Make a list of the things you want to talk about. For example, if you're considering taking an herbal supplement, you might want to talk about the following topics:

  - Why I want to take the supplement

  - How I found out about it

  - Is it safe for me to take? Will it interact with any of my medications?

  - Is it likely to help me?

  - What else should I know about it? Where can I find more information?

  - Should I try this? If not, why not? Might something else be better?

- Take a notepad or tape recorder with you. Listen carefully and keep a record of what you find out. You may want to ask a family member or friend to accompany you, so you can compare notes after your visit.

- If something is unclear to you, or if you want more information, don't be afraid to ask. Your health care providers may not be able to answer every question, but they can help you find the answers.

Chapter 7

Insurance Issues and Paying for CAM Treatment

If you are using (or thinking about using) complementary and alternative medicine (CAM), you may have financial questions about paying for treatment.

How do people pay for CAM treatments?

They pay for CAM treatments in one or both of these ways:

- **Out-of-pocket:** Most people must pay for CAM services and products themselves.

- **Insurance:** Not all health insurance plans offer CAM coverage, however. When they do, the coverage varies by state and is often limited. Examples of CAM therapies that are sometimes covered by insurance are chiropractic, acupuncture, massage therapy, biofeedback, and naturopathy. Consumers' interest in CAM coverage is prompting more insurance companies and managed care organizations to consider offering this coverage as an option.

What are some questions to ask about paying for CAM treatment?

Some questions to ask a CAM practitioner or his office staff include the following:

Excerpted from "Paying for CAM Treatment," by the National Center for Complementary and Alternative Medicine (NCCAM, nccam.nih.gov), part of the National Institutes of Health, August 2008.

- What does the first appointment cost?
- What do followup appointments cost?
- How many appointments does someone with my condition typically need?
- Are there any additional costs (such as for tests, equipment, or supplements)?

If you have a health insurance plan, some other questions might include the following:

- Do you accept this insurance?
- What has your experience been with coverage by this insurance company for my condition?
- Do I file the claim forms, or do you take care of that?

If it would be difficult for you to pay the full fee at each visit, you can ask these questions:

- Could you arrange a payment plan over time?
- Do you offer a sliding-scale fee? (Sliding-scale fees are determined by people's income and ability to pay.)

What types of CAM coverage do employers offer?

If an employer offers CAM coverage, it usually has one or more of the following aspects:

- **Deductibles that may be higher than those for conventional care:** A deductible is a total dollar amount that you must pay before the insurer begins making any payment for treatment.
- **Policy riders:** A rider is an amendment that modifies the policy's coverage in some way (for example, by increasing or decreasing its benefits). You may be able to purchase a rider for CAM coverage.
- **A contracted network of providers:** Some insurers contract with a group of CAM providers who agree to offer their services at a lower rate to members than to nonmembers. You pay out-of-pocket, but at a discounted rate.

Employers negotiate with insurance companies for their rates and services, usually once a year. The Agency for Healthcare Research and Quality, part of the federal government, has publications on choosing and using a health insurance plan.

What are some important things to find out about my plan's coverage of CAM?

First, it is important to read your plan to find out whether it discusses coverage of the therapy in which you are interested. If anything about the coverage is not clear or you have questions, contact the insurance company before you decide about having treatment. Examples of questions that people often ask company representatives include the following:

- Is this treatment covered for my health condition?

- Does this care need to be:

  - preauthorized or preapproved;

  - ordered by a prescription; or

  - ordered through a referral from my primary care provider?

- Do I have to see a practitioner in your network in order to be covered?

- Do I have any coverage if I go out-of-network?

- Are there any limits and requirements—for example, on the number of visits or the amount you will pay?

- What do I have to pay out-of-pocket?

It is a good idea to keep detailed records about all contacts you have with the insurance company, including notes on calls and copies of bills, claims, and letters. This will help you if a dispute arises about a claim.

Does my state have any laws about CAM coverage?

Each state and U.S. territory, as well as the District of Columbia, has a department of insurance (check the government pages, or blue pages, of your phone book). This department regulates the insurance industry within its region, enforces pertinent laws, and assists consumers. The services vary, but every office responds to consumer inquiries on insurance.

If you are seeking CAM treatment from a practitioner, there is likely to be at least one professional association for the specialty— for example, associations for chiropractors. Many of these associations monitor insurance coverage and reimbursement in their field. You can search for them on the internet or ask a reference librarian for help.

41

Which insurance companies cover CAM?

Your state insurance department may be able to help you with this question. Many of these departments provide consumer publications, such as profiles and ratings of companies. (They do not provide recommendations or advice on specific companies.) An insurance broker (an agent who sells policies for a variety of companies) may also be a resource.

My insurance company denied my claim for CAM treatment. Is there anything I can do?

Yes, there are some things you can do:

- Know your plan, including what it does, and does not, cover.

- Check whether the CAM practitioner's office or your insurance company has made a coding error. To do this, compare the codes on the practitioner's bill with the codes on the document you received from the insurance company.

- If you think your insurer may have made a mistake processing your claim, you can request a review.

- The insurance company should also have a process for appealing coverage decisions.

- You can ask the CAM practitioner if there is anything she can do, such as writing a letter on your behalf.

If the problem is still not resolved, contact your state insurance department.

What are FSAs and HSAs, and can they help me with CAM expenses?

An FSA (short for flexible spending arrangement or flexible spending account) is a benefit offered by some employers. An FSA allows you to set aside pretax dollars each pay period for health-related expenses (some employers also make contributions). You submit receipts for yourself, your spouse, and/or your dependents to the FSA administrator for health-related expenses that were not covered some other way (for example, by insurance). You are then reimbursed for qualifying expenses (check your plan's language on this), such as deductibles, medical appointments, tests, and medicines.

An HSA (short for health savings account) is another type of tax-exempt account. It is for people who participate in a high-deductible health plan (also called a catastrophic health plan). In an HSA, you—not your employer—establish and maintain the account (although some employers make contributions). You can also invest your HSA funds to earn tax-deductible interest.

The Internal Revenue Service (IRS) has further information on these accounts. The IRS does not allow the same expenses to be reimbursed through an FSA or HSA and also claimed as tax deductions.

Can I deduct CAM treatments on my income tax return?

In tax year 2007, the IRS allowed taxpayers to deduct medical expenses for a limited number of CAM services and products, such as acupuncture and chiropractic care. These expenses were generally allowed for taxpayers and their spouses and dependents. Note that people cannot deduct the same medical expenses from their taxes and an FSA or HSA.

Can the federal government help me with expenses for CAM?

The federal government helps with at least some of the health expenses of people who are eligible for federal health benefit programs—usually because they meet one or more of the following conditions:

- They have a low income and limited resources.

- They do not have other medical insurance.

- They have a disability or certain medical conditions.

- They are part of a population that has difficulty obtaining medical care.

- They are at least 65 years old.

- They have served in the military.

That assistance may be direct (through payments) or indirect (through benefits like medical care at public clinics). Examples of programs that may provide some CAM coverage under some circumstances (as of July 2008) include the following:

- The Department of Veterans Affairs (for chiropractic care and acupuncture)

- Medicare, which covers chiropractic but does not cover what it calls "alternative therapies," giving as examples acupuncture, chelation therapy, biofeedback, and holistic medicine

43

- Medicaid, depending on your state's guidelines

GovBenefits and USA.gov are two internet resources that explain federal health benefit programs. GovBenefits has a test you can take about qualifying for programs. State and local departments of health or social services also have financial assistance programs for eligible residents, and you can contact them directly to inquire.

Does NCCAM provide financial help for CAM treatment?

Financial help for treatment does not fit under NCCAM's mission. NCCAM does sponsor clinical trials (research studies in people) of some CAM treatments. To find out what therapies are being studied and whether you might qualify to participate, go to nccam.nih.gov/clinicaltrials, or contact the NCCAM Clearinghouse.

Are there any other potential sources of financial assistance?

If treatment (whether CAM or conventional) for a disease or condition is creating a financial crisis for you and your family, you might find it helpful to contact nonprofit organizations that focus on the disease or condition. To locate them, try an internet search or check directories at your local library.

If you are receiving care at a hospital or clinic, ask if a social worker or patient advocate could advise you.

Chapter 8

Health Fraud Awareness

Health fraud is the deceptive sale or advertising of products that claim to be effective against medical conditions or otherwise beneficial to health, but which have not been proven safe and effective for those purposes.

In addition to wasting billions of consumers' dollars each year, health scams can lead patients to delay proper treatment and cause serious—and even fatal—injuries.

Since the 1990s, peddlers of fraudulent "health" products have used the internet as a primary tool to hawk their wares. This has kept the U.S. Food and Drug Administration (FDA) and other agencies busier than ever in protecting the public from health fraud.

Since June 2008, FDA has warned consumers not to use bogus cancer-treatment products marketed online by 28 U.S. companies. These products include tablets, teas, tonics, salves, and creams sold under more than 180 different brand names.

And since December 2008, FDA has warned about more than 70 weight loss products containing unapproved pharmaceutical ingredients and chemicals not listed on the labels. Some of these ingredients present serious health risks when taken in dosages recommended on the product label.

From "FDA 101: Health Fraud Awareness," by the U.S. Food and Drug Administration (FDA, www.fda.gov), May 2009.

Common Types of Health Fraud

Cancer fraud: Among the many long-running cancer scams is the Hoxsey Cancer Treatment, an herbal regimen that has no proven benefit. Another scam involves products called black salves. These are offered with the false promise of drawing cancer out from the skin, but they are potentially corrosive to tissues.

Cancer requires individualized treatment by a specialized physician. No single device, remedy, or treatment can treat all types of cancer.

Patients looking to try an experimental cancer treatment should enroll in a legitimate clinical study. For more information, visit the National Cancer Institute Clinical Trials website www.cancer.gov/CLINICALTRIALS.

HIV/AIDS fraud: There are legitimate treatments that can help people with the human immunodeficiency virus (HIV). While early treatment of HIV can delay progression to AIDS [acquired immunodeficiency syndrome], there is currently no cure for the disease.

Relying on unproven products and treatments can be dangerous and cause delays in seeking legitimate medical treatments that have been proven in clinical trials to improve quality of life.

Safe, reliable testing to determine whether you have HIV can be done by a medical professional.

To date, there is one FDA-approved testing system that allows individuals to test themselves at home. It is an HIV collection system that tests only for HIV-1, which is the cause of the majority of the world's HIV infections.

The test, sold either as The Home Access HIV-1 Test System or The Home Access Express HIV-1 Test System, allows blood samples to be sent to a laboratory for testing with an FDA approved HIV-1 test.

Arthritis fraud: The U.S. Federal Trade Commission says consumers spend about $2 billion annually on unproven arthritis remedies that are not backed by adequate science.

For current, accurate information on arthritis treatments and alternative therapies, visit the Arthritis Foundation website at www.arthritis.org.

Fraudulent "diagnostic" tests: Doctors often use in vitro diagnostic (IVD) tests—in tandem with a physical examination and a medical history—to get a picture of a patient's overall health.

These tests involve blood, urine, or other specimen samples taken from the body. They help diagnose or measure many conditions, including pregnancy, hepatitis, fertility, HIV, cholesterol, and blood sugar.

It's rare that the use of only one of these tests can provide a meaningful diagnosis. You can buy IVD tests in stores, through the mail, or online. Many of these tests are regulated by FDA and sold legally. However, many others are marketed illegally and do not meet FDA's regulatory requirements. These tests may not work or may be harmful.

To find out whether FDA has cleared or approved an IVD test for a particular purpose, call FDA at 888-463-6332, or your local FDA district office www.fda.gov/Safety/ReportaProblem/ConsumerComplaintCoordinators/default.htm.

Bogus dietary supplements: The array of dietary supplements—including vitamins and minerals, amino acids, enzymes, herbs, animal extracts, and others—has grown tremendously.

Although the benefits of some of these have been documented, the advantages of others are unproven. For example, claims that a supplement allows you to eat all you want and lose weight effortlessly are false.

Claims to treat diseases cause products to be considered drugs. Firms wanting to make such claims legally must follow FDA's premarket New Drug Approval process to show that the products are safe and effective.

Weight loss fraud: Since 2003, FDA has worked with national and international partners to take hundreds of compliance actions against companies pushing bogus and misleading weight loss schemes.

FDA has recently enhanced efforts to stop sales and importation of—and to warn consumers about—weight loss products that contain dangerous prescription drug ingredients that are not listed on the label.

Sexual enhancement product fraud: FDA has warned consumers about numerous illegal drugs promoted and sold online for treating erectile dysfunction and for enhancing sexual performance.

Although they are marketed as "dietary supplements," these products are really illegal drugs that contain potentially harmful ingredients that are not listed on the label.

Diabetes fraud: FDA has taken numerous compliance actions against sales of fraudulent diabetes "treatments" promoted with bogus claims such as the following:

- "Drop your blood sugar 50 points in 30 days"
- "Eliminate insulin resistance"
- "Prevent the development of type 2 diabetes"
- "Reduce or eliminate the need for diabetes drugs or insulin"

Influenza (flu) scams: Federal agencies have come across contaminated, counterfeit, and subpotent influenza products.

FDA, with U.S. Customs and Border Protection, has intercepted products claimed to be generic versions of the influenza drug Tamiflu, but which actually contained vitamin C and other substances not shown to be effective in treating or preventing influenza.

Don't Be a Victim

It's ultimately up to the buyer to beware of potential health fraud. Know of the potential for health fraud and learn about the common techniques and gimmicks that fraudulent marketers use to gain your attention and trust.

For instance, testimonials from people who say they have used the product may sound convincing, but these can easily be made up. These "testimonials" are not a substitute for scientific proof.

Also, never diagnose or treat yourself with questionable products. Always check with your health care professional before using new medical products.

Be wary of these red flags:

- Claims that a product is a quick, effective cure-all or a diagnostic tool for a wide variety of ailments
- Suggestions that a product can treat or cure diseases
- Promotions using words such as "scientific breakthrough," "miraculous cure," "secret ingredient," and "ancient remedy"
- Text with impressive-sounding terms such as: "hunger stimulation point" and "thermogenesis" for a weight loss product
- Undocumented case histories by consumers or doctors claiming amazing results
- Limited availability and advance payment requirements
- Promises of no-risk, money-back guarantees
- Promises of an "easy" fix
- Claims that the product is "natural" or "non-toxic" (which doesn't necessarily mean safe)

Don't be fooled by professional-looking websites. Avoid websites that fail to list the company's name, physical address, phone number, or other contact information. For more tips for online buying, visit www.fda.gov/buyonlineguide.

Report Problems

If you find a person or company that you think is illegally selling human drugs, animal drugs, medical devices, biological products, foods, dietary supplements, or cosmetics, report it to FDA.

To report problems with FDA-regulated products, visit www.fda .gov/opacom/backgrounders/complain.html.

To report unlawful sales of medical products on the internet, visit www.fda.gov/oc/buyonline/buyonlineform.htm.

Chapter 9

Use Caution Buying Medical Products Online

Get prescription drugs fast—no doctor needed! Cure cancer with herbs! Zap your pain away with an amazing device! Absolutely safe—pull out your credit card now, and get rock-bottom prices.

It's not hard to find statements like these floating around in cyberspace. "And if they sound too good to be true, it's because they usually are," says Rich Cleland, assistant director of the Division of Advertising Practices at the Federal Trade Commission (FTC).

Many legitimate websites bring customers health products with the benefits of convenience, privacy and, sometimes, cheaper prices. "But consumers need to be aware that the internet has also created a marketplace for unapproved medical products, illegal prescribing, and products marketed with fraudulent health claims," says William Hubbard, former associate commissioner for policy and planning at the Food and Drug Administration.

"And the unique qualities of the internet, including its broad reach, relative anonymity, and the ease of creating and removing websites, pose challenges for enforcing federal and state laws," Hubbard says. "Many sites are connected to other sites and have multiple links, which makes investigations more complex. And there are jurisdictional challenges because the regulatory and enforcement issues cross state, federal, and international lines."

Excerpted from "Use Caution Buying Medical Products Online," by the U.S. Food and Drug Administration (FDA, www.fda.gov), May 1, 2009.

Government agencies work together to shut down illegal websites and prosecute criminals, but enforcement resources are limited. "Consumers need to take some responsibility for recognizing suspicious sites and turning the other way," Hubbard says. So how can you spot the red flags? Here's a guide to help you protect your health and your wallet.

Dietary Supplements

Dietary supplements are products taken as a supplement to the diet. Examples are vitamins, minerals, herbs, botanicals, and amino acids, the individual building blocks of proteins needed for all life. Dietary supplements are classified as foods and not drugs.

Problem sites: Websites cannot claim that dietary supplements will prevent, treat, or cure any disease. This would make the product an unapproved and illegal drug. Also, websites can't make claims that a dietary supplement will have an effect on any structure or function of the body when the claims are not substantiated.

"Websites selling dietary supplements with false or unsubstantiated claims sometimes use testimonials and advertisements touting a quick, miracle cure," says the FTC's Cleland. "And some sites claim a product will cure it all—heart disease, cancer, arthritis, you name it."

Cleland says he sees a lot of miracle claims for major diseases and weight loss. "Criminals also prey on people's fears about terrorism," he adds. After the anthrax attacks in 2001, some sites falsely claimed that dietary supplements such as colloidal silver and oregano oil could protect against biological and chemical contamination.

Risks: "In promoting some products, companies are telling patients not to undergo surgery, chemotherapy, or other needed treatment," says Cleland. "So we are concerned about people forgoing legitimate medical treatment."

Consumers also have to worry about ingesting harmful substances. Companies may call a product "natural," but that doesn't mean it's safe. And dietary supplements are intended to supplement diets, not replace them. Too much of some nutrients can cause problems. There is also a danger of dietary supplements interacting with other drugs you may be taking. The prescription medicine warfarin, the herbal supplement gingko biloba, aspirin, and vitamin E all can thin the blood, so taking any of them together can increase the potential for internal bleeding.

Regulation: Under the Dietary Supplement Health and Education Act of 1994 (DSHEA), dietary supplements are products that are intended to supplement the diet and that contain one or more of the following dietary ingredients: a vitamin, a mineral, an herb or other botanical, an amino acid, a dietary substance that supplements the diet by increasing the total daily intake, or a concentrate, metabolite, constituent, extract, or combination of these ingredients.

Dietary supplement manufacturers must notify the FDA at least 75 days before marketing products containing some "new dietary ingredients." This includes providing the agency with safety information about the supplement. New dietary ingredients are those that were not marketed as dietary supplements before Oct. 15, 1994.

Except for those dietary supplements containing new dietary ingredients, the safety and labeling of most dietary supplements is monitored only after they reach the marketplace. The FDA evaluates the safety of dietary supplements after they are on the market, overseeing safety, manufacturing, and product information on the labeling. The FTC regulates the advertising of dietary supplements under the FTC Act, which prohibits deceptive claims in advertising.

Under DSHEA, the FDA generally has responsibility for showing a dietary supplement is unsafe before it can take action to restrict the product's use. For example, in 2004, the FDA banned the use of ephedrine alkaloids in dietary supplements because the substances pose an unreasonable risk of illness or injury. Ephedrine alkaloids in dietary supplements have been linked to cardiovascular problems.

"If the FDA can establish that claims are false or misleading, or if a firm is making drug claims for a dietary supplement, the agency can take action using any of our enforcement tools, such as warning letters, cyber letters, seizure of products, and criminal prosecution," says Jennifer Thomas, who leads the dietary supplement and labeling enforcement team in the FDA's Center for Food Safety and Applied Nutrition, Office of Compliance.

Consumers should be wary of claims related to diseases or conditions that are prominent in the news. For example, when severe acute respiratory syndrome (SARS) was in the news in 2003, the FDA found several dietary supplement products promoted on the internet for treating or preventing SARS. The FDA took action against 10 of these firms, as there was no evidence of safety or effectiveness of the products for use against SARS.

Enforcement examples: Since 2003, the FDA has taken action against street drug alternative products called "Black Beauties" and "Yellow Jackets," seizing millions of dollars' worth of these products. Although labeled and marketed as dietary supplements, such products are actually unapproved drugs and cannot be sold as dietary supplements.

In February 2004, the FDA warned consumers against purchasing a liquid product called "Green Hornet." Although it was promoted on the internet and sold in stores as a dietary supplement, the product was actually an illegal drug because it was promoted as an herbal version of Ecstasy. After taking the product, four teenagers were rushed to the hospital with seizures, excessive heart rates, severe body rashes, and high blood pressure.

In March 2004, the FDA and the FTC announced that SeaSilver USA Inc. and Americaloe Inc. of Carlsbad, California, signed a consent decree of permanent injunction and agreed to stop manufacturing a bogus cure-all liquid supplement called SeaSilver and other products.

In June 2004, the FDA announced the sentencing of a man who swindled cancer patients by heavily advertising and selling Laetrile, also known as vitamin B-17 or apricot pits. Although he purported it to be a dietary supplement, Laetrile is actually an unapproved drug. The highly toxic product hasn't shown any effect on treating cancer.

The FDA issued a warning letter to Cellular Wellness Foundation in September 2004, citing claims made on its website that the product Cellular Tea was effective in treating serious diseases such as cancer.

In 2004, the FDA issued warning letters to 25 firms that promote their products on the internet with claims that the products are useful for weight loss. The claims are not supported by scientific evidence.

In July 2004, the U.S. District Court for the District of New Jersey found that three products sold as dietary supplements and a cosmetic by Lane Labs-USA Inc. and its president Andrew J. Lane are in fact unapproved new drugs because they were being marketed as treatments for cancer, HIV, and skin cancer without FDA approval. The court permanently enjoined Lane and the company from distributing the products—Benefin, MGN-3, and SkinAnswer—unless they are first either approved for marketing by the FDA or distributed pursuant to an investigational new drug application for purposes of conducting a clinical trial. The court also ordered the defendants to pay restitution to purchasers of the three products since Sept. 22, 1999. The defendants appealed the court's decision.

Tips: Consumers who choose to buy dietary supplements on the internet should consider who operates the website and what evidence is provided to substantiate claims.

Dietary supplement makers are responsible for making sure that their products are safe before they go on the market and that claims on labels are accurate, truthful, and substantiated with adequate scientific evidence. By law, supplement manufacturers are allowed to use these types of claims, when appropriate:

- Nutrient-content claims such as "high in calcium" or "excellent source of vitamin C" may be used.

- Health claims that show a link between the supplement and reduced risk of a disease or health condition, when the use of the claim has been approved by the FDA, may be used. For example, women who get adequate amounts of the B vitamin folic acid during pregnancy have a decreased risk of having a baby with a neural tube defect.

- Qualified health claims, which are for dietary supplements only, may be used. This type of claim came about as a result of a 1999 decision by the U.S. Court of Appeals for the District of Columbia Circuit in the case of Pearson v. Shalala. The court's ruling requires the FDA to allow appropriately qualified health claims that would be misleading without such qualification. These qualified claims are based on the weight of the scientific evidence. An example of this type of claim is "Supportive but not conclusive research shows that consumption of EPA (eicosapentaenoic acid) and DHA (docosahexaenoic acid) omega-3 fatty acids may reduce the risk of coronary heart disease."

- Claims regarding a benefit related to a classical nutrient deficiency disease, such as vitamin C and scurvy, may be used.

- Claims that a dietary supplement has an effect on the structure or function of the body, when such claims are supported by scientific evidence, may be used. An example of such a claim is "calcium builds strong bones" for a supplement that contains calcium.

- Claims that describe general well-being from consumption of the product may be used.

The FDA recommends that consumers contact their health care providers before using dietary supplements. This is especially important for people who are pregnant or breast-feeding, chronically ill, older, younger than 18, or taking prescription or over-the-counter medicines.

Reporting Problems

To report a problem with a website selling human drugs, animal drugs, medical devices, biological products, foods, dietary supplements, or cosmetics, see the following:

- If the problem involves a serious or life-threatening situation, call your health care professional immediately for medical advice. To report the situation to the FDA, call 301-443-1240.

- If the problem involves a serious reaction or problem, contact your health care professional for advice. To fill out the FDA's MedWatch reporting form, go to www.fda.gov/medwatch.

- For problems that do not involve a serious or life-threatening reaction, fill out the form at www.fda.gov/oc/buyonline/buyonlineform.htm.

- To report e-mails or websites promoting medical products that might be illegal, forward the material to webcomplaints @ora.fda.gov.

- To report false claims to the Federal Trade Commission, call 877-382-4357. If you lose your money, contact the credit card company, your state attorney general's office, or the Better Business Bureau.

Part Two

Alternative Medicine Systems

Chapter 10

What Are Whole Medical Systems?

Whole medical systems involve complete systems of theory and practice that have evolved independently from or parallel to allopathic (conventional) medicine. Many are traditional systems of medicine that are practiced by individual cultures throughout the world. Major Eastern whole medical systems include traditional Chinese medicine (TCM), and Ayurveda, one of India's traditional systems of medicine. Major Western whole medical systems include homeopathy and naturopathy. Other systems have been developed by Native American, African, Middle Eastern, Tibetan, and Central and South American cultures.

Traditional Chinese Medicine

TCM is a complete system of healing that dates back to 200 B.C. in written form. Korea, Japan, and Vietnam have all developed their own unique versions of traditional medicine based on practices originating in China. In the TCM view, the body is a delicate balance of two opposing and inseparable forces: yin and yang. Yin represents the cold, slow, or passive principle, while yang represents the hot, excited, or active principle. Among the major assumptions in TCM are that health is achieved by maintaining the body in a "balanced state" and that disease is due to an internal imbalance of yin and yang. This imbalance leads to blockage in the flow of qi (or vital energy) and of blood along

Excerpted from "Whole Medical Systems: An Overview," by the National Center for Complementary and Alternative Medicine (NCCAM, nccam.nih.gov), part of the National Institutes of Health, March 2007.

pathways known as meridians. TCM practitioners typically use herbs, acupuncture, and massage to help unblock qi and blood in patients in an attempt to bring the body back into harmony and wellness.

Treatments in TCM are typically tailored to the subtle patterns of disharmony in each patient and are based on an individualized diagnosis. The diagnostic tools differ from those of conventional medicine. There are three main therapeutic modalities:

1. Acupuncture and moxibustion (moxibustion is the application of heat from the burning of the moxa at the acupuncture point)

2. Chinese Materia Medica (the catalogue of natural products used in TCM)

3. Massage and manipulation

Although TCM proposes that natural products catalogued in Chinese Materia Medica or acupuncture can be used alone to treat virtually any illness, quite often they are used together and sometimes in combination with other modalities (e.g., massage, moxibustion, diet changes, or exercise).

Acupuncture

The report from a Consensus Development Conference on Acupuncture held at the National Institutes of Health (NIH) in 1997 states that acupuncture is being "widely" practiced—by thousands of acupuncturists, physicians, dentists, and other practitioners—for relief or prevention of pain and for various other health conditions. In terms of the evidence at that time, acupuncture was considered to have potential clinical value for nausea/vomiting and dental pain, and limited evidence suggested its potential in the treatment of other pain disorders, paralysis and numbness, movement disorders, depression, insomnia, breathlessness, and asthma.

Preclinical studies have documented acupuncture's effects, but they have not been able to fully explain how acupuncture works within the framework of the Western system of medicine.

It is proposed that acupuncture produces its effects by the conduction of electromagnetic signals at a greater-than-normal rate, thus aiding the activity of pain-killing biochemicals, such as endorphins and immune system cells at specific sites in the body. In addition, studies have shown that acupuncture may alter brain chemistry by changing the release of neurotransmitters and neurohormones and affecting the parts of the central nervous system related to sensation and involuntary body functions, such as immune reactions and processes whereby a person's blood pressure, blood flow, and body temperature are regulated.

Chinese Materia Medica

Chinese Materia Medica is a standard reference book of information on medicinal substances that are used in Chinese herbal medicine. Herbs or botanicals usually contain dozens of bioactive compounds. Many factors—such as geographic location, harvest season, post-harvest processing, and storage—could have a significant impact on the concentration of bioactive compounds. In many cases, it is not clear which of these compounds underlie an herb's medical use. Moreover, multiple herbs are usually used in combinations called formulas in TCM, which makes the standardization of herbal preparations very difficult. Further complicating research on TCM herbs, herbal compositions and the quantity of individual herbs in a classic formula are usually adjusted in TCM practice according to individualized diagnoses.

In the past decades, major efforts have been made to study the effects and effectiveness of single herbs and of combinations of herbs used in classic TCM formulas. The following are examples of such work:

- *Artemisia annua*: Ancient Chinese physicians identified that this herb controls fevers. In the 1970s, scientists extracted the chemical artemisinin from Artemisia annua. Artemisinin is the starting material for the semi-synthetic artemisinins that are proven to treat malaria and are widely used.

- *Tripterygium wilfordii Hook F* (**Chinese Thunder God vine**): Thunder God vine has been used in TCM for the treatment of autoimmune and inflammatory diseases. The first small randomized, placebo-controlled trial of a Thunder God vine extract in the United States showed a significant dose-dependent response in patients with rheumatoid arthritis. In larger, uncontrolled studies, however, renal, cardiac, hematopoietic, and reproductive toxicities of Thunder God vine extracts have been observed.

Ayurvedic Medicine

Ayurveda, which literally means "the science of life," is a natural healing system developed in India. Ayurvedic texts claim that the sages who developed India's original systems of meditation and yoga developed the foundations of this medical system. It is a comprehensive system of medicine that places equal emphasis on the body, mind, and spirit, and strives to restore the innate harmony of the individual. Some of the primary Ayurvedic treatments include diet, exercise, meditation, herbs, massage, exposure to sunlight, and controlled breathing. In

India, Ayurvedic treatments have been developed for various diseases (e.g., diabetes, cardiovascular conditions, and neurological disorders). However, a survey of the Indian medical literature indicates that the quality of the published clinical trials generally falls short of contemporary methodological standards with regard to criteria for randomization, sample size, and adequate controls.

Naturopathy

Naturopathy is a system of healing, originating from Europe, that views disease as a manifestation of alterations in the processes by which the body naturally heals itself. It emphasizes health restoration as well as disease treatment. The term "naturopathy" literally translates as "nature disease." Today naturopathy, or naturopathic medicine, is practiced throughout Europe, Australia, New Zealand, Canada, and the United States. There are six principles that form the basis of naturopathic practice in North America (not all are unique to naturopathy):

1. The healing power of nature

2. Identification and treatment of the cause of disease

3. The concept of "first do no harm"

4. The doctor as teacher

5. Treatment of the whole person

6. Prevention

The core modalities supporting these principles include diet modification and nutritional supplements, herbal medicine, acupuncture and Chinese medicine, hydrotherapy, massage and joint manipulation, and lifestyle counseling. Treatment protocols combine what the practitioner deems to be the most suitable therapies for the individual patient.

As of this writing, virtually no research studies on naturopathy as a complete system of medicine have been published. A limited number of studies on botanicals in the context of use as naturopathic treatments have been published. For example, in a study of 524 children, echinacea did not prove effective in treating colds. In contrast, a smaller, double-blind trial of an herbal extract solution containing echinacea, propolis (a resinous product collected from beehives), and vitamin C for ear pain in 171 children concluded that the extract may be beneficial for ear pain associated with acute otitis media. A naturopathic extract known as Otikon Otic Solution (containing *Allium sativum*, *Verbascum thapsus, Calendula flores,* and *Hypericum perforatum* in olive oil) was found as effective as anesthetic ear drops and was proven appropriate for the management of acute otitis media-associated ear pain. Another study looked at the clinical effectiveness and cost-effectiveness of naturopathic cranberry tablets—versus cranberry juice and versus a placebo—as prophylaxis against urinary tract infections (UTIs). Compared with the placebo, both cranberry juice and cranberry tablets decreased the number of UTIs. Cranberry tablets proved to be the most cost-effective prevention for UTIs.

Homeopathy

Homeopathy is a complete system of medical theory and practice. Its founder, German physician Samuel Christian Hahnemann (1755–1843), hypothesized that one can select therapies on the basis of how closely symptoms produced by a remedy match the symptoms of the patient's disease. He called this the "principle of similars." Hahnemann proceeded to give repeated doses of many common remedies to healthy volunteers and carefully record the symptoms they produced. This procedure is called a "proving" or, in modern homeopathy, a "human pathogenic trial." As a result of this experience, Hahnemann developed his treatments for sick patients by matching the symptoms produced by a drug to symptoms in sick patients. Hahnemann emphasized from the beginning carefully examining all aspects of a person's health status, including emotional and mental states, and tiny idiosyncratic characteristics.

Since homeopathy is administered in minute or potentially nonexistent material dosages, there is an *a priori* skepticism in the scientific community about its efficacy. Nonetheless, the medical literature provides evidence of ongoing research in the field. Studies of homeopathy's effectiveness involve three areas of research:

1. Comparisons of homeopathic remedies and placebos

2. Studies of homeopathy's effectiveness for particular clinical conditions

3. Studies of the biological effects of potencies, especially ultra-high dilutions

Five systematic reviews and meta-analyses evaluated clinical trials of the effectiveness of homeopathic remedies as compared with placebo. The reviews found that, overall, the quality of clinical research in homeopathy is low. But when high-quality studies were selected for analysis, a surprising number showed positive results.

Overall, clinical trial results are contradictory, and systematic reviews and meta-analyses have not found homeopathy to be a definitively proven treatment for any medical conditions.

Summary

While whole medical systems differ in their philosophical approaches to the prevention and treatment of disease, they share a number of common elements. These systems are based on the belief that one's body has the power to heal itself. Healing often involves marshalling multiple techniques that involve the mind, body, and spirit. Treatment is often individualized and dependent on the presenting symptoms. To date, NCCAM's research efforts have focused on individual therapies with adequate experimental rationale and not on evaluating whole systems of medicine as they are commonly practiced.

Chapter 11

Ayurvedic Medicine

Ayurvedic medicine (also called Ayurveda) is one of the world's oldest medical systems. It originated in India and has evolved there over thousands of years. In the United States, Ayurvedic medicine is considered complementary and alternative medicine (CAM)—more specifically, a CAM whole medical system. Many therapies used in Ayurvedic medicine are also used on their own as CAM—for example, herbs, massage, and specialized diets.

Background

Ayurvedic medicine, also called Ayurveda, originated in India several thousand years ago. The term "Ayurveda" combines the Sanskrit words ayur (life) and veda (science or knowledge). Thus, Ayurveda means "the science of life."

In the United States, Ayurvedic medicine is considered a type of CAM and a whole medical system. As with other such systems, it is based on theories of health and illness and on ways to prevent, manage, or treat health problems.

Ayurvedic medicine aims to integrate and balance the body, mind, and spirit; thus, some view it as "holistic." This balance is believed to lead to happiness and health, and to help prevent illness. Ayurvedic medicine also treats specific physical and mental health problems. A chief aim of

From "Ayurvedic Medicine: An Introduction," by the National Center for Complementary and Alternative Medicine (NCCAM, nccam.nih.gov), part of the National Institutes of Health, July 2009.

Ayurvedic practices is to cleanse the body of substances that can cause disease, thus helping to reestablish harmony and balance.

Ayurvedic Medicine in India

Ayurvedic medicine, as practiced in India, is one of the oldest systems of medicine in the world. Many Ayurvedic practices predate written records and were handed down by word of mouth. Two ancient books, written in Sanskrit more than 2,000 years ago, are considered the main texts on Ayurvedic medicine—*Caraka Samhita* and *Sushruta Samhita*. The texts describe eight branches of Ayurvedic medicine:

- Internal medicine
- Surgery
- Treatment of head and neck disease
- Gynecology, obstetrics, and pediatrics
- Toxicology
- Psychiatry
- Care of the elderly and rejuvenation
- Sexual vitality

Ayurvedic medicine continues to be practiced in India, where nearly 80 percent of the population uses it exclusively or combined with conventional (Western) medicine. It is also practiced in Bangladesh, Sri Lanka, Nepal, and Pakistan.

Most major cities in India have an Ayurvedic college and hospital. The Indian government began systematic research on Ayurvedic practices in 1969, and that work continues.

Use in the United States

According to the 2007 National Health Interview Survey, which included a comprehensive survey of CAM use by Americans, more than 200,000 U.S. adults had used Ayurvedic medicine in the previous year.

Underlying Concepts

Ayurvedic medicine has several key foundations that pertain to health and disease. These concepts have to do with universal interconnectedness, the body's constitution (prakriti), and life forces (doshas).

Interconnectedness: Ideas about the relationships among people, their health, and the universe form the basis for how Ayurvedic practitioners think about problems that affect health. Ayurvedic medicine holds that the following statements are true:

- All things in the universe (both living and nonliving) are joined together.

- Every human being contains elements that can be found in the universe.

- Health will be good if one's mind and body are in harmony, and one's interaction with the universe is natural and wholesome.

- Disease arises when a person is out of harmony with the universe. Disruptions can be physical, emotional, spiritual, or a combination of these.

Constitution (prakriti): Ayurvedic medicine also has specific beliefs about the body's constitution. Constitution refers to a person's general health, the likelihood of becoming out of balance, and the ability to resist and recover from disease or other health problems.

The constitution is called the prakriti. The prakriti is a person's unique combination of physical and psychological characteristics and the way the body functions to maintain health. It is influenced by such factors as digestion and how the body deals with waste products. The prakriti is believed to be unchanged over a person's lifetime.

Life forces (doshas): Important characteristics of the prakriti are the three life forces or energies called doshas, which control the activities of the body. A person's chances of developing certain types of diseases are thought to be related to the way doshas are balanced, the state of the physical body, and mental or lifestyle factors.

Ayurvedic medicine holds the following beliefs about the three doshas:

- Each dosha is made up of two of five basic elements: ether (the upper regions of space), air, fire, water, and earth.

- Each dosha has a particular relationship to bodily functions and can be upset for different reasons.

- Each person has a unique combination of the three doshas, although one dosha is usually prominent. Doshas are constantly being formed and reformed by food, activity, and bodily processes.

- Each dosha has its own physical and psychological characteristics.

- An imbalance of a dosha will produce symptoms that are unique to that dosha. Imbalances may be caused by a person's age, unhealthy lifestyle, or diet; too much or too little mental and physical exertion; the seasons; or inadequate protection from the weather, chemicals, or germs.

The doshas are known by their original Sanskrit names: vata, pitta, and kapha.

The vata dosha combines the elements ether and air. It is considered the most powerful dosha because it controls very basic body processes such as cell division, the heart, breathing, discharge of waste, and the mind. Vata can be aggravated by, for example, fear, grief, staying up late at night, eating dry fruit, or eating before the previous meal is digested. People with vata as their main dosha are thought to be especially susceptible to skin and neurological conditions, rheumatoid arthritis, heart disease, anxiety, and insomnia.

The pitta dosha represents the elements fire and water. Pitta controls hormones and the digestive system. A person with a pitta imbalance may experience negative emotions such as anger and may have physical symptoms such as heartburn within 2 or 3 hours of eating. Pitta is upset by, for example, eating spicy or sour food, fatigue, or spending too much time in the sun. People with a predominantly pitta constitution are thought to be susceptible to hypertension, heart disease, infectious diseases, and digestive conditions such as Crohn disease.

The kapha dosha combines the elements water and earth. Kapha helps to maintain strength and immunity and to control growth. An imbalance of the kapha dosha may cause nausea immediately after eating. Kapha is aggravated by, for example, greed, sleeping during the daytime, eating too many sweet foods, eating after one is full, and eating and drinking foods and beverages with too much salt and water (especially in the springtime). Those with a predominant kapha dosha are thought to be vulnerable to diabetes, cancer, obesity, and respiratory illnesses such as asthma.

Treatment

Ayurvedic treatment is tailored to each person's constitution. Practitioners expect patients to be active participants because many Ayurvedic treatments require changes in diet, lifestyle, and habits.

The patient's dosha balance: Ayurvedic practitioners first determine the patient's primary dosha and the balance among the three doshas by doing the following:

- Asking about diet, behavior, lifestyle practices, recent illnesses (including reasons and symptoms), and resilience (ability to recover quickly from illness or setbacks)

- Observing such physical characteristics as teeth and tongue, skin, eyes, weight, and overall appearance

- Checking the patient's urine, stool, speech and voice, and pulse (each dosha is thought to make a particular kind of pulse)

Treatment practices: Ayurvedic treatment goals include eliminating impurities, reducing symptoms, increasing resistance to disease, and reducing worry and increasing harmony in the patient's life. The practitioner uses a variety of methods to achieve these goals:

- Eliminating impurities: A process called panchakarma is intended to cleanse the body by eliminating ama. Ama is described as an undigested food that sticks to tissues, interferes with normal functioning of the body, and leads to disease. Panchakarma focuses on eliminating ama through the digestive tract and the respiratory system. Enemas, massage, medical oils administered in a nasal spray, and other methods may be used.

- Reducing symptoms: The practitioner may suggest various options, including physical exercises, stretching, breathing exercises, meditation, massage, lying in the sun, and changing the diet. The patient may take certain herbs—often with honey, to make them easier to digest. Sometimes diets are restricted to certain foods. Very small amounts of metal and mineral preparations, such as gold or iron, also may be given.

- Increasing resistance to disease: The practitioner may combine several herbs, proteins, minerals, and vitamins in tonics to improve digestion and increase appetite and immunity. These tonics are based on formulas from ancient texts.

- Reducing worry and increasing harmony: Ayurvedic medicine emphasizes mental nurturing and spiritual healing. Practitioners may recommend avoiding situations that cause worry and using techniques that promote release of negative emotions.

Use of plants: Ayurvedic treatments rely heavily on herbs and other plants—including oils and common spices. Currently, more than 600 herbal formulas and 250 single plant drugs are included in the "pharmacy" of Ayurvedic treatments. Historically, Ayurvedic medicine has grouped plant compounds into categories according to their effects (for example, healing, promoting vitality, or relieving pain). The compounds are described in texts issued by national medical agencies in India. Sometimes, botanicals are mixed with metals or other naturally occurring substances to make formulas prepared according to specific Ayurvedic text procedures; such preparations involve several herbs and herbal extracts and precise heat treatment.

Practitioner Training and Certification

Many practitioners study in India, where there are more than 150 undergraduate and 30 postgraduate colleges for Ayurvedic medicine. Training can take 5 years or longer. Students who receive their Ayurvedic training in India can earn either a bachelor's degree (Bachelor of Ayurvedic Medicine and Surgery, BAMS) or doctoral degree (Doctor of Ayurvedic Medicine and Surgery, DAMS) there. After graduation, some Ayurvedic practitioners choose to provide services in the United States or other countries.

The United States has no national standard for training or certifying Ayurvedic practitioners, although a few states have approved Ayurvedic schools as educational institutions.

Concerns about Ayurvedic Medications

Ayurvedic practice involves the use of medications that typically contain herbs, metals, minerals, or other materials. Health officials in India and other countries have taken steps to address some concerns about these medications. Concerns relate to toxicity, formulations, interactions, and scientific evidence.

Toxicity: Ayurvedic medications have the potential to be toxic. Many materials used in them have not been thoroughly studied in either Western or Indian research. In the United States, Ayurvedic medications are regulated as dietary supplements. As such, they are not required to meet the safety and efficacy standards for conventional medicines. An NCCAM-funded study published in 2004 found that of 70 Ayurvedic remedies purchased over-the-counter (all manufactured in South Asia), 14 contained lead, mercury, and/or arsenic at levels that could be harmful. Also in 2004, the Centers for Disease Control and Prevention reported that 12 cases of lead poisoning occurring over a recent 3-year period were linked to the use of Ayurvedic medications.

Formulations: Most Ayurvedic medications consist of combinations of herbs and other medicines. It can be challenging to know which components are having an effect and why.

Interactions: Whenever two or more medications are used, there is the potential for them to interact with each other. As a result, the effectiveness of at least one may increase or decrease in the body.

Scientific evidence: Most clinical trials (i.e., studies in people) of Ayurvedic approaches have been small, had problems with research designs, lacked appropriate control groups, or had other issues that affected how meaningful the results were. Therefore, scientific evidence for the effectiveness of Ayurvedic practices varies, and more rigorous research is needed to determine which practices are safe and effective.

Other Points to Consider about Using Ayurvedic Medicine

- Tell your health care providers about any complementary and alternative practices you use, including Ayurvedic medicine. Give them a full picture of what you do to manage your health. This will help to ensure coordinated and safe care.

- Women who are pregnant or nursing, or people who are thinking of using Ayurvedic therapy to treat a child, should be especially sure to consult their health care provider.

- It is important to make sure that any diagnosis of a disease or condition has been made by a provider who has substantial conventional medical training and experience with managing that disease or condition.

- Proven conventional treatments should not be replaced with an unproven CAM treatment.

- It is better to use Ayurvedic remedies under the supervision of an Ayurvedic medicine practitioner than to try to treat yourself.

- Before using Ayurvedic treatment, ask about the practitioner's training and experience.

- Find out whether any rigorous scientific studies have been done on the therapies in which you are interested.

Chapter 12

Other Indigenous Medical Systems

Chapter Contents

Section 12.1—Traditional Chinese Medicine 74

Section 12.2—Native American Medicine 78

Section 12.1

Traditional Chinese Medicine

From "Traditional Chinese Medicine: An Introduction," from the National Center for Complementary and Alternative Medicine (NCCAM, nccam.nih.gov), part of the National Institutes of Health, March 2009.

Traditional Chinese medicine (TCM) originated in ancient China and has evolved over thousands of years. TCM practitioners use herbs, acupuncture, and other methods to treat a wide range of conditions. In the United States, TCM is considered part of complementary and alternative medicine (CAM).

Background

Traditional Chinese medicine, which encompasses many different practices, is rooted in the ancient philosophy of Taoism and dates back more than 5,000 years. Today, TCM is practiced side by side with Western medicine in many of China's hospitals and clinics.

TCM is widely used in the United States. Although the exact number of people who use TCM in the United States is unknown, it was estimated in 1997 that some 10,000 practitioners served more than 1 million patients each year. According to the 2007 National Health Interview Survey, which included questions on the use of various CAM therapies, an estimated 3.1 million U.S. adults had used acupuncture in the previous year. In addition, according to this same survey, approximately 17 percent of adults use natural products, including herbs, making it the most commonly used therapy. In another survey, more than one third of the patients at six large acupuncture clinics said they also received Chinese herbal treatments at the clinics.

Underlying Concepts

Underlying the practice of TCM is a unique view of the world and the human body that is different from Western medicine concepts. This view is based on the ancient Chinese perception of humans as microcosms of the larger, surrounding universe—interconnected with nature and subject to its forces. The human body is regarded as an organic entity in which the various organs, tissues, and other parts have distinct functions but are all interdependent. In this view, health and disease relate to balance of the functions.

The theoretical framework of TCM has a number of key components:

- Yin-yang theory—the concept of two opposing, yet complementary, forces that shape the world and all life—is central to TCM.

- In the TCM view, a vital energy or life force called qi circulates in the body through a system of pathways called meridians. Health is an ongoing process of maintaining balance and harmony in the circulation of qi.

- The TCM approach uses eight principles to analyze symptoms and categorize conditions: cold/heat, interior/exterior, excess/deficiency, and yin/yang (the chief principles). TCM also uses the theory of five elements—fire, earth, metal, water, and wood—to explain how the body works; these elements correspond to particular organs and tissues in the body.

These concepts are documented in the *Huang Di Nei Jing* (Inner Canon of the Yellow Emperor), the classic Chinese medicine text.

Treatment

TCM emphasizes individualized treatment. Practitioners traditionally used four methods to evaluate a patient's condition: observing (especially the tongue), hearing/smelling, asking/interviewing, and touching/palpating (especially the pulse).

TCM practitioners use a variety of therapics in an effort to promote health and treat disease. The most commonly used are Chinese herbal medicine and acupuncture.

- **Chinese herbal medicine:** The Chinese materia medica (a pharmacological reference book used by TCM practitioners) contains hundreds of medicinal substances—primarily plants, but also some minerals and animal products—classified by their perceived action in the body. Different parts of plants such as the leaves, roots, stems, flowers, and seeds are used. Usually, herbs are combined in formulas and given as teas, capsules, tinctures, or powders.

- **Acupuncture:** By stimulating specific points on the body, most often by inserting thin metal needles through the skin, practitioners seek to remove blockages in the flow of qi.

Other TCM therapies include moxibustion (burning moxa—a cone or stick of dried herb, usually mugwort—on or near the skin, sometimes in conjunction with acupuncture); cupping (applying a heated cup to the skin to create a slight suction); Chinese massage; mind-body therapies such as qi gong and tai chi; and dietary therapy.

Status of TCM Research

In spite of the widespread use of TCM in China and its use in the West, scientific evidence of its effectiveness is, for the most part, limited. TCM's complexity and underlying conceptual foundations present challenges for researchers seeking evidence on whether and how it works. Most research has focused on specific modalities, primarily acupuncture and Chinese herbal remedies.

Acupuncture research has produced a large body of scientific evidence. Studies suggest that it may be useful for a number of different conditions, but additional research is still needed.

Chinese herbal medicine has also been studied for a wide range of conditions. Most of the research has been done in China. Although there is evidence that herbs may be effective for some conditions, most studies have been methodologically flawed, and additional, better designed research is needed before any conclusions can be drawn.

Examples of TCM Uses and Studies

Both acupuncture and Chinese herbal medicine have been used and studied for a wide range of conditions:

- Acupuncture
  - Back pain
  - Depression
  - Chemotherapy-induced nausea
  - Osteoarthritis
- Chinese herbal medicine
  - Cancer
  - Heart disease
  - Diabetes
  - HIV/AIDS [human immunodeficiency virus/acquired immunodeficiency syndrome]

Safety

The U.S. Food and Drug Administration (FDA) regulations for dietary supplements (including manufactured herbal products) are not the same as those for prescription or over-the-counter drugs; in general, the regulations for dietary supplements are less strict. Some Chinese herbal treatments may be safe, but others may not. There have been reports of products being contaminated with drugs, toxins, or heavy metals or not containing the listed ingredients. Some of the herbs are very powerful, can interact with drugs, and may have serious side effects. For example, the Chinese herb ephedra (ma huang) has been linked to serious health complications, including heart attack and stroke. In 2004, the FDA banned the sale of ephedra-containing dietary supplements used for weight loss and performance enhancement, but the ban does not apply to TCM remedies or to herbal teas.

Acupuncture is considered safe when performed by an experienced practitioner using sterile needles.

Training, Licensing, and Certification

Most states license acupuncture, but states vary in their inclusion of other TCM components (e.g., herbal medicine) in the licenses they issue. The federally recognized Accreditation Commission for Acupuncture and Oriental Medicine (ACAOM) accredits schools that teach acupuncture and TCM, and about one third of the states that license acupuncture require graduation from an ACAOM-accredited school. The National Certification Commission for Acupuncture and Oriental Medicine (NCCAOM) offers separate certification programs in acupuncture, Chinese herbology, and Oriental bodywork. Almost all licensing states require completion of NCCAOM's national written exam; some states also require a practical exam.

If You Are Thinking about Using TCM

- Look for published research studies on TCM for the health condition that interests you.

- If you are thinking about trying TCM herbal remedies, it is better to use these products under the supervision of a medical professional trained in herbal medicine than to try to treat yourself.

- Ask about the training and experience of the TCM practitioner you are considering.

- Do not use TCM as a replacement for effective conventional care or as a reason to postpone seeing a doctor about a medical problem.

- If you are pregnant or nursing, or are thinking of using TCM to treat a child, you should be especially sure to consult your health care provider.

- Tell all your health care providers about any complementary and alternative practices you use. Give them a full picture of what you do to manage your health. This will help ensure coordinated and safe care.

NCCAM-Funded Research

Recent NCCAM-supported studies have been investigating the following:

- TCM for endometriosis-related pelvic pain, irritable bowel syndrome, and temporomandibular (jaw) disorders

- Chinese herbal medicines for food allergies and for osteoarthritis of the knee

- Consistency of TCM practitioners' diagnosis and herbal prescriptions for rheumatoid arthritis patients

Section 12.2

Native American Medicine

Reprinted with permission from the website of the John Moores University of California–San Diego Cancer Center, http://cancer.ucsd.edu. © 2002 University of California–San Diego. All rights reserved. Reviewed by David A. Cooke, MD, FACP, December 25, 2009.

This treatment modality is thought to manage symptoms of cancer, side effects from conventional therapies, and/or control pain. Native American healing should be used with, not in place of, standard cancer therapy.

What does Native American healing involve?

Native American healing combines religion, community ritual, spirituality, and herbal medicine to treat illness. Because of their Eurasian ancestry, many of the beliefs of Native Americans have their roots in ancient Indian (Ayurvedic) and Chinese medicine. Native American tribes share a common belief in the interconnectedness of people, the community, the environment and the spiritual world.

Harmony must exist amongst them for good health to dominant a community. Native American healers believe that illness results from spiritual imbalances within the individual and the community. The community relies upon medicine men and women, or shamanic healers, who are thought to be able to contact the spiritual world to heal illness and fight disease. Native American tradition focuses on four elements of healing:

1. Symbolic ritual—to communicate with the spiritual world and enlist its aid in healing

2. Shamanic healers—offer prayers to appease spirits so that they will treat illness and restore health

3. Purification of the body—to rid the body of impurities and restore a spiritually pure state

4. Use of herbs as medicine

How is Native American healing thought to manage specific symptoms of cancer, side effects of conventional therapies, and/or control pain?

The heavy dependence on spiritual communication and meditation may reduce stress and anxiety, bring about peace of mind, and produce a sense of wholeness among patients. Native American knowledge of herbs is extensive and many have value in treating a variety of ills, symptoms of disease, side effects of conventional treatment, and reduction of pain.

What has been proven about the benefit of Native American healing?

Formal research of the healing ceremonies and traditions of Native Americans is almost nonexistent even though claims have been made regarding cures of a variety of ailments, including cancer. However, the community-based approach to health care may provide comfort to patients who enjoy the sense of sharing a common purpose and history with a large group of people. Other health benefits may be the result of the placebo response. According to the American Cancer Society, "although Native American healing has not been shown to cure disease, anecdotal reports suggest that it can reduce pain and stress, and improve quality of life." However, it should not be relied on to cure cancer, or used instead of modern, science-based treatment.

What is the potential risk or harm of Native American healing?

Many purification rituals have side effects. Sweat lodges may cause patients to become dehydrated. An herbal tea called "Black Drink" causes patients to vomit.

How much does Native American healing cost?

Information on cost is unavailable.

For Additional Information

Association of American Indian Physicians
1225 Sovereign Row, Suite 103
Oklahoma City, OK 73108
Phone: 405-946-7072
Website: www.aaip.org

Institute for Traditional Medicine
2017 SE Hawthorne Boulevard
Portland, OR 97214
Phone: 503-233-4907
Website: www.itmonline.org

Chapter 13

Acupuncture

Acupuncture is among the oldest healing practices in the world. As part of traditional Chinese medicine, acupuncture aims to restore and maintain health through the stimulation of specific points on the body. In the United States, where practitioners incorporate healing traditions from China, Japan, Korea, and other countries, acupuncture is considered part of complementary and alternative medicine (CAM).

About Acupuncture

The term "acupuncture" describes a family of procedures involving the stimulation of anatomical points on the body using a variety of techniques. The acupuncture technique that has been most often studied scientifically involves penetrating the skin with thin, solid, metallic needles that are manipulated by the hands or by electrical stimulation.

Practiced in China and other Asian countries for thousands of years, acupuncture is one of the key components of traditional Chinese medicine. In TCM, the body is seen as a delicate balance of two opposing and inseparable forces: yin and yang. Yin represents the cold, slow, or passive principle, while yang represents the hot, excited, or active principle. According to TCM, health is achieved by maintaining the body in a "balanced state"; disease is due to an internal imbalance of yin and

---

Excerpted from "Acupuncture: An Introduction," by the National Center for Complementary and Alternative Medicine (NCCAM, nccam.nih.gov), part of the National Institutes of Health, December 2007.

yang. This imbalance leads to blockage in the flow of qi (vital energy) along pathways known as meridians. Qi can be unblocked, according to TCM, by using acupuncture at certain points on the body that connect with these meridians. Sources vary on the number of meridians, with numbers ranging from 14 to 20. One commonly cited source describes meridians as 14 main channels "connecting the body in a weblike interconnecting matrix" of at least 2,000 acupuncture points.

Acupuncture became better known in the United States in 1971, when *New York Times* reporter James Reston wrote about how doctors in China used needles to ease his pain after surgery. American practices of acupuncture incorporate medical traditions from China, Japan, Korea, and other countries.

Acupuncture Use in the United States

The report from a Consensus Development Conference on Acupuncture held at the National Institutes of Health (NIH) in 1997 stated that acupuncture is being "widely" practiced—by thousands of physicians, dentists, acupuncturists, and other practitioners—for relief or prevention of pain and for various other health conditions. According to the 2007 National Health Interview Survey, which included a comprehensive survey of CAM use by Americans, an estimated 3.1 million U.S. adults and 150,000 children had used acupuncture in the previous year. Between the 2002 and 2007 NHIS, acupuncture use among adults increased by three-tenths of 1 percent (approximately 1 million people).

Acupuncture Side Effects and Risks

The U.S. Food and Drug Administration (FDA) regulates acupuncture needles for use by licensed practitioners, requiring that needles be manufactured and labeled according to certain standards. For example, the FDA requires that needles be sterile, nontoxic, and labeled for single use by qualified practitioners only.

Relatively few complications from the use of acupuncture have been reported to the FDA, in light of the millions of people treated each year and the number of acupuncture needles used. Still, complications have resulted from inadequate sterilization of needles and from improper delivery of treatments. Practitioners should use a new set of disposable needles taken from a sealed package for each patient and should swab treatment sites with alcohol or another disinfectant before inserting needles. When not delivered properly, acupuncture can cause serious adverse effects, including infections and punctured organs.

Status of Acupuncture Research

There have been many studies on acupuncture's potential health benefits for a wide range of conditions. Summarizing earlier research, the 1997 NIH Consensus Statement on Acupuncture found that, overall, results were hard to interpret because of problems with the size and design of the studies.

In the years since the Consensus Statement was issued, the National Center for Complementary and Alternative Medicine (NCCAM) has funded extensive research to advance scientific understanding of acupuncture. Some recent NCCAM-supported studies have looked at the following:

- Whether acupuncture works for specific health conditions such as chronic low-back pain, headache, and osteoarthritis of the knee

- How acupuncture might work, such as what happens in the brain during acupuncture treatment

- Ways to better identify and understand the potential neurological properties of meridians and acupuncture points

- Methods and instruments for improving the quality of acupuncture research

Finding a Qualified Practitioner

Health care providers can be a resource for referral to acupuncturists, and some conventional medical practitioners—including physicians and dentists—practice acupuncture. In addition, national acupuncture organizations (which can be found through libraries or search engines) may provide referrals to acupuncturists.

- Check a practitioner's credentials. Most states require a license to practice acupuncture; however, education and training standards and requirements for obtaining a license to practice vary from state to state. Although a license does not ensure quality of care, it does indicate that the practitioner meets certain standards regarding the knowledge and use of acupuncture.

- Do not rely on a diagnosis of disease by an acupuncture practitioner who does not have substantial conventional medical training. If you have received a diagnosis from a doctor, you may wish to ask your doctor whether acupuncture might help.

What to Expect from Acupuncture Visits

During your first office visit, the practitioner may ask you at length about your health condition, lifestyle, and behavior. The practitioner will want to obtain a complete picture of your treatment needs and behaviors that may contribute to your condition. Inform the acupuncturist about all treatments or medications you are taking and all medical conditions you have.

Acupuncture needles are metallic, solid, and hair-thin. People experience acupuncture differently, but most feel no or minimal pain as the needles are inserted. Some people feel energized by treatment, while others feel relaxed. Improper needle placement, movement of the patient, or a defect in the needle can cause soreness and pain during treatment. This is why it is important to seek treatment from a qualified acupuncture practitioner.

Treatment may take place over a period of several weeks or more.

Treatment Costs

Ask the practitioner about the estimated number of treatments needed and how much each treatment will cost. Some insurance companies may cover the costs of acupuncture, while others may not. It is important to check with your insurer before you start treatment to see whether acupuncture is covered for your condition and, if so, to what extent.

Chapter 14

Homeopathy

Homeopathy, also known as homeopathic medicine, is a whole medical system that was developed in Germany more than 200 years ago and has been practiced in the United States since the early 19th century. Homeopathy is used for wellness and prevention and to treat many diseases and conditions.

Overview

The term homeopathy comes from the Greek words homeo, meaning similar, and pathos, meaning suffering or disease. Homeopathy seeks to stimulate the body's ability to heal itself by giving very small doses of highly diluted substances. This therapeutic method was developed by German physician Samuel Christian Hahnemann at the end of the 18th century. Hahnemann articulated two main principles:

- **The principle of similars** (or "like cures like") states that a disease can be cured by a substance that produces similar symptoms in healthy people. This idea, which can be traced back to Hippocrates, was further developed by Hahnemann after he repeatedly ingested cinchona bark, a popular treatment for malaria, and found that he developed the symptoms of the disease. Hahnemann theorized that if a substance could cause disease symptoms in a healthy person, small amounts could cure a sick person who had similar symptoms.

Excerpted from "Homeopathy: An Introduction," by the National Center for Complementary and Alternative Medicine (NCCAM, nccam.nih.gov), part of the National Institutes of Health, July 2009.

85

- **The principle of dilutions** (or "law of minimum dose") states that the lower the dose of the medication, the greater its effectiveness. In homeopathy, substances are diluted in a stepwise fashion and shaken vigorously between each dilution. This process, referred to as "potentization," is believed to transmit some form of information or energy from the original substance to the final diluted remedy. Most homeopathic remedies are so dilute that no molecules of the healing substance remain; however, in homeopathy, it is believed that the substance has left its imprint or "essence," which stimulates the body to heal itself (this theory is called the "memory of water").

Homeopaths treat people based on genetic and personal health history, body type, and current physical, emotional, and mental symptoms. Patient visits tend to be lengthy. Treatments are "individualized" or tailored to each person—it is not uncommon for different people with the same condition to receive different treatments.

Homeopathic remedies are derived from natural substances that come from plants, minerals, or animals. Common remedies include red onion, arnica (mountain herb), and stinging nettle plant.

Use in the United States

According to the 2007 National Health Interview Survey, which included a comprehensive survey of complementary and alternative medicine (CAM) use by Americans, an estimated 3.9 million U.S. adults and approximately 900,000 children used homeopathy in the previous year.

People use homeopathy for a range of health concerns, from wellness and prevention, to the treatment of diseases and conditions such as allergies, asthma, chronic fatigue syndrome, depression, digestive disorders, ear infections, headaches, and skin rashes.

Regulation of Homeopathic Treatments

Homeopathic remedies are prepared according to the guidelines of the *Homeopathic Pharmacopeia of the United States (HPUS),* which was written into law in the Federal Food, Drug, and Cosmetic Act in 1938. Homeopathic remedies are regulated in the same manner as nonprescription, over-the-counter (OTC) drugs. However, because homeopathic products contain little or no active ingredients, they do not have to undergo the same safety and efficacy testing as prescription and new OTC drugs.

The U.S. Food and Drug Administration (FDA) does require that homeopathic remedies meet certain legal standards for strength, purity, and packaging. The labels on the remedies must include at least one major indication (i.e., medical problem to be treated), a list of ingredients, the dilution, and safety instructions. In addition, if a homeopathic remedy claims to treat a serious disease such as cancer, it needs to be sold by prescription. Only products for self-limiting conditions (minor health problems like a cold or headache that go away on their own) can be sold without a prescription.

The Status of Homeopathy Research

Most analyses of the research on homeopathy have concluded that there is little evidence to support homeopathy as an effective treatment for any specific condition, and that many of the studies have been flawed. However, there are some individual observational studies, randomized placebo-controlled trials, and laboratory research that report positive effects or unique physical and chemical properties of homeopathic remedies.

Research Challenges

Homeopathy is difficult to study using current scientific methods because highly diluted substances (known as ultra-high dilutions or UHDs) cannot be readily measured, making it difficult to design or replicate studies. In addition, homeopathic treatments are highly individualized and there is no uniform prescribing standard for homeopaths. There are hundreds of different homeopathic remedies, which can be prescribed in a variety of different dilutions to treat thousands of symptoms. On the other hand, many aspects of the interactions between the homeopathic practitioner and his or her patients may be quite beneficial, and can be studied more easily.

Controversies Regarding Homeopathy

Homeopathy is a controversial area of CAM because a number of its key concepts are not consistent with established laws of science (particularly chemistry and physics). Critics think it is implausible that a remedy containing a miniscule amount of an active ingredient (sometimes not a single molecule of the original compound) can have any biological effect—beneficial or otherwise. For these reasons, critics argue that continuing the scientific study of homeopathy is not worthwhile. Others point to observational and anecdotal evidence that homeopathy does work and argue that it should not be rejected just because science has not been able to explain it.

Side Effects and Risks

Although the side effects and risks of homeopathic treatments are not well researched outside of observational studies, some general points can be made about the safety of these treatments:

- A systematic review found that homeopathic remedies in high dilution, taken under the supervision of trained professionals, are generally considered safe and unlikely to cause severe adverse reactions.

- Liquid homeopathic remedies may contain alcohol. The FDA allows higher levels of alcohol in these remedies than it allows in conventional drugs. However, no adverse effects from alcohol levels have been reported to the FDA.

- Homeopaths expect some of their patients to experience homeopathic aggravation (a temporary worsening of existing symptoms after taking a homeopathic prescription). Researchers have not found much evidence of this reaction in clinical studies; however, research on homeopathic aggravations is scarce.

- Homeopathic remedies are not known to interfere with conventional drugs; however, if you are considering using homeopathic remedies, you should discuss this with your health care provider first.

Licensing and Certification

There are currently no uniform licensing or professional standards for the practice of homeopathy in the United States; the licensing of homeopaths varies from state to state. Usually, a homeopathic practitioner is licensed in a medical profession, such as conventional or osteopathic medicine. Homeopathy is also part of the medical education for naturopathy.

Licensure as a homeopathic physician is available only to medical doctors and doctors of osteopathy in Arizona, Connecticut, and Nevada. Arizona and Nevada also license homeopathic assistants, who are allowed to perform medical services under the supervision of a homeopathic physician. Some states explicitly include homeopathy within the scope of practice of chiropractic, naturopathy, physical therapy, dentistry, nursing, and veterinary medicine.

National certification may be obtained through organizations such as the Council for Homeopathic Certification, American Board of Homeotherapeutics, and the Homeopathic Academy of Naturopathic

Physicians. The U.S. Department of Education, which officially recognizes some CAM organizations for certification purposes, has not recognized these organizations; however, members of the homeopathic community consider certification a way to help set education and competency standards for practicing homeopathy.

If You Are Thinking about Using Homeopathy

- Do not use homeopathy as a replacement for proven conventional care or to postpone seeing a doctor about a medical problem.

- Look for published research studies on homeopathy for the health condition you are interested in.

- If you are considering using homeopathy and decide to seek treatment from a homeopath, ask about the training and experience of the practitioner you are considering.

- Women who are pregnant or nursing, or people who are thinking of using homeopathy to treat a child, should consult their health care provider.

Tell your health care providers about any complementary and alternative practices you use. Give them a full picture of all you do to manage your health. This will ensure coordinated and safe care.

NCCAM-Funded Research

NCCAM-supported exploratory grants have sought to understand patient and provider perspectives on homeopathic treatment and have explored the effectiveness of homeopathic remedies with various succussions (vigorous shaking) and dilutions.

Chapter 15

Naturopathy

Naturopathy, also called naturopathic medicine, is a whole medical system—one of the systems of healing and beliefs that have evolved over time in different cultures and parts of the world. Naturopathy is rooted in health care approaches that were popular in Europe, especially in Germany, in the 19th century, but it also includes therapies (both ancient and modern) from other traditions. In naturopathy, the emphasis is on supporting health rather than combating disease.

A Brief Description of Naturopathy

Naturopathy is a whole medical system that has its roots in Germany. It was developed further in the late 19th and early 20th centuries in the United States, where today it is part of complementary and alternative medicine (CAM). The word naturopathy comes from Greek and Latin and literally translates as "nature disease."

A central belief in naturopathy is that nature has a healing power (a principle called vis medicatrix naturae). Another belief is that living organisms (including the human body) have the power to maintain (or return to) a state of balance and health, and to heal themselves. Practitioners of naturopathy prefer to use treatment approaches that they consider to be the most natural and least invasive, instead of using drugs and more invasive procedures.

Excerpted from "An Introduction to Naturopathy," by the National Center for Complementary and Alternative Medicine (NCCAM, nccam.nih.gov), part of the National Institutes of Health, April 2007.

Naturopathy was named and popularized in the United States by Benedict Lust, who was born in Germany in the late 1800s. When Lust became seriously ill with what he believed was tuberculosis, he was treated by a priest and healer in Germany named Sebastian Kneipp. Kneipp's treatment was based on various healing approaches and philosophies that were popular in Europe, including the following:

- Hydrotherapy (water treatments)

- The "nature cure" movement, which focused on restoring health through a return to nature

This movement advocated therapies such as gentle exercise, herbal medications, wholesome dietary approaches, and exposure to sun and air.

Lust found his health much improved from Kneipp's treatment, and when he immigrated to the United States at the turn of the 20th century, he was dedicated to popularizing it. He gave it the name naturopathy, led the way in developing it as a medical system in the United States, and founded the first naturopathic college and professional association. In naturopathy's early years, other therapies were added to its practice—for example, homeopathy and manipulation (a hands-on therapy).

Naturopathy's popularity reached its peak in the United States in the 1920s and 1930s. However, its use began to decline when drugs (such as antibiotics) and other developments in conventional medicine moved to the forefront of health care. Naturopathy began to reemerge in the 1970s, with increased consumer interest in "holistic" health approaches and the founding of new naturopathic medical colleges. Today, naturopathy is practiced in a number of countries, including the United States, Canada, Great Britain, Australia, and New Zealand.

Americans' Use of Naturopathy

In a national survey on Americans' use of CAM, published in 2004, just under 1 percent of the 31,000 survey respondents had used naturopathy. These respondents reported that they used it because of the following reasons:

- They believed that naturopathy combined with conventional medicine would help (62 percent).

- They believed that conventional medical treatments would not help (53 percent).

- They thought naturopathy would be interesting to try (44 percent).

- They thought that conventional medicine was too expensive (28 percent).

- They were referred to naturopathy by a conventional medical professional (17 percent).

Source: Barnes PM, Powell-Griner E, McFann K, Nahin RL. Complementary and alternative medicine use among adults: United States, 2002. CDC Advance Data Report #343. 2004.

Key Principles

The practice of naturopathy is based on six key principles:

1. Promote the healing power of nature.

2. First do no harm. Naturopathic practitioners choose therapies with the intent to keep harmful side effects to a minimum and not suppress symptoms.

3. Treat the whole person. Practitioners believe a person's health is affected by many factors, such as physical, mental, emotional, genetic, environmental, and social ones. Practitioners consider all these factors when choosing therapies and tailor treatment to each patient.

4. Treat the cause. Practitioners seek to identify and treat the causes of a disease or condition, rather than its symptoms. They believe that symptoms are signs that the body is trying to fight disease, adapt to it, or recover from it.

5. Prevention is the best cure. Practitioners teach ways of living that they consider most healthy and most likely to prevent illness.

6. The physician is a teacher. Practitioners consider it important to educate their patients in taking responsibility for their own health.

Who Provides Naturopathy?

In the United States, professionals who practice naturopathy generally fall into one of several groups. (The terms used by some practitioners vary and may depend on the legal situation in the states where they practice.)

Naturopathic Physicians

Naturopathic physicians are educated and trained in a 4-year, graduate-level program at one of the four U.S. naturopathic medical schools accredited by the Council on Naturopathic Medical Education. Admission requirements include a bachelor's degree and standard premedical courses. The study program includes basic sciences, naturopathic therapies and techniques, diagnostic techniques and tests, specialty courses, clinical sciences, and clinical training. Graduates receive the degree of N.D. (Doctor of Naturopathic Medicine). Post-doctoral training is not required, but graduates may pursue it.

Depending on where they wish to practice, naturopathic physicians may also need to be licensed. A number of states, the District of Columbia, and two U.S. territories have such licensing requirements, most often consisting of graduation from a 4-year naturopathic medical college and passing the national standardized board examination (known as the NPLEX [Naturopathic Physicians Licensing Examinations]). The scope of practice varies by state and jurisdiction. For example, some states allow naturopathic physicians with special training to prescribe drugs, perform minor surgery, practice acupuncture, and/or assist in childbirth.

Traditional Naturopaths

The second major group of practitioners are traditional naturopaths, or simply naturopaths. They emphasize education in naturopathic approaches to a healthy lifestyle, strengthening and cleansing the body, and noninvasive treatments. Prescription drugs, x-rays, and surgery are several of the practices that traditional naturopaths do not use. Education and training for these practitioners typically consists of correspondence courses, an apprenticeship, and/or self-teaching. Admission requirements for schools can range from none, to a high school diploma, to specific degrees and coursework. Programs vary in length and content. They are not accredited by agencies recognized for accreditation purposes by the U.S. Department of Education. Traditional naturopaths are not subject to licensing.

Conventional Providers with Naturopathic Training

This group consists of licensed conventional medical providers (such as doctors of medicine, doctors of osteopathy, dentists, and nurses) who pursue additional training in naturopathic treatments, and possibly other holistic therapies. Education and training programs for this purpose also vary.

What Practitioners Do in Treating Patients

A first visit to a naturopathic practitioner is usually an extended appointment. The practitioner will interview the patient at length about his health history, reasons for the visit, and lifestyle (such as diet, stress, alcohol and tobacco use, sleep, and exercise). The practitioner may perform examinations and, if in her scope of practice, order diagnostic and screening tests. Toward the end of the appointment, a management plan is set up to address the patient's general health and problems with illness. Referrals to other health care providers may be made, if appropriate. Practitioners may deliver some naturopathic treatments in their offices, such as hydrotherapy or manipulation. Examples of additional treatments include the following:

- Dietary changes (for example, eating more whole and unprocessed foods)
- Vitamins, minerals, and other dietary supplements
- Herbal medicine
- Counseling and education on lifestyle changes
- Homeopathy
- Hydrotherapy (for example, applying hot water, then cold water)
- Manual and body-based therapies such as manipulation and mobilization
- Exercise therapy
- Mind-body therapies such as yoga and meditation

Some practitioners use other treatments as well.

Side Effects and Risks

Naturopathy appears to be a generally safe health care approach, especially if used as complementary (rather than alternative) medicine, but several qualifying points are important:

- Naturopathy is not a complete substitute for conventional medical care.
- Some therapies used in naturopathy have the potential to be harmful if not used properly or under the direction of a trained practitioner. For example, herbs can cause side effects on their own and interact with prescription or over-the-counter medicines. Restrictive or other unconventional diets can be unsafe for some people.

- Some practitioners of naturopathy do not recommend using all or some of the childhood vaccinations that are standard practice in conventional medicine.

- The education and training of practitioners of naturopathy vary widely.

Naturopathy as a whole medical system is challenging to study. Rigorous research on this whole medical system is taking place but is at an early stage.

Some Other Points to Consider

- Tell your health care providers about any complementary and alternative practices you use. Give them a full picture of what you do to manage your health. This will help ensure coordinated and safe care.

- Naturopathic physicians are trained to know that herbs and some dietary supplements can potentially interact with drugs, and to avoid those combinations. To do so, they need to be informed of all drugs (whether prescription or over-the-counter) and supplements that you are taking.

- Talk to the practitioner about the following:
  - His education and training and any licensing or certification
  - Any special medical conditions you have and whether the practitioner has had any specialized training or experience in them
  - Costs and whether the services are covered by your medical insurance plan

Some Points of Controversy

As in other fields of CAM, there are some controversies in naturopathy.

- Practitioners of naturopathy do not always agree on educational requirements or how naturopathy should be practiced and regulated.

- A number of beliefs and practices in naturopathy do not follow the scientific approach of conventional medicine.

- Practitioners are divided on whether this system of medicine should be studied using conventional medical research approaches.

NCCAM-Funded Research in Naturopathy

Some recent NCCAM-supported projects have been studying the following:

- CAM approaches, including naturopathic treatments, for women with temporomandibular disorder, a condition in which the joints connecting the skull to the lower jaw become inflamed

- A naturopathic dietary approach as a complementary treatment for type 2 diabetes

- The mushroom *Trametes versicolor,* for its effects as a complementary immune therapy in women with breast cancer

- The costs and effects of naturopathic care, compared with conventional care, for low-back pain

- Herbal and dietary approaches for menopausal symptoms

Part Three

Dietary Supplements

Chapter 16

Questions and Answers about Dietary Supplements

What is a dietary supplement?

As defined by Congress in the Dietary Supplement Health and Education Act, which became law in 1994, a dietary supplement is a product (other than tobacco) that:

- is intended to supplement the diet;

- contains one or more dietary ingredients (including vitamins; minerals; herbs or other botanicals; amino acids; and other substances) or their constituents;

- is intended to be taken by mouth as a pill, capsule, tablet, or liquid; and

- is labeled on the front panel as being a dietary supplement.

What is a new dietary ingredient?

A new dietary ingredient is a dietary ingredient that was not sold in the United States in a dietary supplement before October 15, 1994.

Excerpted from "Dietary Supplements: Background Information," by the Office of Dietary Supplements (ODS, ods.od.nih.gov), part of the National Institutes of Health, July 9, 2009.

Are dietary supplements different from foods and drugs?

Although dietary supplements are regulated by the U.S. Food and Drug Administration (FDA) as foods, they are regulated differently from other foods and from drugs. Whether a product is classified as a dietary supplement, conventional food, or drug is based on its intended use. Most often, classification as a dietary supplement is determined by the information that the manufacturer provides on the product label or in accompanying literature, although many food and dietary supplement product labels do not include this information.

What claims can manufacturers make for dietary supplements and drugs?

The types of claims that can be made on the labels of dietary supplements and drugs differ. Drug manufacturers may claim that their product will diagnose, cure, mitigate, treat, or prevent a disease. Such claims may not legally be made for dietary supplements.

The label of a dietary supplement or food product may contain one of three types of claims: a health claim, nutrient content claim, or structure/function claim. Health claims describe a relationship between a food, food component, or dietary supplement ingredient, and reducing risk of a disease or health-related condition. Nutrient content claims describe the relative amount of a nutrient or dietary substance in a product. A structure/function claim is a statement describing how a product may affect the organs or systems of the body and it can not mention any specific disease.

Structure/function claims do not require FDA approval but the manufacturer must provide FDA with the text of the claim within 30 days of putting the product on the market. Product labels containing such claims must also include a disclaimer that reads, "This statement has not been evaluated by the FDA. This product is not intended to diagnose, treat, cure, or prevent any disease."

How does FDA regulate dietary supplements?

In addition to regulating label claims, FDA regulates dietary supplements in other ways. Supplement ingredients sold in the United States before October 15, 1994, are not required to be reviewed by FDA for their safety before they are marketed because they are presumed to be safe based on their history of use by humans. For a new dietary ingredient (one not sold as a dietary supplement before 1994) the manufacturer must notify FDA of its intent to market a dietary supplement containing the new dietary ingredient and provide information on how it determined that reasonable evidence exists for safe human use of the product. FDA can either refuse to allow new ingredients into or remove existing ingredients from the marketplace for safety reasons.

Manufacturers do not have to provide FDA with evidence that dietary supplements are effective or safe; however, they are not permitted to market unsafe or ineffective products. Once a dietary supplement is marketed, FDA has to prove that the product is not safe in order to restrict its use or remove it from the market. In contrast, before being allowed to market a drug product, manufacturers must obtain FDA approval by providing convincing evidence that it is both safe and effective.

The label of a dietary supplement product is required to be truthful and not misleading. If the label does not meet this requirement, FDA may remove the product from the marketplace or take other appropriate actions.

What information is required on a dietary supplement label?

FDA requires that certain information appear on the dietary supplement label. General information includes the following:

- Name of product (including the word "supplement" or a statement that the product is a supplement)
- Net quantity of contents
- Name and place of business of manufacturer, packer, or distributor
- Directions for use

The Supplement Facts panel includes the following information:

- Serving size, list of dietary ingredients, amount per serving size (by weight), percent of Daily Value (%DV), if established
- If the dietary ingredient is a botanical, the scientific name of the plant or the common or usual name standardized in the reference *Herbs of Commerce, 2nd Edition* (2000 edition) and the name of the plant part used
- If the dietary ingredient is a proprietary blend (i.e., a blend exclusive to the manufacturer), the total weight of the blend and the components of the blend in order of predominance by weight

Other ingredients that must be listed include nondietary ingredients such as fillers, artificial colors, sweeteners, flavors, or binders; listed by weight in descending order of predominance and by common name or proprietary blend.

The label of the supplement may contain a cautionary statement but the lack of a cautionary statement does not mean that no adverse effects are associated with the product.

Does a label indicate the quality of a dietary supplement product?

It is difficult to determine the quality of a dietary supplement product from its label. The degree of quality control depends on the manufacturer, the supplier, and others in the production process.

In 2007, the FDA issued Good Manufacturing Practices (GMPs) for dietary supplements, a set of requirements and expectations by which dietary supplements must be manufactured, prepared, and stored to ensure quality. Manufacturers are expected to guarantee the identity, purity, strength, and composition of their dietary supplements. For example, the GMPs aim to prevent the inclusion of the wrong ingredients, the addition of too much or too little of a dietary ingredient, the possibility of contamination (by pesticides, heavy metals such as lead, bacteria, etc.), and the improper packaging and labeling of a product. Large companies are required to comply with FDA's dietary supplement GMPs now, and the smallest companies by June 2010.

Are dietary supplements standardized?

Standardization is a process that manufacturers may use to ensure batch-to-batch consistency of their products. In some cases, standardization involves identifying specific chemicals (known as markers) that can be used to manufacture a consistent product. The standardization process can also provide a measure of quality control.

Dietary supplements are not required to be standardized in the United States. In fact, no legal or regulatory definition exists in the United States for standardization as it applies to dietary supplements. Because of this, the term "standardization" may mean many different things. Some manufacturers use the term standardization incorrectly to refer to uniform manufacturing practices; following a recipe is not sufficient for a product to be called standardized. Therefore, the presence of the word "standardized" on a supplement label does not necessarily indicate product quality.

What methods are used to evaluate the health benefits and safety of a dietary supplement?

Scientists use several approaches to evaluate dietary supplements for their potential health benefits and safety risks, including their history of use and laboratory studies using cell or animal studies. Studies involving people (individual case reports, observational studies, and clinical trials) can provide information that is relevant to how dietary supplements are used. Researchers may conduct a systematic review to summarize and evaluate a group of clinical trials that meet certain criteria. A meta-analysis is a review that includes a statistical analysis of data combined from many studies.

What safety advice should people know about dietary supplements?

- The information in this text does not replace medical advice.

- Before taking a dietary supplement, consult a doctor or other health care provider—especially if you have a disease or medical condition, take any medications, are pregnant or nursing, or are planning to have an operation.

- Before treating a child with a dietary supplement, consult with a doctor or other health care provider.

- Like drugs, dietary supplements have chemical and biological activity. They may have side effects. They may interact with certain medications. These interactions can cause problems and can even be dangerous.

- If you have any unexpected reactions to a dietary supplement, inform your doctor or other health care provider.

Chapter 17

Botanical Dietary Supplements

What is a botanical?

A botanical is a plant or plant part valued for its medicinal or therapeutic properties, flavor, and/or scent. Herbs are a subset of botanicals. Products made from botanicals that are used to maintain or improve health may be called herbal products, botanical products, or phytomedicines.

In naming botanicals, botanists use a Latin name made up of the genus and species of the plant. Under this system the botanical black cohosh is known as *Actaea racemosa L.*, where "L" stands for Linneaus, who first described the type of plant specimen. In this text, we do not include such initials because they do not appear on most products used by consumers.

Can botanicals be dietary supplements?

To be classified as a dietary supplement, a botanical must meet the definition given below. Many botanical preparations meet the definition.

As defined by Congress in the Dietary Supplement Health and Education Act, which became law in 1994, a dietary supplement is a product (other than tobacco) that:

- is intended to supplement the diet;

Excerpted from "Botanical Dietary Supplements: Background Information," by the Office of Dietary Supplements (ODS, ods.od.nih.gov), part of the National Institutes of Health, July 9, 2009.

- contains one or more dietary ingredients (including vitamins; minerals; herbs or other botanicals; amino acids; and other substances) or their constituents;

- is intended to be taken by mouth as a pill, capsule, tablet, or liquid; and

- is labeled on the front panel as being a dietary supplement.

How are botanicals commonly sold and prepared?

Botanicals are sold in many forms: as fresh or dried products; liquid or solid extracts; and tablets, capsules, powders, and tea bags. For example, fresh ginger root is often found in the produce section of food stores; dried ginger root is sold packaged in tea bags, capsules, or tablets; and liquid preparations made from ginger root are also sold. A particular group of chemicals or a single chemical may be isolated from a botanical and sold as a dietary supplement, usually in tablet or capsule form. An example is phytoestrogens from soy products.

Common preparations include teas, decoctions, tinctures, and extracts:

- A tea, also known as an infusion, is made by adding boiling water to fresh or dried botanicals and steeping them. The tea may be drunk either hot or cold.

- Some roots, bark, and berries require more forceful treatment to extract their desired ingredients. They are simmered in boiling water for longer periods than teas, making a decoction, which also may be drunk hot or cold.

- A tincture is made by soaking a botanical in a solution of alcohol and water. Tinctures are sold as liquids and are used for concentrating and preserving a botanical. They are made in different strengths that are expressed as botanical-to-extract ratios (i.e., ratios of the weight of the dried botanical to the volume or weight of the finished product).

- An extract is made by soaking the botanical in a liquid that removes specific types of chemicals. The liquid can be used as is or evaporated to make a dry extract for use in capsules or tablets.

Are botanical dietary supplements standardized?

Standardization is a process that manufacturers may use to ensure batch-to-batch consistency of their products. In some cases, standardization involves identifying specific chemicals (also known as markers) that can be used to manufacture a consistent product. The standardization process can also provide a measure of quality control.

Dietary supplements are not required to be standardized in the United States. In fact, no legal or regulatory definition exists for standardization in the United States as it applies to botanical dietary supplements. Because of this, the term "standardization" may mean many different things. Some manufacturers use the term standardization incorrectly to refer to uniform manufacturing practices; following a recipe is not sufficient for a product to be called standardized. Therefore, the presence of the word "standardized" on a supplement label does not necessarily indicate product quality.

Ideally, the chemical markers chosen for standardization would also be the compounds that are responsible for a botanical's effect in the body. In this way, each lot of the product would have a consistent health effect. However, the components responsible for the effects of most botanicals have not been identified or clearly defined. For example, the sennosides in the botanical senna are known to be responsible for the laxative effect of the plant, but many compounds may be responsible for valerian's relaxing effect.

Are botanical dietary supplements safe?

Many people believe that products labeled "natural" are safe and good for them. This is not necessarily true because the safety of a botanical depends on many things, such as its chemical makeup, how it works in the body, how it is prepared, and the dose used.

The action of botanicals range from mild to powerful (potent). A botanical with mild action may have subtle effects. Chamomile and peppermint, both mild botanicals, are usually taken as teas to aid digestion and are generally considered safe for self-administration. Some mild botanicals may have to be taken for weeks or months before their full effects are achieved. For example, valerian may be effective as a sleep aid after 14 days of use but it is rarely effective after just one dose. In contrast a powerful botanical produces a fast result. Kava, as one example, is reported to have an immediate and powerful action affecting anxiety and muscle relaxation.

The dose and form of a botanical preparation also play important roles in its safety. Teas, tinctures, and extracts have different strengths. The same amount of a botanical may be contained in a cup of tea, a few teaspoons of tincture, or an even smaller quantity of an extract. Also, different preparations vary in the relative amounts and concentrations of chemical removed from the whole botanical. For example, peppermint tea is generally considered safe to drink but peppermint oil is much more concentrated and can be toxic if used incorrectly. It is important to follow the manufacturer's suggested directions for using a botanical and not exceed the recommended dose without the advice of a health care provider.

Does a label indicate the quality of a botanical dietary supplement product?

It is difficult to determine the quality of a botanical dietary supplement product from its label. The degree of quality control depends on the manufacturer, the supplier, and others in the production process.

In 2007, the FDA issued Good Manufacturing Practices (GMPs) for dietary supplements, a set of requirements and expectations by which dietary supplements must be manufactured, prepared, and stored to ensure quality. Manufacturers are expected to guarantee the identity, purity, strength, and composition of their dietary supplements. For example, the GMPs aim to prevent the inclusion of the wrong ingredients, the addition of too much or too little of a dietary ingredient, the possibility of contamination (by pesticides, heavy metals such as lead, bacteria, etc.), and the improper packaging and labeling of a product. Large companies are required to comply with FDA's dietary supplement GMPs now, and the smallest companies by June 2010.

What methods are used to evaluate the health benefits and safety of a botanical dietary supplement?

Scientists use several approaches to evaluate botanical dietary supplements for their potential health benefits and safety risks, including their history of use and laboratory studies using cell or animal studies. Studies involving people (individual case reports, observational studies, and clinical trials) can provide information that is relevant to how botanical dietary supplements are used.

Researchers may conduct a systematic review to summarize and evaluate a group of clinical trials that meet certain criteria. A meta-analysis is a review that includes a statistical analysis of data combined from many studies.

Chapter 18

Using Dietary Supplements Wisely

Many people take dietary supplements in an effort to be well and stay healthy. With so many dietary supplements available and so many claims made about their health benefits, how can a consumer decide what's safe and effective? This text provides a general overview of dietary supplements, discusses safety considerations, and suggests sources for additional information.

About Dietary Supplements

Dietary supplements were defined in a law passed by Congress in 1994 called the Dietary Supplement Health and Education Act (DSHEA). According to DSHEA, a dietary supplement is a product that:

- is intended to supplement the diet;

- contains one or more dietary ingredients (including vitamins, minerals, herbs or other botanicals, amino acids, and certain other substances) or their constituents;

- is intended to be taken by mouth, in forms such as tablet, capsule, powder, softgel, gelcap, or liquid;

- is labeled as being a dietary supplement.

Excerpted from text by the National Center for Complementary and Alternative Medicine (NCCAM, nccam.nih.gov), part of the National Institutes of Health, February 2009.

Herbal supplements are one type of dietary supplement. An herb is a plant or plant part (such as leaves, flowers, or seeds) that is used for its flavor, scent, and/or therapeutic properties. "Botanical" is often used as a synonym for "herb." An herbal supplement may contain a single herb or mixtures of herbs.

Research has shown that some uses of dietary supplements are effective in preventing or treating diseases. For example, scientists have found that folic acid (a vitamin) prevents certain birth defects, and a regimen of vitamins and zinc can slow the progression of the age-related eye disease macular degeneration. Also, calcium and vitamin D supplements can be helpful in preventing and treating bone loss and osteoporosis (thinning of bone tissue).

Research has also produced some promising results suggesting that other dietary supplements may be helpful for other health conditions (e.g., omega-3 fatty acids for coronary disease), but in most cases, additional research is needed before firm conclusions can be drawn.

Dietary Supplement Use in the United States

A national survey conducted in 2007 found that 17.7 percent of American adults had used "natural products" (i.e., dietary supplements other than vitamins and minerals) in the past 12 months. The most popular products used by adults for health reasons in the past 30 days were fish oil/omega 3/DHA [docosahexaenoic acid] (37.4%), glucosamine (19.9%), echinacea (19.8%), flaxseed oil or pills (15.9%), and ginseng (14.1%). In another, earlier national survey covering all types of dietary supplements, approximately 52 percent of adult respondents said they had used some type of supplement in the last 30 days; the most commonly reported were multivitamins/multiminerals (35%), vitamins E and C (12–13%), calcium (10%), and B-complex vitamins (5%).

Federal Regulation of Dietary Supplements

The federal government regulates dietary supplements through the U.S. Food and Drug Administration (FDA). The regulations for dietary supplements are not the same as those for prescription or over-the-counter drugs. In general, the regulations for dietary supplements are less strict.

- A manufacturer does not have to prove the safety and effectiveness of a dietary supplement before it is marketed. A manufacturer is permitted to say that a dietary supplement addresses a nutrient deficiency, supports health, or is linked to a particular body function (e.g., immunity), if there is research to support the claim. Such a claim must be followed by the words "This statement has not been evaluated by the Food and Drug Administration. This product is not intended to diagnose, treat, cure, or prevent any disease."

- Manufacturers are expected to follow certain "good manufac- turing practices" (GMPs) to ensure that dietary supplements are processed consistently and meet quality standards. Require- ments for GMPs went into effect in 2008 for large manufacturers and are being phased in for small manufacturers through 2010.

- Once a dietary supplement is on the market, the FDA monitors safety. If it finds a product to be unsafe, it can take action against the manufacturer and/or distributor, and may issue a warning or require that the product be removed from the marketplace.

Also, once a dietary supplement is on the market, the FDA moni- tors product information, such as label claims and package inserts. The Federal Trade Commission (FTC) is responsible for regulating product advertising; it requires that all information be truthful and not misleading.

The federal government has taken legal action against a number of dietary supplement promoters or websites that promote or sell dietary supplements because they have made false or deceptive statements about their products or because marketed products have proven to be unsafe.

Sources of Science-Based Information

It's important to look for reliable sources of information on dietary supplements so you can evaluate the claims that are made about them. The most reliable information on dietary supplements is based on the results of rigorous scientific testing.

To get reliable information on a particular dietary supplement, try the following:

- Ask your health care providers. Even if they do not know about a specific dietary supplement, they may be able to access the latest medical guidance about its uses and risks.

- Look for scientific research findings on the dietary supplement. The National Center for Complementary and Alternative Medi- cine (NCCAM) and the NIH Office of Dietary Supplements, as well as other federal agencies, have free publications, clearing- houses, and information on their websites.

Safety Considerations

If you are thinking about or are using a dietary supplement, here are some points to keep in mind.

Tell your health care providers about any complementary and alternative practices you use, including dietary supplements. Give them a full picture of what you do to manage your health. This will help ensure coordinated and safe care. It is especially important to talk to your health care provider if you are considering the following:

- Talk to your provider if you are thinking about replacing your regular medication with one or more dietary supplements.

- Talk to your provider if you are thinking about taking any medications (whether prescription or over-the-counter), as some dietary supplements have been found to interact with medications.

- Talk to your provider if you are planning to have surgery. Certain dietary supplements may increase the risk of bleeding or affect the response to anesthesia.

- Talk to your provider if you are pregnant or nursing a baby, or are considering giving a child a dietary supplement. Most dietary supplements have not been tested in pregnant women, nursing mothers, or children.

If you are taking a dietary supplement, read the label instructions. Talk to your health care provider if you have any questions, particularly about the best dosage for you to take. If you experience any side effects that concern you, stop taking the dietary supplement, and contact your health care provider. You can also report your experience to the FDA's MedWatch program. Consumer safety reports on dietary supplements are an important source of information for the FDA.

Keep in mind that although many dietary supplements (and some prescription drugs) come from natural sources, "natural" does not always mean "safe." For example, the herbs comfrey and kava can cause serious harm to the liver. Also, a manufacturer's use of the term "standardized" (or "verified" or "certified") does not necessarily guarantee product quality or consistency.

Be aware that an herbal supplement may contain dozens of compounds and that its active ingredients may not be known. Researchers are studying many of these products in an effort to identify active ingredients and understand their effects in the body. Also consider the possibility that what's on the label may not be what's in the bottle. Analyses of dietary supplements sometimes find differences between labeled and actual ingredients. Here are some examples:

- An herbal supplement may not contain the correct plant species.

- The amount of the active ingredient may be lower or higher than the label states. That means you may be taking less—or more—of the dietary supplement than you realize.

- The dietary supplement may be contaminated with other herbs, pesticides, or metals, or even adulterated with unlabeled ingredients such as prescription drugs.

For current information from the federal government on the safety of particular dietary supplements, check the "Dietary Supplements: Warnings and Safety Information" section of the FDA website at www.fda.gov/Food/DietarySupplements/Alerts/default.htm or the "Alerts and Advisories" section of the NCCAM website at nccam.nih.gov/news/alerts.

Dietary Supplements Research at the National Institutes of Health

NCCAM, which is part of the National Institutes of Health (NIH), is the federal government's lead agency for studying all types of CAM. As part of that role, the Center sponsors a wide array of research to see how dietary supplements might affect the body and tests their use in clinical trials. In fiscal year 2007, NCCAM supported more than 200 research projects studying dietary supplements, including herbs and botanicals.

Also within NIH, the Office of Dietary Supplements (ODS) focuses specifically on dietary supplements, seeking to strengthen knowledge by supporting and evaluating research, disseminating results, and educating the public.

NCCAM and ODS collaborate to fund dietary supplement research centers focused on botanicals, known collectively as the NIH Botanical Research Centers Program. Scientists at the centers conduct basic research and other studies on botanicals and help to select products to be tested in clinical trials. The centers are advancing the scientific base of knowledge about botanicals, making it possible to better evaluate their safety and effectiveness.

NCCAM also sponsors a number of Centers of Excellence for Research on CAM, including centers studying antioxidant therapies, botanicals for autoimmune and inflammatory diseases, grape-derived polyphenols for Alzheimer disease, and botanicals for pancreatic diseases and for colorectal cancer.

Chapter 19

Adolescents and Supplement Use

Teens striving to shape their bodies or improve their athletic performance may be tempted to use dietary or sports supplements. These products, readily available and often touted as natural, may seem like perfect—or at least harmless—solutions. Yet, supplements can cause problems. While some simply fail to deliver what they promise, supplements also can actually be dangerous. So, monitor your teen's use of supplements and guide her toward safe ways to boost her physical fitness.

Wide Variety

Vitamins and minerals may be the most familiar dietary supplements. However, they include many other substances such as herbals, botanicals, amino acids, and enzymes. Dietary and nutritional supplements also come in many forms such as tablets, capsules, powders, energy bars, or drinks.

Sports and bodybuilding supplements promise more power, improved performance, and better health. While your teen may know better than to take steroids, which are illegal, he may think it is okay to use other legal substances. However, most supplements have not been studied thoroughly, especially for the effects on teenage athletes.

From "Supplements: Added Risk, Doubtful Benefit," by the Substance Abuse and Mental Health Services Administration (SAMHSA, samhsa.gov), part of the U.S. Department of Health and Human Services, February 26, 2007.

Little Control

The U.S. Food and Drug Administration (FDA) does not approve dietary supplements as safe and effective. Manufacturers and distributors are responsible for making sure that their products are safe and that claims about them are correct. The FDA acts only when it finds that a dietary supplement product carries a high risk of illness or injury. Some problems become clear over time through reports of tragedies or through the results of studies that often take years to conduct.

In 2004, the FDA banned the supplement ephedra, also known as ephedrine or ma huang. Ephedra was labeled as a fat burner because it acts as a stimulant, speeding up the nervous system and increasing metabolism. The FDA found that ephedra is risky, especially for people suffering from heart disease and high blood pressure.

Ephedra had been controversial before the FDA declared it illegal. Beginning in the 1990s, several organizations governing sports banned the drug. The United States military banned ephedra from commissaries and military exchanges in 2002 after the deaths of military personnel who were taking the drug. Ephedra drew added attention when the drug was linked to the death of 23-year-old Baltimore Orioles pitcher Steve Bechler in 2003.

Uncertain Effects

Because many supplements have not been studied scientifically, we cannot be sure how well they work or if they are dangerous. Supplements that are safe for most people who use them may be risky for others. Groups at increased risk include women who are pregnant or nursing a baby and people who have medical conditions such as diabetes, hypertension, or heart disease.

Likewise, a supplement that is safe when taken by itself may cause problems if combined with other medications. Even well-known products such as vitamin supplements, which are widely used and generally considered safe for teens and children, can cause problems under certain conditions. For example, combining supplements and medications that thin the blood can increase the potential for internal bleeding. In addition, vitamins, minerals, herbals, or other supplements can be dangerous for people having surgery. To avoid harmful drug reactions, doctors may ask patients to stop taking these substances 2 or 3 weeks before surgery.

Need for Caution

With so many supplements on the market, each claiming to be effective, knowing which products are safe for a teen to take is difficult. So, if you have a teenager who is driven to win or who frets about her shape, talk with a doctor or pharmacist before she takes a supplement. Including your teen in the discussion will help her understand the seriousness of protecting her health.

Better yet, urge him to hit the gym and reach for those fruits and veggies. Keep nutritious food on hand and plan well-balanced meals. By definition, a supplement is an "add-on," which cannot take the place of making healthy choices related to diet and exercise.

Chapter 20

Tips for Older Dietary Supplement Users

Can dietary supplements help older consumers?

Even if you eat a wide variety of foods, how can you be sure that you are getting all the vitamins, minerals, and other nutrients you need as you get older? If you are over 50, your nutritional needs may change. Informed food choices are the first place to start, making sure you get a variety of foods while watching your calorie intake. Supplements and fortified foods may also help you get appropriate amounts of nutrients. To help you make informed decisions, talk to your doctor and/or registered dietitian. They can work together with you to determine if your intake of a specific nutrient might be too low or too high and then decide how you can achieve a balance between the foods and nutrients you personally need.

What are dietary supplements?

Today's dietary supplements are not only vitamins and minerals. They also include other less-familiar substances, such as herbals, botanicals, amino acids, enzymes, and animal extracts. Some dietary supplements are well understood and established, but others need further study. Whatever your choice, supplements should not replace the variety of foods important to a healthful diet.

Excerpted from text by the U.S. Food and Drug Administration (FDA, www.fda .gov), May 7, 2009.

Unlike drugs, dietary supplements are not preapproved by the government for safety or effectiveness before marketing. Also, unlike drugs, supplements are not intended to treat, diagnose, prevent, or cure diseases. But some supplements can help assure that you get an adequate dietary intake of essential nutrients; others may help you reduce your risk of disease. Some older people, for example, are tired due to low iron levels. In that case, their doctor may recommend an iron supplement.

At times, it can be confusing to tell the difference between a dietary supplement, a food, or over-the-counter (OTC) medicines. This is because supplements, by law, come in a variety of forms that resemble these products, such as tablets, capsules, powders, energy bars, or drinks. One way to know if a product is a dietary supplement is to look for the Supplement Facts label on the product.

Are there any risks, especially to older consumers?

While certain products may be helpful to some older individuals, there may be circumstances when these products may not benefit your health or when they may create unexpected risks. Many supplements contain active ingredients that have strong biological effects in the body. This could make them unsafe in some situations and hurt or complicate your health. For example:

- **Are you taking both medicines and supplements? Are you substituting one for the other?** Taking a combination of supplements, using these products together with medications (whether prescription or over-the-counter), or substituting them in place of medicines your doctor prescribes could lead to harmful, even life-threatening results. Be alert to any advisories about these products. Coumadin (a prescription medicine), ginkgo biloba (an herbal supplement), aspirin (an over-the-counter drug), and vitamin E (a vitamin supplement) can each thin the blood. Taking any of these products alone or together can increase the potential for internal bleeding or stroke. Another example is St. John's wort that may reduce the effectiveness of prescription drugs for heart disease, depression, seizures, certain cancers, or HIV [human immunodeficiency virus].

- **Are you planning surgery?** Some supplements can have unwanted effects before, during, and after surgery. It is important to fully inform your healthcare professional, including your pharmacist, about the vitamins, minerals, herbals, and any other supplements you are taking, especially before surgery. You may be asked to stop taking these products at least 2–3 weeks ahead of the procedure to avoid potentially dangerous supplement/drug interactions—such as changes in heart rate, blood pressure, or bleeding risk that could adversely affect the outcome of your surgery.

- **Is taking more of a good thing better?** Some people might think that if a little is good, taking a lot is even better. But taking too much of some nutrients, even vitamins and minerals, can also cause problems. Depending on the supplement, your age, and the status of your health, taking more than 100% of the Daily Value (DV) of certain vitamins and minerals, e.g., vitamin A, vitamin D, and iron (from supplements and food sources like vitamin-fortified cereals and drinks) may actually harm your health. Large amounts can also interfere with how your medicines work.

Remember: Your combined intake from all supplements (including multivitamins, single supplements, and combination products) plus fortified foods, like some cereals and drinks, could cause health problems.

Why speak to my healthcare provider about dietary supplements?

You and your health professionals (doctors, nurses, registered dietitians, pharmacists, and other caregivers) are a team working toward a common goal—to develop a personalized health plan for you. Your doctor and other members of the health team can help monitor your medical condition and overall health, especially if any problems develop. Although they may not immediately have answers to your questions, these health professionals have access to the most current research on dietary supplements.

There are numerous resources that provide information about dietary supplements. These include TV, radio, newspapers, magazines, store clerks, friends, family, or the internet. It is important to question recommendations from people who have no formal training in nutrition, botanicals, or medicine. While some of these sources, like the web, may seem to offer a wealth of accurate information, these same sources may contain misinformation that may not be obvious. Given the abundance and conflicting nature of information now available about supplements, it is more important than ever to partner with your healthcare team to sort the reliable information from the questionable.

How will I be able to spot false claims?

Be savvy! Although the benefits of some dietary supplements have been documented, the claims of others may be unproven. If something sounds too good to be true, it usually is. Here are some signs of a false claim:

- It makes statements that the product is a quick and effective "cure-all." For example: "Extremely beneficial in treatment of rheumatism, arthritis, infections, prostate problems, ulcers, cancer, heart trouble, hardening of the arteries, and more."

- It makes statements that suggest the product can treat or cure diseases. For example: "shrinks tumors" or "cures impotency." Actually, these are drug claims and should not be made for dietary supplements.

- It makes statements that claim the product is "totally safe," "all natural," or has "definitely no side effects."

- It includes promotions that use words like "scientific breakthrough," "miraculous cure," "exclusive product," "secret ingredient," or "ancient remedy." For example: "A scientific breakthrough formulated by using proven principles of natural health-based medical science."

- It includes text that uses overly impressive-sounding terms, like those for a weight-loss product: "hunger stimulation point" and "thermogenesis."

- It uses personal testimonials by consumers or doctors claiming amazing results. For example: "My husband has Alzheimer disease. He began eating a teaspoonful of this product each day. And now in just 22 days, he mowed the grass, cleaned out the garage, and weeded the flower beds; we take our morning walk together again."

- It has limited availability and requires advance payment. For example: "Hurry. This offer will not last. Send us a check now to reserve your supply."

- It promises no-risk "money-back guarantees." For example: "If after 30 days you have not lost at least 4 pounds each week, your uncashed check will be returned to you."

What are the key "points to ponder" before I buy?

- **Think twice about chasing the latest headline.** Sound health advice is generally based on research over time, not a single study. Be wary of results claiming a "quick fix" that depart from scientific research and established dietary guidance. Keep in mind that science does not generally proceed by dramatic breakthroughs, but rather by taking many small steps, slowly building toward scientific agreement.

- **We may think, "Even if a product may not help me, it at least won't hurt me."** It's best not to assume that this will always be true. Some product ingredients, including nutrients and plant components, can be toxic based on their activity in your body. Some products may become harmful when consumed in high enough amounts, for a long enough time, or in combination with certain other substances.

- **The term 'natural' does not always mean safe.** Do not assume this term assures wholesomeness or that these products have milder effects, making them safer to use than prescribed drugs. For example, many weight-loss products claim to be "natural" or "herbal" but this doesn't necessarily make them safe. The products' ingredients may interact with drugs or may be dangerous for people with certain medical conditions.

- **Spend your money wisely.** Some supplement products may be expensive and may not work, given your specific condition. Be wary of substituting a product or therapy for prescription medicines. Be sure to talk with your healthcare team to help you determine what is best for your overall health.

Remember: Safety first. Resist the pressure to decide "on the spot" about trying an untested product or treatment. Ask for more information and consult your doctor, nurse, dietitian, pharmacist, and/or caregiver about whether the product is right for you and safe for you to use.

Who is responsible for ensuring the safety and efficacy of dietary supplements?

Unlike prescription and over-the-counter medicines, dietary supplement products are not reviewed by the government before they are marketed. Under the law, manufacturers of dietary supplements are responsible for making sure their products are safe before they go to market. If you want to know more about the product you are purchasing, check with the manufacturer to find out if the firm can provide the following information:

- Information to support the claims for their products

- Information on the safety or efficacy of the ingredients in the product

- Adverse event reports from consumers using their products

What is FDA's responsibility?

FDA has the responsibility to take action against unsafe dietary supplement products after they reach the market. The agency may also take legal action against dietary supplement manufacturers if FDA can prove that claims on marketed dietary supplements are false and misleading.

What if I think I have had a reaction to a dietary supplement?

Adverse effects from the use of dietary supplements should be reported to the FDA's MedWatch Program. You, your healthcare provider, or anyone should report a serious adverse event or illness directly to FDA if you believe it is related to the use of any dietary supplement product by calling FDA at 800-FDA-1088, faxing to 800-FDA-0178, or reporting online. FDA would like to know whenever you think a product caused you a serious problem, even if you are not sure that the product was the cause, and even if you do not visit a doctor or clinic.

What's the bottom line?

- Dietary supplements are intended to supplement the diet, not to cure, prevent, or treat diseases or replace the variety of foods important to a healthful diet.

- Supplements can help you meet daily requirements for certain nutrients, but when you combine drugs and foods, too much of some nutrients can also cause problems.

- Many factors play a role in deciding if a supplement is right for you, including possible drug interactions and side effects.

- Do not self-diagnose any health condition. Together, you and your healthcare team can make the best decision for optimal health.

Ask yourself the following questions and talk to your doctor, nurse, dietitian, pharmacist, and/or caregiver about dietary supplements.

- Is taking a dietary supplement an important part of my total diet?

- Are there any precautions or warnings I should know about (e.g., is there an amount or "upper limit" I should not go above)?

- Are there any known side effects (e.g., loss of appetite, nausea, headaches, etc.)? Do they apply to me?

- Are there any foods, medicines (prescription or over-the counter), or other supplements I should avoid while taking this product?

- If I am scheduled for surgery, should I be concerned about the dietary supplements I am taking?
- What is this product for?
- What are its intended benefits?
- How, when, and for how long should I take it?

What are some examples of products marketed as dietary supplements?

Because many products are marketed as dietary supplements, it is important to remember that supplements include botanical/herbal as well as vitamin/mineral products. The list* in the following text gives some examples of products you may see sold as dietary supplements. It is not possible to list them all here. Note: the examples provided do not represent either an endorsement or approval by FDA or any coalition members.

Vitamins, minerals, and nutrients include the following:

- Multiple vitamin/mineral
- Vitamin C
- Vitamin E
- Fiber
- Zinc
- Beta-carotene

- Vitamin B complex
- Vitamin D
- Calcium
- Folic acid
- Iron
- Omega-3 fatty acids

Botanicals and other substances include the following:

- Acidophilus
- Ginger
- Echinacea
- *Ginkgo biloba*
- St. John's wort
- Glucosamine and/or chondroitin sulfate

- Black cohosh
- Evening primrose oil
- Garlic
- Fish oil
- Saw palmetto

*Adapted from *A Healthcare Professional's Guide to Evaluating Dietary Supplements, the American Dietetic Association & American Pharmaceutical Association Special Report.* (2000).

Chapter 21

Vitamin A and Carotenoids

Vitamin A: What is it?

Vitamin A is a group of compounds that play an important role in vision, bone growth, reproduction, cell division, and cell differentiation (in which a cell becomes part of the brain, muscle, lungs, blood, or other specialized tissue.). Vitamin A helps regulate the immune system, which helps prevent or fight off infections by making white blood cells that destroy harmful bacteria and viruses. Vitamin A also may help lymphocytes (a type of white blood cell) fight infections more effectively.

Vitamin A promotes healthy surface linings of the eyes and the respiratory, urinary, and intestinal tracts. When those linings break down, it becomes easier for bacteria to enter the body and cause infection. Vitamin A also helps the skin and mucous membranes function as a barrier to bacteria and viruses.

In general, there are two categories of vitamin A, depending on whether the food source is an animal or a plant.

Vitamin A found in foods that come from animals is called preformed vitamin A. It is absorbed in the form of retinol, one of the most usable (active) forms of vitamin A. Sources include liver, whole milk, and some fortified food products. Retinol can be made into retinal and retinoic acid (other active forms of vitamin A) in the body.

Vitamin A that is found in colorful fruits and vegetables is called provitamin A carotenoid. They can be made into retinol in the body. In

---

Excerpted from text by the Office of Dietary Supplements (ODS, ods.od.nih.gov), part of the National Institutes of Health, April 23, 2006.

the United States, approximately 26% of vitamin A consumed by men and 34% of vitamin A consumed by women is in the form of provitamin A carotenoids. Common provitamin A carotenoids found in foods that come from plants are beta-carotene, alpha-carotene, and beta-cryptoxanthin. Among these, beta-carotene is most efficiently made into retinol. Alpha-carotene and beta-cryptoxanthin are also converted to vitamin A, but only half as efficiently as beta-carotene.

Of the 563 identified carotenoids, fewer than 10% can be made into vitamin A in the body. Lycopene, lutein, and zeaxanthin are carotenoids that do not have vitamin A activity but have other health promoting properties. The Institute of Medicine (IOM) encourages consumption of all carotenoid-rich fruits and vegetables for their health-promoting benefits.

Some provitamin A carotenoids have been shown to function as antioxidants in laboratory studies; however, this role has not been consistently demonstrated in humans. Antioxidants protect cells from free radicals, which are potentially damaging by-products of oxygen metabolism that may contribute to the development of some chronic diseases.

What foods provide vitamin A?

Retinol is found in foods that come from animals such as whole eggs, milk, and liver. Most fat-free milk and dried nonfat milk solids sold in the United States are fortified with vitamin A to replace the amount lost when the fat is removed. Fortified foods such as fortified breakfast cereals also provide vitamin A. Provitamin A carotenoids are abundant in darkly colored fruits and vegetables. The 2000 National Health and Nutrition Examination Survey (NHANES) indicated that major dietary contributors of retinol are milk, margarine, eggs, beef liver and fortified breakfast cereals, whereas major contributors of provitamin A carotenoids are carrots, cantaloupes, sweet potatoes, and spinach.

Vitamin A in foods that come from animals is well absorbed and used efficiently by the body. Vitamin A in foods that come from plants is not as well absorbed as animal sources of vitamin A.

What are recommended intakes of vitamin A?

Recommendations for vitamin A are provided in the Dietary Reference Intakes (DRIs) developed by the Institute of Medicine (IOM). DRI is the general term for a set of reference values used for planning and assessing nutrient intake in healthy people. Three important types of reference values included in the DRIs are Recommended Dietary Allowances (RDA), Adequate Intakes (AI), and Tolerable Upper Intake

Levels (UL). The RDA recommends the average daily dietary intake level that is sufficient to meet the nutrient requirements of nearly all (97% to 98%) healthy individuals in each age and gender group. An AI is set when there are insufficient scientific data to establish an RDA. AIs meet or exceed the amount needed to maintain nutritional adequacy in nearly all people. The UL, on the other hand, is the maximum daily intake unlikely to result in adverse health effects.

The NHANES III survey (1988–1994) found that most Americans consume recommended amounts of vitamin A. More recent NHANES data (1999–2000) show average adult intakes to be about 3,300 IU per day, which also suggests that most Americans get enough vitamin A.

There is no RDA for beta-carotene or other provitamin A carotenoids. The IOM states that consuming 3 mg to 6 mg of beta-carotene daily (equivalent to 833 IU to 1,667 IU vitamin A) will maintain blood levels of beta-carotene in the range associated with a lower risk of chronic diseases. A diet that provides five or more servings of fruits and vegetables per day and includes some dark green and leafy vegetables and deep yellow or orange fruits should provide sufficient beta-carotene and other carotenoids.

What are some current issues and controversies about vitamin A?

Vitamin A, beta carotene, and cancer: Dietary intake studies suggest an association between diets rich in beta-carotene and vitamin A and a lower risk of many types of cancer. A higher intake of green and yellow vegetables or other food sources of beta carotene and/or vitamin A may decrease the risk of lung cancer. However, a number of studies that tested the role of beta-carotene supplements in cancer prevention did not find them to protect against the disease. In the Alpha-Tocopherol Beta-Carotene (ATBC) Cancer Prevention Study, more than 29,000 men who regularly smoked cigarettes were randomized to receive 20 mg beta-carotene alone, 50 mg alpha-tocopherol alone, supplements of both, or a placebo for 5 to 8 years. Incidence of lung cancer was 18% higher among men who took the beta-carotene supplement. Eight percent more men in this group died, as compared to those receiving other treatments or placebo. Similar results were seen in the Carotene and Retinol Efficacy Trial (CARET), a lung cancer chemoprevention study that provided subjects with supplements of 30 mg beta-carotene and 25,000 IU retinyl palmitate (a form of vitamin A) or a placebo. This study was stopped after researchers discovered that subjects receiving beta-carotene had a 46% higher risk of dying from lung cancer.

The IOM states that "beta-carotene supplements are not advisable for the general population," although they also state that this advice "does not pertain to the possible use of supplemental beta-carotene as a provitamin A source for the prevention of vitamin A deficiency in populations with inadequate vitamin A."

Vitamin A and osteoporosis: Osteoporosis, a disorder characterized by porous and weak bones, is a serious health problem for more than 10 million Americans, 80% of whom are women. Another 18 million Americans have decreased bone density which precedes the development of osteoporosis. Many factors increase the risk for developing osteoporosis, including being female, thin, inactive, at advanced age, and having a family history of osteoporosis. An inadequate dietary intake of calcium, cigarette smoking, and excessive intake of alcohol also increase the risk.

Researchers are now examining a potential new risk factor for osteoporosis: an excess intake of vitamin A. Animal, human, and laboratory research suggests an association between greater vitamin A intake and weaker bones. Worldwide, the highest incidence of osteoporosis occurs in northern Europe, a population with a high intake of vitamin A. However, decreased biosynthesis of vitamin D associated with lower levels of sun exposure in this population may also contribute to this finding.

One small study of nine healthy individuals in Sweden found that the amount of vitamin A in one serving of liver may impair the ability of vitamin D to promote calcium absorption. To further test the association between excess dietary intakes of vitamin A and increased risk for hip fractures, researchers in Sweden compared bone mineral density and retinol intake in approximately 250 women with a first hip fracture to 875 age-matched controls. They found that a dietary retinol intake greater than 1,500 mcg/day (more than twice the recommended intake for women) was associated with reduced bone mineral density and increased risk of hip fracture as compared to women who consumed less than 500 mcg/day.

This issue was also examined by researchers with the Nurses Health Study, who looked at the association between vitamin A intake and hip fractures in over 72,000 postmenopausal women. Women who consumed the most vitamin A in foods and supplements (3,000 mcg or more per day as retinol equivalents, which is over three times the recommended intake) had a significantly increased risk of experiencing a hip fracture as compared to those consuming the least amount (less than 1,250 mcg/day). The effect was lessened by use of estrogens. These observations raise questions about the effect of retinol because retinol intakes greater than 2,000 mcg/day were associated with an increased risk of hip fracture as compared to intakes less than 500 mcg.

A longitudinal study in more than 2,000 Swedish men compared blood levels of retinol to the incidence of fractures in men. The investigators found that the risk of fractures was greatest in men with the highest blood levels of retinol (more than 75 mcg per deciliter [dL]). Men with blood retinol levels in the 99th percentile (greater than 103 mcg per dL) had an overall risk of fracture that exceeded the risk among men with lower levels of retinol by a factor of seven. High vitamin A intake, however, does not necessarily equate to high blood levels of retinol. Age, gender, hormones, and genetics also influence these levels. Researchers did not find any association between blood levels of beta-carotene and risk of hip fracture. Researchers' findings, which are consistent with the results of animal, in vitro (laboratory), and epidemiologic studies, suggest that intakes above the UL, or approximately two times that of the RDA for vitamin A, may pose subtle risks to bone health that require further study.

The Centers for Disease Control and Prevention (CDC) reviewed data from NHANES III (1988–94) to determine whether there was any association between bone mineral density and blood levels of retinyl esters, a form of vitamin A. No significant associations between blood levels of retinyl esters and bone mineral density in 5,800 subjects were found.

There is no evidence of an association between beta-carotene intake, especially from fruits and vegetables, and increased risk of osteoporosis. Current evidence points to a possible association with vitamin A as retinol only. If you have specific questions regarding your intake of vitamin A and risk of osteoporosis, discuss this information with your physician or other qualified healthcare provider to determine what's best for your personal health.

What are the health risks of too much vitamin A?

Hypervitaminosis A refers to high storage levels of vitamin A in the body that can lead to toxic symptoms. There are four major adverse effects of hypervitaminosis A: birth defects, liver abnormalities, reduced bone mineral density that may result in osteoporosis (see the previous section), and central nervous system disorders.

Toxic symptoms can also arise after consuming very large amounts of preformed vitamin A over a short period of time. Signs of acute toxicity include nausea and vomiting, headache, dizziness, blurred vision, and muscular uncoordination. Although hypervitaminosis A can occur when large amounts of liver are regularly consumed, most cases result from taking excess amounts of the nutrient in supplements.

133

The IOM has established Tolerable Upper Intake Levels (ULs) for vitamin A that apply to healthy populations. The UL was established to help prevent the risk of vitamin A toxicity. The risk of adverse health effects increases at intakes greater than the UL. The UL does not apply to malnourished individuals receiving vitamin A either periodically or through fortification programs as a means of preventing vitamin A deficiency. It also does not apply to individuals being treated with vitamin A by medical doctors for diseases such as retinitis pigmentosa.

Retinoids are compounds that are chemically similar to vitamin A. Over the past 15 years, synthetic retinoids have been prescribed for acne, psoriasis, and other skin disorders. Isotretinoin (Roaccutane® or Accutane®) is considered an effective anti-acne therapy. At very high doses, however, it can be toxic, which is why this medication is usually saved for the most severe forms of acne. The most serious consequence of this medication is birth defects. It is extremely important for sexually active females who may become pregnant and who take these medications to use an effective method of birth control. Women of childbearing age who take these medications are advised to undergo monthly pregnancy tests to make sure they are not pregnant.

What are the health risks of too many carotenoids?

Provitamin A carotenoids such as beta-carotene are generally considered safe because they are not associated with specific adverse health effects. Their conversion to vitamin A decreases when body stores are full. A high intake of provitamin A carotenoids can turn the skin yellow, but this is not considered dangerous to health.

Clinical trials that associated beta-carotene supplements with a greater incidence of lung cancer and death in current smokers raise concerns about the effects of beta-carotene supplements on long-term health; however, conflicting studies make it difficult to interpret the health risk. For example, the Physicians Health Study compared the effects of taking 50 mg beta-carotene every other day to a placebo in over 22,000 male physicians and found no adverse health effects. Also, a trial that tested the ability of four different nutrient combinations to help prevent the development of esophageal and gastric cancers in 30,000 men and women in China suggested that after five years those participants who took a combination of beta-carotene, selenium, and vitamin E had a 13% reduction in cancer deaths. In one lung cancer trial, men who consumed more than 11 grams/day of alcohol (approximately one drink per day) were more likely to show an adverse response to beta-carotene supplements, which may suggest a potential relationship between alcohol and beta-carotene.

The IOM did not set ULs for carotene or other carotenoids. Instead, it concluded that beta-carotene supplements are not advisable for the general population. As stated earlier, however, they may be appropriate as a provitamin A source for the prevention of vitamin A deficiency in specific populations.

Vitamin A intakes and healthful diets: According to the 2005 Dietary Guidelines for Americans, "Nutrient needs should be met primarily through consuming foods. Foods provide an array of nutrients and other compounds that may have beneficial effects on health. In certain cases, fortified foods and dietary supplements may be useful sources of one or more nutrients that otherwise might be consumed in less than recommended amounts. However, dietary supplements, while recommended in some cases, cannot replace a healthful diet." For more information about building a healthful diet, refer to the Dietary Guidelines for Americans (http://www.health.gov/dietaryguidelines/dga2005/document/pdf/DGA2005.pdf) and the U.S. Department of Agriculture's food guidance system (My Pyramid; http://www.mypyramid.gov).

Chapter 22

Vitamin B$_6$

Vitamin B$_6$: What is it?

Vitamin B$_6$ is a water-soluble vitamin that exists in three major chemical forms: pyridoxine, pyridoxal, and pyridoxamine. It performs a wide variety of functions in your body and is essential for your good health. For example, vitamin B$_6$ is needed for more than 100 enzymes involved in protein metabolism. It is also essential for red blood cell metabolism. The nervous and immune systems need vitamin B$_6$ to function efficiently, and it is also needed for the conversion of tryptophan (an amino acid) to niacin (a vitamin).

Hemoglobin within red blood cells carries oxygen to tissues. Your body needs vitamin B$_6$ to make hemoglobin. Vitamin B$_6$ also helps increase the amount of oxygen carried by hemoglobin. A vitamin B$_6$ deficiency can result in a form of anemia that is similar to iron deficiency anemia.

An immune response is a broad term that describes a variety of biochemical changes that occur in an effort to fight off infections. Calories, protein, vitamins, and minerals are important to your immune defenses because they promote the growth of white blood cells that directly fight infections. Vitamin B$_6$, through its involvement in protein metabolism and cellular growth, is important to the immune system. It helps maintain the health of lymphoid organs (thymus, spleen, and lymph nodes) that make your white blood cells. Animal studies show that a vitamin B$_6$ deficiency can decrease your antibody production and suppress your immune response.

Excerpted from text by the Office of Dietary Supplements (ODS, ods.od.nih.gov), part of the National Institutes of Health, August 24, 2007.

Vitamin B$_6$ also helps maintain your blood glucose (sugar) within a normal range. When caloric intake is low your body needs vitamin B$_6$ to help convert stored carbohydrate or other nutrients to glucose to maintain normal blood sugar levels. While a shortage of vitamin B$_6$ will limit these functions, supplements of this vitamin do not enhance them in well-nourished individuals.

What foods provide vitamin B$_6$?

Vitamin B$_6$ is found in a wide variety of foods including fortified cereals, beans, meat, poultry, fish, and some fruits and vegetables.

What is the Recommended Dietary Allowance for vitamin B$_6$ for adults?

The Recommended Dietary Allowance (RDA) is the average daily dietary intake level that is sufficient to meet the nutrient requirements of nearly all (97 to 98 percent) healthy individuals in each life-stage and gender group.

The 1998 RDAs for vitamin B$_6$ for adults, in milligrams, are 1.3 mg for men and women 19–50. Men 51 and older should get 1.7 mg and women 51 and older should get 1.5 mg. Pregnant women should get 1.9 mg and lactating women need 2.0 mg of this vitamin.

Results of two national surveys, the National Health and Nutrition Examination Survey (NHANES III 1988–94) and the Continuing Survey of Food Intakes by Individuals (1994–96 CSFII), indicated that diets of most Americans meet current intake recommendations for vitamin B$_6$.

What are some current issues and controversies about vitamin B$_6$?

Vitamin B$_6$ and the nervous system: Vitamin B$_6$ is needed for the synthesis of neurotransmitters such as serotonin and dopamine. These neurotransmitters are required for normal nerve cell communication. Researchers have been investigating the relationship between vitamin B$_6$ status and a wide variety of neurologic conditions such as seizures, chronic pain, depression, headache, and Parkinson disease.

Lower levels of serotonin have been found in individuals suffering from depression and migraine headaches. So far, however, vitamin B$_6$ supplements have not proved effective for relieving these symptoms. One study found that a sugar pill was just as likely as vitamin B$_6$ to relieve headaches and depression associated with low dose oral contraceptives.

Alcohol abuse can result in neuropathy, abnormal nerve sensations in the arms and legs. A poor dietary intake contributes to this neuropathy and dietary supplements that include vitamin B$_6$ may prevent or decrease its incidence.

Vitamin B$_6$ and carpal tunnel syndrome: Vitamin B$_6$ was first recommended for carpal tunnel syndrome almost 30 years ago. Several popular books still recommend taking 100 to 200 milligrams (mg) of vitamin B$_6$ daily to treat carpal tunnel syndrome, even though scientific studies do not indicate it is effective. Anyone taking large doses of vitamin B$_6$ supplements for carpal tunnel syndrome needs to be aware that the Institute of Medicine recently established an upper tolerable limit of 100 mg per day for adults. There are documented cases in the literature of neuropathy caused by excessive vitamin B$_6$ taken for treatment of carpal tunnel syndrome.

Vitamin B$_6$ and premenstrual syndrome: Vitamin B$_6$ has become a popular remedy for treating the discomforts associated with premenstrual syndrome (PMS). Unfortunately, clinical trials have failed to support any significant benefit. One recent study indicated that a sugar pill was as likely to relieve symptoms of PMS as vitamin B$_6$. In addition, vitamin B$_6$ toxicity has been seen in increasing numbers of women taking vitamin B$_6$ supplements for PMS. One review indicated that neuropathy was present in 23 of 58 women taking daily vitamin B$_6$ supplements for PMS whose blood levels of B$_6$ were above normal. There is no convincing scientific evidence to support recommending vitamin B$_6$ supplements for PMS.

Vitamin B$_6$ and interactions with medications: There are many drugs that interfere with the metabolism of vitamin B$_6$. Isoniazid, which is used to treat tuberculosis, and L-DOPA [L-3,4-dihydroxyphenylalanine], which is used to treat a variety of neurologic problems such as Parkinson disease, alter the activity of vitamin B$_6$. There is disagreement about the need for routine vitamin B$_6$ supplementation when taking isoniazid. Acute isoniazid toxicity can result in coma and seizures that are reversed by vitamin B$_6$, but in a group of children receiving isoniazid, no cases of neurological or neuropsychiatric problems were observed regardless of whether or not they took a vitamin B$_6$ supplement. Some doctors recommend taking a supplement that provides 100% of the RDA for B$_6$ when isoniazid is prescribed, which is usually enough to prevent symptoms of vitamin B$_6$ deficiency. It is important to consult with a physician about the need for a vitamin B$_6$ supplement when taking isoniazid.

What is the relationship between vitamin B_6, homocysteine, and heart disease?

A deficiency of vitamin B_6, folic acid, or vitamin B_{12} may increase your level of homocysteine, an amino acid normally found in your blood. There is evidence that an elevated homocysteine level is an independent risk factor for heart disease and stroke. The evidence suggests that high levels of homocysteine may damage coronary arteries or make it easier for blood clotting cells called platelets to clump together and form a clot. However, there is currently no evidence available to suggest that lowering homocysteine level with vitamins will reduce your risk of heart disease. Clinical intervention trials are needed to determine whether supplementation with vitamin B_6, folic acid, or vitamin B_{12} can help protect you against developing coronary heart disease.

What is the health risk of too much vitamin B_6?

Too much vitamin B_6 can result in nerve damage to the arms and legs. This neuropathy is usually related to high intake of vitamin B_6 from supplements, and is reversible when supplementation is stopped.

According to the Institute of Medicine, "Several reports show sensory neuropathy at doses lower than 500 mg per day." As previously mentioned, the Food and Nutrition Board of the Institute of Medicine has established an upper tolerable intake level (UL) for vitamin B_6 of 100 mg per day for all adults. "As intake increases above the UL, the risk of adverse effects increases."

Vitamin B_6 intakes and healthful diets: Vitamin B_6 is found in a wide variety of foods. Foods such as fortified breakfast cereals, fish including salmon and tuna fish, meats such as pork and chicken, bananas, beans and peanut butter, and many vegetables will contribute to your vitamin B_6 intake.

According to the 2005 Dietary Guidelines for Americans, "Nutrient needs should be met primarily through consuming foods. Foods provide an array of nutrients and other compounds that may have beneficial effects on health. In certain cases, fortified foods and dietary supplements may be useful sources of one or more nutrients that otherwise might be consumed in less than recommended amounts. However, dietary supplements, while recommended in some cases, cannot replace a healthful diet."

The Dietary Guidelines for Americans describes a healthy diet as one that does the following:

- Emphasizes a variety of fruits, vegetables, whole grains, and fat-free or low-fat milk and milk products

- Includes lean meats, poultry, fish, beans, eggs, and nuts
- Is low in saturated fats, trans fats, cholesterol, salt (sodium), and added sugars
- Stays within your daily calorie needs

For more information about building a healthful diet, refer to the Dietary Guidelines for Americans and the U.S. Department of Agriculture's food guidance system, MyPyramid.

Chapter 23

Vitamin B$_{12}$

Vitamin B$_{12}$ is a water-soluble vitamin that is naturally present in some foods, added to others, and available as a dietary supplement and a prescription medication. Vitamin B$_{12}$ exists in several forms and contains the mineral cobalt, so compounds with vitamin B$_{12}$ activity are collectively called "cobalamins." Methylcobalamin and 5-deoxyadenosylcobalamin are the forms of vitamin B$_{12}$ that are active in human metabolism.

Vitamin B$_{12}$ is required for proper red blood cell formation, neurological function, and DNA [deoxyribonucleic acid] synthesis. Vitamin B$_{12}$ functions as a cofactor for methionine synthase and L-methylmalonyl-CoA mutase. Methionine synthase catalyzes the conversion of homocysteine to methionine. Methionine is required for the formation of S-adenosylmethionine, a universal methyl donor for almost 100 different substrates, including DNA, RNA [ribonucleic acid], hormones, proteins, and lipids. L-methylmalonyl-CoA mutase converts L-methylmalonyl-CoA to succinyl-CoA in the degradation of propionate, an essential biochemical reaction in fat and protein metabolism. Succinyl-CoA is also required for hemoglobin synthesis.

Vitamin B$_{12}$, bound to protein in food, is released by the activity of hydrochloric acid and gastric protease in the stomach. When synthetic vitamin B$_{12}$ is added to fortified foods and dietary supplements, it is already in free form and, thus, does not require this separation step. Free vitamin B$_{12}$ then combines with intrinsic factor, a glycoprotein secreted by the stomach's parietal cells, and the resulting complex

Excerpted from text by the Office of Dietary Supplements (ODS, ods.od.nih.gov), part of the National Institutes of Health, October 12, 2009.

143

undergoes absorption within the distal ileum by receptor-mediated endocytosis. Approximately 56% of a 1 mcg oral dose of vitamin B_{12} is absorbed, but absorption decreases drastically when the capacity of intrinsic factor is exceeded (at 1–2 mcg of vitamin B_{12}).

Pernicious anemia is an autoimmune disease that affects the gastric mucosa and results in gastric atrophy. This leads to the destruction of parietal cells, achlorhydria, and failure to produce intrinsic factor, resulting in vitamin B_{12} malabsorption. If pernicious anemia is left untreated, it causes vitamin B_{12} deficiency, leading to megaloblastic anemia and neurological disorders, even in the presence of adequate dietary intake of vitamin B_{12}.

Dietary Supplements

In dietary supplements, vitamin B_{12} is usually present as cyano-cobalamin, a form that the body readily converts to the active forms methylcobalamin and 5-deoxyadenosylcobalamin. Dietary supplements can also contain methylcobalamin and other forms of vitamin B_{12}.

Existing evidence does not suggest any differences among forms with respect to absorption or bioavailability. However the body's ability to absorb vitamin B_{12} from dietary supplements is largely limited by the capacity of intrinsic factor. For example, only about 10 mcg of a 500 mcg oral supplement is actually absorbed in healthy people.

In addition to oral dietary supplements, vitamin B_{12} is available in sublingual preparations as tablets or lozenges. These preparations are frequently marketed as having superior bioavailability, although evidence suggests no difference in efficacy between oral and sublingual forms.

Vitamin B_{12} and Health

Cardiovascular Disease

Cardiovascular disease is the most common cause of death in industrialized countries, such as the United States, and is on the rise in developing countries. Risk factors for cardiovascular disease include elevated low-density lipoprotein (LDL) levels, high blood pressure, low high-density lipoprotein (HDL) levels, obesity, and diabetes.

Elevated homocysteine levels have also been identified as an independent risk factor for cardiovascular disease. Homocysteine is a sulfur-containing amino acid derived from methionine that is normally present in blood. Elevated homocysteine levels are thought to promote thrombogenesis, impair endothelial vasomotor function, promote lipid peroxidation, and induce vascular smooth muscle proliferation. Evidence from retrospective, cross-sectional, and prospective studies links elevated homocysteine levels with coronary heart disease and stroke.

Vitamin B$_{12}$, folate, and vitamin B$_6$ are involved in homocysteine metabolism. In the presence of insufficient vitamin B$_{12}$, homocysteine levels can rise due to inadequate function of methionine synthase. Results from several randomized controlled trials indicate that combinations of vitamin B$_{12}$ and folic acid supplements with or without vitamin B$_6$ decrease homocysteine levels in people with vascular disease or diabetes and in young adult women. In another study, older men and women who took a multivitamin/multimineral supplement for 8 weeks experienced a significant decrease in homocysteine levels.

Evidence supports a role for folic acid and vitamin B$_{12}$ supplements in lowering homocysteine levels, but results from several large prospective studies have not shown that these supplements decrease the risk of cardiovascular disease. In the Women's Antioxidant and Folic Acid Cardiovascular Study, women at high risk of cardiovascular disease who took daily supplements containing 1 mg vitamin B$_{12}$, 2.5 mg folic acid, and 50 mg vitamin B$_6$ for 7.3 years did not have a reduced risk of major cardiovascular events, despite lowered homocysteine levels. The Heart Outcomes Prevention Evaluation (HOPE) 2 trial, which included 5,522 patients older than 54 years with vascular disease or diabetes, found that daily treatment with 2.5 mg folic acid, 50 mg vitamin B$_6$, and 1 mg vitamin B$_{12}$ for an average of 5 years reduced homocysteine levels and the risk of stroke but did not reduce the risk of major cardiovascular events. In the Western Norway B Vitamin Intervention Trial, which included 3,096 patients undergoing coronary angiography, daily supplements of 0.4 mg vitamin B$_{12}$ and 0.8 mg folic acid with or without 40 mg vitamin B$_6$ for 1 year reduced homocysteine levels by 30% but did not affect total mortality or the risk of major cardiovascular events during 38 months of follow-up. The Norwegian Vitamin (NORVIT) trial and the Vitamin Intervention for Stroke Prevention trial had similar results.

The American Heart Association has concluded that the available evidence is inadequate to support a role for B vitamins in reducing cardiovascular risk.

Dementia and Cognitive Function

Researchers have long been interested in the potential connection between vitamin B$_{12}$ deficiency and dementia. A deficiency in vitamin B$_{12}$ causes an accumulation of homocysteine in the blood and might decrease levels of substances needed to metabolize neurotransmitters. Observational studies show positive associations between elevated homocysteine levels and the incidence of both Alzheimer disease and dementia. Low vitamin B_{12} status has also been positively associated with cognitive decline.

Despite evidence that vitamin B12 lowers homocysteine levels and correlations between low vitamin B12 levels and cognitive decline, research has not shown that vitamin B12 has an independent effect on cognition. In one randomized, double-blind, placebo-controlled trial, 195 subjects aged 70 years or older with no or moderate cognitive impairment received 1,000 mcg vitamin B12, 1,000 mcg vitamin B12 plus 400 mcg folic acid, or placebo for 24 weeks. Treatment with vitamin B12 plus folic acid reduced homocysteine concentrations by 36%, but neither vitamin B12 treatment nor vitamin B12 plus folic acid treatment improved cognitive function.

Women at high risk of cardiovascular disease who participated in the Women's Antioxidant and Folic Acid Cardiovascular Study were randomly assigned to receive daily supplements containing 1 mg vitamin B12, 2.5 mg folic acid and 50 mg vitamin B6, or placebo. After a mean of 1.2 years, B-vitamin supplementation did not affect mean cognitive change from baseline compared with placebo. However, in a subset of women with low baseline dietary intake of B vitamins, supplementation significantly slowed the rate of cognitive decline. In a trial conducted by the Alzheimer's Disease Cooperative Study consortium that included individuals with mild-to-moderate Alzheimer disease, daily supplements of 1 mg vitamin B12, 5 mg folic acid, and 25 mg vitamin B6 for 18 months did not slow cognitive decline compared with placebo. Another study found similar results in 142 individuals at risk of dementia who received supplements of 2 mg folic acid and 1 mg vitamin B12 for 12 weeks.

The authors of two Cochrane reviews and a systematic review of randomized trials of the effects of B vitamins on cognitive function concluded that insufficient evidence is available to show whether vitamin B12 alone or in combination with vitamin B6 or folic acid has an effect on cognitive function or dementia. Additional large clinical trials of vitamin B12 supplementation are needed to assess whether vitamin B12 has a direct effect on cognitive function and dementia.

Energy and Endurance

Due to its role in energy metabolism, vitamin B12 is frequently promoted as an energy enhancer and an athletic performance and endurance booster. These claims are based on the fact that correcting the megaloblastic anemia caused by vitamin B12 deficiency should improve the associated symptoms of fatigue and weakness. However, vitamin B12 supplementation appears to have no beneficial effect on performance in the absence of a nutritional deficit.

Chapter 24

Vitamin D

Vitamin D is a fat-soluble vitamin that is naturally present in very few foods, added to others, and available as a dietary supplement. It is also produced endogenously when ultraviolet rays from sunlight strike the skin and trigger vitamin D synthesis. Vitamin D obtained from sun exposure, food, and supplements is biologically inert and must undergo two hydroxylations in the body for activation. The first occurs in the liver and converts vitamin D to 25-hydroxyvitamin D [25(OH)D], also known as calcidiol. The second occurs primarily in the kidney and forms the physiologically active 1,25-dihydroxyvitamin D [1,25(OH)2D], also known as calcitriol.

Vitamin D is essential for promoting calcium absorption in the gut and maintaining adequate serum calcium and phosphate concentrations to enable normal mineralization of bone and prevent hypocalcemic tetany. It is also needed for bone growth and bone remodeling by osteoblasts and osteoclasts. Without sufficient vitamin D, bones can become thin, brittle, or misshapen. Vitamin D sufficiency prevents rickets in children and osteomalacia in adults. Together with calcium, vitamin D also helps protect older adults from osteoporosis.

Vitamin D has other roles in human health, including modulation of neuromuscular and immune function and reduction of inflammation. Many genes encoding proteins that regulate cell proliferation, differentiation, and apoptosis are modulated in part by vitamin D. Many

Excerpted from text by the Office of Dietary Supplements (ODS, ods.od.nih.gov), part of the National Institutes of Health, November 13, 2009.

laboratory-cultured human cells have vitamin D receptors and some convert 25(OH)D to 1,25(OH)2D. It remains to be determined whether cells with vitamin D receptors in the intact human carry out this conversion.

Dietary Supplements

In supplements and fortified foods, vitamin D is available in two forms, D_2 (ergocalciferol) and D_3 (cholecalciferol). Vitamin D_2 is manufactured by the UV irradiation of ergosterol in yeast, and vitamin D_3 is manufactured by the irradiation of 7-dehydrocholesterol from lanolin and the chemical conversion of cholesterol. The two forms have traditionally been regarded as equivalent based on their ability to cure rickets, but evidence has been offered that they are metabolized differently. Vitamin D_3 could be more than three times as effective as vitamin D_2 in raising serum 25(OH)D concentrations and maintaining those levels for a longer time, and its metabolites have superior affinity for vitamin D-binding proteins in plasma. Because metabolite receptor affinity is not a functional assessment, as the earlier results for the healing of rickets were, further research is needed on the comparative physiological effects of both forms. Many supplements are being reformulated to contain vitamin D_3 instead of vitamin D_2. Both forms (as well as vitamin D in foods and from cutaneous synthesis) effectively raise serum 25(OH)D levels. According to NHANES (National Health and Nutrition Survey) data from 2005-2006, only 29% of adult men and 17% of adult women (ages 19 and older) had intakes of vitamin D from food alone that exceeded their AIs. Overall in the U.S. population, only about one third of individuals 1 year of age and older had vitamin D intakes from food exceeding their respective AIs. However, dietary supplements as well as foods contribute vitamin D, so both sources must be included to obtain a true picture of total intakes. In 2005–2006, 37% of people in the United States reported the use of a dietary supplement containing vitamin D. Total intake estimates of vitamin D from both food and supplements are currently being tabulated by the Office of Dietary Supplements.

Vitamin D and Health

Optimal serum concentrations of 25(OH)D for bone and general health throughout life have not been established and are likely to vary at each stage of life, depending on the physiological measures selected. The three-fold range of cut points that have been proposed by various experts, from 16 to 48 ng/mL (40 to 120 nmol/L), reflect differences in the functional endpoints chosen (e.g., serum concentrations of parathyroid hormone or bone fractures), as well as differences in the analytical methods used.

In March 2007, a group of vitamin D and nutrition researchers published a controversial and provocative editorial contending that the desirable concentration of 25(OH)D is greater than or equal to ng/mL (greater than or equal to 75 nmol/L). They noted that supplemental intakes of 400 IU/day of vitamin D increase 25(OH)D concentrations by only 2.8–4.8 ng/mL (7–12 nmol/L) and that daily intakes of approximately 1,700 IU are needed to raise these concentrations from 20 to 32 ng/mL (50 to 80 nmol/L).

Osteoporosis: More than 25 million adults in the United States have or are at risk of developing osteoporosis, a disease characterized by fragile bones that significantly increases the risk of bone fractures. Osteoporosis is most often associated with inadequate calcium intakes (generally <1,000-1,200 mg/day), but insufficient vitamin D contributes to osteoporosis by reducing calcium absorption. Although rickets and osteomalacia are extreme examples of the effects of vitamin D deficiency, osteoporosis is an example of a long-term effect of calcium and vitamin D insufficiency. Adequate storage levels of vitamin D maintain bone strength and might help prevent osteoporosis in older adults, nonambulatory individuals who have difficulty exercising, postmenopausal women, and individuals on chronic steroid therapy.

Normal bone is constantly being remodeled. During menopause, the balance between these processes changes, resulting in more bone being resorbed than rebuilt. Hormone therapy with estrogen and progesterone might be able to delay the onset of osteoporosis. However, some medical groups and professional societies recommend that postmenopausal women consider using other agents to slow or stop bone resorption because of the potential adverse health effects of hormone therapy.

Most supplementation trials of the effects of vitamin D on bone health also include calcium, so it is not possible to isolate the effects of each nutrient. The authors of a recent evidence-based review of research concluded that supplements of both vitamin D_3 (at 700–800 IU/day) and calcium (500–1,200 mg/day) decreased the risk of falls, fractures, and bone loss in elderly individuals aged 62–85 years. The decreased risk of fractures occurred primarily in elderly women aged 85 years, on average, and living in a nursing home. Women should consult their healthcare providers about their needs for vitamin D (and calcium) as part of an overall plan to prevent or treat osteoporosis.

African Americans have lower levels of 25(OH)D than Caucasians, yet they develop fewer osteoporotic fractures. This suggests that factors other than vitamin D provide protection. African Americans have an advantage in bone density from early childhood, a function of their more efficient calcium economy, and have a lower risk of fracture even when they have the same bone density as Caucasians. They also have a higher prevalence of obesity, and the resulting higher estrogen levels in obese women might protect them from bone loss. Further reducing the risk of osteoporosis in African Americans are their lower levels of bone-turnover markers, shorter hip-axis length, and superior renal calcium conservation. However, despite this advantage in bone density, osteoporosis is a significant health problem among African Americans as they age.

Cancer: Laboratory and animal evidence as well as epidemiologic data suggest that vitamin D status could affect cancer risk. Strong biological and mechanistic bases indicate that vitamin D plays a role in the prevention of colon, prostate, and breast cancers. Emerging epidemiologic data suggest that vitamin D has a protective effect against colon cancer, but the data are not as strong for a protective effect against prostate and breast cancer, and are variable for cancers at other sites. Studies do not consistently show a protective effect or no effect, however. One study of Finnish smokers, for example, found that subjects in the highest quintile of baseline vitamin D status have a three-fold higher risk of developing pancreatic cancer.

Vitamin D emerged as a protective factor in a prospective, cross-sectional study of 3,121 adults aged greater than or equal to 50 years (96% men) who underwent a colonoscopy. The study found that 10% had at least one advanced cancerous lesion. Those with the highest vitamin D intakes (>645 IU/day) had a significantly lower risk of these lesions. However, the Women's Health Initiative, in which 36,282 postmenopausal women of various races and ethnicities were randomly assigned to receive 400 IU vitamin D plus 1,000 mg calcium daily or a placebo, found no significant differences between the groups in the incidence of colorectal cancers over 7 years. More recently, a clinical trial focused on bone health in 1,179 postmenopausal women residing in rural Nebraska found that subjects supplemented daily with calcium (1,400–1,500 mg) and vitamin D3 (1,100 IU) had a significantly lower incidence of cancer over 4 years compared to women taking a placebo. The small number of cancers reported (50) precludes generalizing about a protective effect from either or both nutrients or for cancers at different sites. This caution is supported by an analysis of 16,618 participants in NHANES III, where total cancer mortality was found to be unrelated to baseline vitamin D status. However, colorectal cancer mortality was inversely related to serum 25(OH)D concentrations.

Further research is needed to determine whether vitamin D inadequacy in particular increases cancer risk, whether greater exposure to the nutrient is protective, and whether some individuals could be at increased risk of cancer because of vitamin D exposure.

Other conditions: A growing body of research suggests that vitamin D might play some role in the prevention and treatment of type 1 and type 2 diabetes, hypertension, glucose intolerance, multiple sclerosis, and other medical conditions. However, most evidence for these roles comes from in vitro, animal, and epidemiological studies, not the randomized clinical trials considered to be more definitive. Until such trials are conducted, the implications of the available evidence for public health and patient care will be debated. A systematic review of health outcomes related to vitamin D and calcium intakes, both alone and in combination, was published in August 2009.

A recent meta-analysis found that use of vitamin D supplements was associated with a reduction in overall mortality from any cause by a statistically significant 7%. The subjects in these trials were primarily healthy, middle aged or elderly, and at high risk of fractures; they took 300–2,000 IU/day of vitamin D supplements.

Chapter 25

Vitamin E

Vitamin E is found naturally in some foods, added to others, and available as a dietary supplement. "Vitamin E" is the collective name for a group of fat-soluble compounds with distinctive antioxidant activities.

Naturally occurring vitamin E exists in eight chemical forms (alpha-, beta-, gamma-, and delta-tocopherol and alpha-, beta-, gamma-, and delta-tocotrienol) that have varying levels of biological activity. Alpha-tocopherol is the only form that is recognized to meet human requirements.

Serum concentrations of vitamin E (alpha-tocopherol) depend on the liver, which takes up the nutrient after the various forms are absorbed from the small intestine. The liver preferentially resecretes only alpha-tocopherol via the hepatic alpha-tocopherol transfer protein; the liver metabolizes and excretes the other vitamin E forms. As a result, blood and cellular concentrations of other forms of vitamin E are lower than those of alpha-tocopherol and have been the subjects of less research.

Antioxidants protect cells from the damaging effects of free radicals, which are molecules that contain an unshared electron. Free radicals damage cells and might contribute to the development of cardiovascular disease and cancer. Unshared electrons are highly energetic and react rapidly with oxygen to form reactive oxygen species (ROS). The body forms ROS endogenously when it converts food to energy, and antioxidants might protect cells from the damaging effects of ROS. The

Excerpted from "Vitamin E Fact Sheet," by the Office of Dietary Supplements (ODS, ods.od.nih.gov), December 15, 2009.

body is also exposed to free radicals from environmental exposures, such as cigarette smoke, air pollution, and ultraviolet radiation from the sun. ROS are part of signaling mechanisms among cells.

Vitamin E is a fat-soluble antioxidant that stops the production of ROS formed when fat undergoes oxidation. Scientists are investigating whether, by limiting free-radical production and possibly through other mechanisms, vitamin E might help prevent or delay the chronic diseases associated with free radicals.

In addition to its activities as an antioxidant, vitamin E is involved in immune function and, as shown primarily by in vitro studies of cells, cell signaling, regulation of gene expression, and other metabolic processes. Alpha-tocopherol inhibits the activity of protein kinase C, an enzyme involved in cell proliferation and differentiation in smooth muscle cells, platelets, and monocytes. Vitamin-E–replete endothelial cells lining the interior surface of blood vessels are better able to resist blood-cell components adhering to this surface. Vitamin E also increases the expression of two enzymes that suppress arachidonic acid metabolism, thereby increasing the release of prostacyclin from the endothelium, which, in turn, dilates blood vessels and inhibits platelet aggregation.

Vitamin E and Health

Many claims have been made about vitamin E's potential to promote health and prevent and treat disease. The mechanisms by which vitamin E might provide this protection include its function as an antioxidant and its roles in anti-inflammatory processes, inhibition of platelet aggregation, and immune enhancement.

A primary barrier to characterizing the roles of vitamin E in health is the lack of validated biomarkers for vitamin E intake and status to help relate intakes to valid predictors of clinical outcomes. This section focuses on four diseases and disorders in which vitamin E might be involved: heart disease, cancer, eye disorders, and cognitive decline.

Coronary Heart Disease

Evidence that vitamin E could help prevent or delay coronary heart disease (CHD) comes from several sources. In vitro studies have found that the nutrient inhibits oxidation of low-density lipoprotein (LDL) cholesterol, thought to be a crucial initiating step for atherosclerosis. Vitamin E might also help prevent the formation of blood clots that could lead to a heart attack or venous thromboembolism.

Several observational studies have associated lower rates of heart disease with higher vitamin E intakes. One study of approximately

90,000 nurses found that the incidence of heart disease was 30% to 40% lower in those with the highest intakes of vitamin E, primarily from supplements. Among a group of 5,133 Finnish men and women followed for a mean of 14 years, higher vitamin E intakes from food were associated with decreased mortality from CHD.

However, randomized clinical trials cast doubt on the efficacy of vitamin E supplements to prevent CHD. For example, the Heart Outcomes Prevention Evaluation (HOPE) study, which followed almost 10,000 patients at high risk of heart attack or stroke for 4.5 years, found that participants taking 400 IU/day of natural vitamin E experienced no fewer cardiovascular events or hospitalizations for heart failure or chest pain than participants taking a placebo. In the HOPE-TOO followup study, almost 4,000 of the original participants continued to take vitamin E or placebo for an additional 2.5 years. HOPE-TOO found that vitamin E provided no significant protection against heart attacks, strokes, unstable angina, or deaths from cardiovascular disease or other causes after 7 years of treatment. Participants taking vitamin E, however, were 13% more likely to experience, and 21% more likely to be hospitalized for, heart failure, a statistically significant but unexpected finding not reported in other large studies.

The HOPE and HOPE-TOO trials provide compelling evidence that moderately high doses of vitamin E supplements do not reduce the risk of serious cardiovascular events among men and women >50 years of age with established heart disease or diabetes. These findings are supported by evidence from the Women's Angiographic Vitamin and Estrogen study, in which 423 postmenopausal women with some degree of coronary stenosis took supplements with 400 IU vitamin E (type not specified) and 500 mg vitamin C twice a day or placebo for >4 years. Not only did the supplements provide no cardiovascular benefits, but all-cause mortality was significantly higher in the women taking the supplements.

The latest published clinical trial of vitamin E's effects on the heart and blood vessels of women included almost 40,000 healthy women greater than or equal to 45 years of age who were randomly assigned to receive either 600 IU of natural vitamin E on alternate days or placebo and who were followed for an average of 10 years. The investigators found no significant differences in rates of overall cardiovascular events (combined nonfatal heart attacks, strokes, and cardiovascular deaths) or all-cause mortality between the groups. However, the study did find two positive and significant results for women taking vitamin E: they had a 24% reduction in cardiovascular death rates, and those greater than or equal to 65 years of age had a 26% decrease in nonfatal heart attack and a 49% decrease in cardiovascular death rates.

The most recent published clinical trial of vitamin E and men's cardiovascular health included almost 15,000 healthy physicians greater than or equal to 50 years of age who were randomly assigned to receive 400 IU synthetic alpha-tocopherol every other day, 500 mg vitamin C daily, both vitamins, or placebo. During a mean followup period of 8 years, intake of vitamin E (and/or vitamin C) had no effect on the incidence of major cardiovascular events, myocardial infarction, stroke, or cardiovascular morality. Furthermore, use of vitamin E was associated with a significantly increased risk of hemorrhagic stroke.

In general, clinical trials have not provided evidence that routine use of vitamin E supplements prevents cardiovascular disease or reduces its morbidity and mortality. However, participants in these studies have been largely middle-aged or elderly individuals with demonstrated heart disease or risk factors for heart disease. Some researchers have suggested that understanding the potential utility of vitamin E in preventing CHD might require longer studies in younger participants taking higher doses of the supplement. Further research is needed to determine whether supplemental vitamin E has any protective value for younger, healthier people at no obvious risk of CHD.

Cancer

Antioxidant nutrients like vitamin E protect cell constituents from the damaging effects of free radicals that, if unchecked, might contribute to cancer development. Vitamin E might also block the formation of carcinogenic nitrosamines formed in the stomach from nitrites in foods and protect against cancer by enhancing immune function. Human trials and surveys that attempted to associate vitamin E intake with cancer incidence have generally been inconclusive.

Some research links higher intakes of vitamin E with a decreased incidence of breast and prostate cancers, but the evidence is inconsistent. For example, an examination of the impact of dietary factors, including vitamin E, on the incidence of postmenopausal breast cancer in >18,000 women found no benefit from the vitamin. Similarly, a prospective cohort study of >29,000 men found no association between dietary or supplemental vitamin E intake and prostate cancer risk, with one exception: among current smokers and men who had quit, vitamin E intakes of more than 400 IU/day were associated with a statistically significant 71% reduction in the risk of advanced prostate cancer. A large randomized clinical trial began in 2001 to determine whether 7–12 years of daily supplementation with synthetic vitamin E (400 IU), with or without selenium (200 mcg), reduces the number of new prostate cancers in healthy men. The trial was discontinued in October 2008 when an analysis found that the supplements, taken alone or together for an average of 5 years, did not prevent prostate cancer. Study staff members will continue to monitor participants' health for an additional 3 years.

One study of women in Iowa provides evidence that higher intakes of vitamin E from foods and supplements could decrease the risk of colon cancer, especially in women <65 years of age. The overall relative risk for the highest quintile of intake (>35.7 IU/day) compared to the lowest quintile (<5.7 IU/day) was 0.32. However, prospective cohort studies of 87,998 women in the Nurses' Health Study and 47,344 men in the Health Professionals Follow-up Study failed to replicate these results.

The American Cancer Society conducted an epidemiologic study examining the association between use of vitamin C and vitamin E supplements and bladder cancer mortality. Of the almost one million adults followed between 1982 and 1998, adults who took supplemental vitamin E for 10 years or longer had a reduced risk of death from bladder cancer; vitamin C supplementation provided no protection.

Both the recently published HOPE-TOO Trial and Women's Health Study evaluated whether vitamin E supplements might protect people from cancer. HOPE-TOO, which followed men and women greater than or equal to 55 years of age with heart disease or diabetes for 7 years, found no significant differences in the number of new cancers or cancer deaths between the groups taking 400 IU/day vitamin E or a placebo. In the Women's Health Study, in which healthy women greater than or equal to 45 years of age received either 600 IU vitamin E every other day or a placebo for 10 years, the supplement did not reduce the risk of developing any form of cancer.

The inconsistent and limited evidence precludes any recommendations about using vitamin E supplements to prevent cancer.

Eye Disorders

Age-related macular degeneration (AMD) and cataracts are among the most common causes of significant vision loss in older people. Their etiologies are usually unknown, but the cumulative effects of oxidative stress have been postulated to play a role. If so, nutrients with antioxidant functions, such as vitamin E, could be used to prevent or treat these conditions.

Prospective cohort studies have found that people with relatively high dietary intakes of vitamin E (e.g., 30 IU/day) have an approximately 20% lower risk of developing AMD than people with low intakes (e.g., <15 IU/day). However, two randomized controlled trials in which participants took supplements of vitamin E (500 IU/day d-alpha-tocopherol in one study and 111 IU/day dl-alpha-tocopheryl acetate combined with 20 mg/day beta-carotene in the other) or a placebo failed to show a protective effect for vitamin E on AMD. The Age-Related Eye Disease Study (AREDS), a large randomized clinical trial, revealed that participants with early-stage AMD could slow the progression of their disease by taking a daily supplement of vitamin E (400 IU dl-alpha-tocopheryl acetate), vitamin C (500 mg), beta-carotene (15 mg), zinc (80 mg), and copper (2 mg) for an average of 6.3 years compared to participants taking a placebo.

Several observational studies have revealed a potential relationship between vitamin E supplements and the risk of cataract formation. One prospective cohort study found that lens clarity was superior in participants who took vitamin E supplements and those with higher blood levels of the vitamin. In another study, long-term use of vitamin E supplements was associated with slower progression of age-related lens opacification. However, in the randomized AREDS study, the use of the vitamin E-containing supplement package had no apparent effect on the development or progression of cataracts over 7 years.

Overall, the available evidence is inconsistent with respect to whether vitamin E supplements, taken alone or in combination with other antioxidants, can reduce the risk of developing AMD or cataracts. However, the formulation of vitamin E, other antioxidants, zinc, and copper used in AREDS holds promise for slowing the progression of AMD in people with early-stage disease. AREDS 2, a followup study, will determine whether a modified combination of dietary supplements can further slow the progression of vision loss from AMD.

Cognitive Decline

The brain has a high oxygen consumption rate and abundant poly-unsaturated fatty acids in the neuronal cell membranes. Researchers hypothesize that if cumulative free-radical damage to neurons over time contributes to cognitive decline and neurodegenerative diseases, such as Alzheimer disease, then ingestion of sufficient or supplemental antioxidants (such as vitamin E) might provide some protection. This hypothesis was supported by the results of a clinical trial in 341 patients with Alzheimer disease of moderate severity who were randomly assigned to receive a placebo, vitamin E (2,000 IU/day dl-alpha-tocopherol), a monoamine oxidase inhibitor (selegiline), or vitamin E and selegiline. Over 2 years, treatment with vitamin E and selegiline, separately or together, significantly delayed functional deterioration and the need for institutionalization compared to placebo. However, participants taking vitamin E experienced significantly more falls.

Vitamin E consumption from foods or supplements was associated with less cognitive decline over 3 years in a prospective cohort study of elderly, free-living individuals aged 65–102 years. However, a clinical trial in primarily healthy older women who were randomly assigned to receive 600 IU d-alpha-tocopherol every other day or a placebo for less than or equal to 4 years found that the supplements provided no apparent cognitive benefits. Another trial in which 769 men and women with mild cognitive impairment were randomly assigned to receive 2,000 IU/day vitamin E (type not specified), a cholinesterase inhibitor (donepezil), or placebo found no significant differences in the progression rate of Alzheimer disease between the vitamin E and placebo groups.

In summary, most research results do not support the use of vitamin E supplements by healthy or mildly impaired individuals to maintain cognitive performance or slow its decline with normal aging. More research is needed to identify the role of vitamin E, if any, in the management of cognitive impairment.

Chapter 26

Folate (Folic Acid)

Folate: What is it?

Folate is a water-soluble B vitamin that occurs naturally in food. Folic acid is the synthetic form of folate that is found in supplements and added to fortified foods.

Folate gets its name from the Latin word "folium" for leaf. A key observation of researcher Lucy Wills nearly 70 years ago led to the identification of folate as the nutrient needed to prevent the anemia of pregnancy. Dr. Wills demonstrated that the anemia could be corrected by a yeast extract. Folate was identified as the corrective substance in yeast extract in the late 1930s, and was extracted from spinach leaves in 1941.

Folate helps produce and maintain new cells. This is especially important during periods of rapid cell division and growth such as infancy and pregnancy. Folate is needed to make DNA [deoxyribonucleic acid] and RNA [ribonucleic acid], the building blocks of cells. It also helps prevent changes to DNA that may lead to cancer. Both adults and children need folate to make normal red blood cells and prevent anemia. Folate is also essential for the metabolism of homocysteine, and helps maintain normal levels of this amino acid.

What foods provide folate?

Leafy green vegetables (like spinach and turnip greens), fruits (like citrus fruits and juices), and dried beans and peas are all natural sources of folate.

Excerpted from "Folate," by the Office of Dietary Supplements (ODS, ods.od.nih .gov), part of the National Institutes of Health, April 15, 2009.

161

In 1996, the Food and Drug Administration (FDA) published regulations requiring the addition of folic acid to enriched breads, cereals, flours, corn meals, pastas, rice, and other grain products. Since cereals and grains are widely consumed in the United States, these products have become a very important contributor of folic acid to the American diet.

What are the Dietary Reference Intakes for folate?

Recommendations for folate are given in the Dietary Reference Intakes (DRIs) developed by the Institute of Medicine of the National Academy of Sciences. Dietary Reference Intakes is the general term for a set of reference values used for planning and assessing nutrient intake for healthy people. Three important types of reference values included in the DRIs are Recommended Dietary Allowances (RDA), Adequate Intakes (AI), and Tolerable Upper Intake Levels (UL). The RDA recommends the average daily intake that is sufficient to meet the nutrient requirements of nearly all (97–98%) healthy individuals in each age and gender group. An AI is set when there is insufficient scientific data available to establish a RDA. AIs meet or exceed the amount needed to maintain a nutritional state of adequacy in nearly all members of a specific age and gender group. The UL, on the other hand, is the maximum daily intake unlikely to result in adverse health effects.

The RDAs for folate are expressed in a term called the Dietary Folate Equivalent. The Dietary Folate Equivalent (DFE) was developed to help account for the differences in absorption of naturally occurring dietary folate and the more bioavailable synthetic folic acid. Table 26.1 lists the RDAs for folate, expressed in micrograms (mcg) of DFE, for children and adults.

Table 26.1. Recommended Dietary Allowances for Folate for Children and Adults

Age (years)	Males and Females (mcg/day)	Pregnancy (mcg/day)	Lactation (mcg/day)
1–3	150	N/A	N/A
4–8	200	N/A	N/A
9–13	300	N/A	N/A
14–18	400	600	500
19+	400	600	500

Note: 1 DFE = 1 mcg food folate = 0.6 mcg folic acid from supplements and fortified foods.

The National Health and Nutrition Examination Survey (NHANES III 1988–94) and the Continuing Survey of Food Intakes by Individuals (1994–96 CSFII) indicated that most individuals surveyed did not consume adequate folate. However, the folic acid fortification program, which was initiated in 1998, has increased folic acid content of commonly eaten foods such as cereals and grains, and as a result most diets in the United States now provide recommended amounts of folate equivalents.

When can folate deficiency occur?

A deficiency of folate can occur when an increased need for folate is not matched by an increased intake, when dietary folate intake does not meet recommended needs, and when folate loss increases. Medications that interfere with the metabolism of folate may also increase the need for this vitamin and risk of deficiency.

Medical conditions that increase the need for folate or result in increased loss of folate include the following:

- Pregnancy and lactation (breastfeeding)

- Alcohol abuse

- Malabsorption

- Kidney dialysis

- Liver disease

- Certain anemias

Medications that interfere with folate utilization include the following:

- Anticonvulsant medications (such as Dilantin, phenytoin, and primidone)

- Metformin (sometimes prescribed to control blood sugar in type 2 diabetes)

- Sulfasalazine (used to control inflammation associated with Crohn disease and ulcerative colitis)

- Triamterene (a diuretic)

- Methotrexate (used for cancer and other diseases such as rheumatoid arthritis)

- Barbiturates (used as sedatives)

163

What are some current issues and controversies about folate?

Folic acid and cardiovascular disease: Cardiovascular disease involves any disorder of the heart and blood vessels that make up the cardiovascular system. Coronary heart disease occurs when blood vessels which supply the heart become clogged or blocked, increasing the risk of a heart attack. Vascular damage can also occur to blood vessels supplying the brain, and can result in a stroke.

Cardiovascular disease is the most common cause of death in industrialized countries such as the United States, and is on the rise in developing countries. The National Heart, Lung, and Blood Institute of the National Institutes of Health has identified many risk factors for cardiovascular disease, including an elevated LDL [low-density lipoprotein]-cholesterol level, high blood pressure, a low HDL [high-density lipoprotein]-cholesterol level, obesity, and diabetes. In recent years, researchers have identified another risk factor for cardiovascular disease, an elevated homocysteine level. Homocysteine is an amino acid normally found in blood, but elevated levels have been linked with coronary heart disease and stroke. Elevated homocysteine levels may impair endothelial vasomotor function, which determines how easily blood flows through blood vessels. High levels of homocysteine also may damage coronary arteries and make it easier for blood clotting cells called platelets to clump together and form a clot, which may lead to a heart attack.

A deficiency of folate, vitamin B_{12}, or vitamin B_6 may increase blood levels of homocysteine, and folate supplementation has been shown to decrease homocysteine levels and to improve endothelial function. At least one study has linked low dietary folate intake with an increased risk of coronary events. The folic acid fortification program in the United States has decreased the prevalence of low levels of folate and high levels of homocysteine in the blood in middle-aged and older adults. Daily consumption of folic-acid fortified breakfast cereal and the use of folic acid supplements has been shown to be an effective strategy for reducing homocysteine concentrations.

Evidence supports a role for supplemental folic acid for lowering homocysteine levels, however this does not mean that folic acid supplements will decrease the risk of cardiovascular disease. Clinical intervention trials are underway to determine whether supplementation with folic acid, vitamin B_{12}, and vitamin B_6 can lower risk of coronary heart disease. It is premature to recommend folic acid supplementation for the prevention of heart disease until results of ongoing randomized, controlled clinical trials positively link increased folic acid intake with decreased homocysteine levels and decreased risk of cardiovascular disease.

Folic acid and cancer: Some evidence associates low blood levels of folate with a greater risk of cancer. Folate is involved in the synthesis, repair, and function of DNA, our genetic map, and there is some evidence that a deficiency of folate can cause damage to DNA that may lead to cancer. Several studies have associated diets low in folate with increased risk of breast, pancreatic, and colon cancer.

Over 88,000 women enrolled in the Nurses' Health Study who were free of cancer in 1980 were followed from 1980 through 1994. Researchers found that women ages 55 to 69 years in this study who took multivitamins containing folic acid for more than 15 years had a markedly lower risk of developing colon cancer. Findings from over 14,000 subjects followed for 20 years suggest that men who do not consume alcohol and whose diets provide the recommended intake of folate are less likely to develop colon cancer. However, associations between diet and disease do not indicate a direct cause. Researchers are continuing to investigate whether enhanced folate intake from foods or folic acid supplements may reduce the risk of cancer. Until results from such clinical trials are available, folic acid supplements should not be recommended to reduce the risk of cancer.

Folic acid and methotrexate for cancer: Folate is important for cells and tissues that rapidly divide. Cancer cells divide rapidly, and drugs that interfere with folate metabolism are used to treat cancer. Methotrexate is a drug often used to treat cancer because it limits the activity of enzymes that need folate.

Unfortunately, methotrexate can be toxic, producing side effects such as inflammation in the digestive tract that may make it difficult to eat normally. Leucovorin is a form of folate that can help "rescue" or reverse the toxic effects of methotrexate. There are many studies underway to determine if folic acid supplements can help control the side effects of methotrexate without decreasing its effectiveness in chemotherapy. It is important for anyone receiving methotrexate to follow a medical doctor's advice on the use of folic acid supplements.

Folic acid and methotrexate for non-cancerous diseases: Low dose methotrexate is used to treat a wide variety of non-cancerous diseases such as rheumatoid arthritis, lupus, psoriasis, asthma, sarcoidosis, primary biliary cirrhosis, and inflammatory bowel disease. Low doses of methotrexate can deplete folate stores and cause side effects that are similar to folate deficiency. Both high folate diets and supplemental folic acid may help reduce the toxic side effects of low dose methotrexate without decreasing its effectiveness. Anyone taking low dose methotrexate for the health problems listed should consult with a physician about the need for a folic acid supplement.

What cautions should I take with folic acid supplements?

Beware of the interaction between vitamin B_{12} and folic acid. Intake of supplemental folic acid should not exceed 1,000 micrograms (mcg) per day to prevent folic acid from triggering symptoms of vitamin B_{12} deficiency. Folic acid supplements can correct the anemia associated with vitamin B_{12} deficiency. Unfortunately, folic acid will not correct changes in the nervous system that result from vitamin B_{12} deficiency. Permanent nerve damage can occur if vitamin B_{12} deficiency is not treated.

It is very important for older adults to be aware of the relationship between folic acid and vitamin B_{12} because they are at greater risk of having a vitamin B_{12} deficiency. If you are 50 years of age or older, ask your physician to check your B_{12} status before you take a supplement that contains folic acid. If you are taking a supplement containing folic acid, read the label to make sure it also contains $B1_2$ or speak with a physician about the need for a B_{12} supplement.

What is the health risk of too much folic acid?

Folate intake from food is not associated with any health risk. The risk of toxicity from folic acid intake from supplements and/or fortified foods is also low. It is a water soluble vitamin, so any excess intake is usually lost in the urine. There is some evidence that high levels of folic acid can provoke seizures in patients taking anticonvulsant medications. Anyone taking such medications should consult with a medical doctor before taking a folic acid supplement.

The Institute of Medicine has established a tolerable upper intake level (UL) for folate from fortified foods or supplements (i.e., folic acid) for ages 1 and above. Intakes above this level increase the risk of adverse health effects. In adults, supplemental folic acid should not exceed the UL to prevent folic acid from triggering symptoms of vitamin B_{12} deficiency. It is important to recognize that the UL refers to the amount of synthetic folate (i.e., folic acid) being consumed per day from fortified foods and/or supplements. There is no health risk, and no UL, for natural sources of folate found in food.

As the 2000 Dietary Guidelines for Americans states, "Different foods contain different nutrients and other healthful substances. No single food can supply all the nutrients in the amounts you need." Green leafy vegetables, dried beans and peas, and many other types of vegetables and fruits provide folate. In addition, fortified foods are a major source of folic acid. It is not unusual to find foods such as some ready-to-eat cereals fortified with 100% of the RDA for folate. The variety of fortified foods available has made it easier for women of childbearing age in the

United States to consume the recommended 400 mcg of folic acid per day from fortified foods and/or supplements. The large numbers of fortified foods on the market, however, also raises the risk of exceeding the UL. This is especially important for anyone at risk of vitamin B_{12} deficiency, which can be triggered by too much folic acid. It is important for anyone who is considering taking a folic acid supplement to first consider whether their diet already includes adequate sources of dietary folate and fortified food sources of folic acid.

Chapter 27

Magnesium

Magnesium: What is it?

Magnesium is the fourth most abundant mineral in the body and is essential to good health. Approximately 50% of total body magnesium is found in bone. The other half is found predominantly inside cells of body tissues and organs. Only 1% of magnesium is found in blood, but the body works very hard to keep blood levels of magnesium constant.

Magnesium is needed for more than 300 biochemical reactions in the body. It helps maintain normal muscle and nerve function, keeps heart rhythm steady, supports a healthy immune system, and keeps bones strong. Magnesium also helps regulate blood sugar levels, promotes normal blood pressure, and is known to be involved in energy metabolism and protein synthesis. There is an increased interest in the role of magnesium in preventing and managing disorders such as hypertension, cardiovascular disease, and diabetes. Dietary magnesium is absorbed in the small intestines. Magnesium is excreted through the kidneys.

What are some current issues and controversies about magnesium?

Magnesium and blood pressure: "Epidemiologic evidence suggests that magnesium may play an important role in regulating blood pressure." Diets that provide plenty of fruits and vegetables, which are

Excerpted from text by the Office of Dietary Supplements (ODS, ods.od.nih .gov), part of the National Institutes of Health, July 13, 2009.

good sources of potassium and magnesium, are consistently associated with lower blood pressure. The DASH study (Dietary Approaches to Stop Hypertension), a human clinical trial, suggested that high blood pressure could be significantly lowered by a diet that emphasizes fruits, vegetables, and low-fat dairy foods. Such a diet will be high in magnesium, potassium, and calcium, and low in sodium and fat.

An observational study examined the effect of various nutritional factors on incidence of high blood pressure in over 30,000 U.S. male health professionals. After 4 years of follow-up, it was found that a lower risk of hypertension was associated with dietary patterns that provided more magnesium, potassium, and dietary fiber. For 6 years, the Atherosclerosis Risk in Communities (ARIC) Study followed approximately 8,000 men and women who were initially free of hypertension. In this study, the risk of developing hypertension decreased as dietary magnesium intake increased in women, but not in men.

Foods high in magnesium are frequently high in potassium and dietary fiber. This makes it difficult to evaluate the independent effect of magnesium on blood pressure. However, newer scientific evidence from DASH clinical trials is strong enough that the Joint National Committee on Prevention, Detection, Evaluation, and Treatment of High Blood Pressure states that diets that provide plenty of magnesium are positive lifestyle modifications for individuals with hypertension. This group recommends the DASH diet as a beneficial eating plan for people with hypertension and for those with "prehypertension" who desire to prevent high blood pressure http://www.nhlbi.nih.gov/health/public/heart/hbp/dash.

Magnesium and diabetes: Diabetes is a disease resulting in insufficient production and/or inefficient use of insulin. Insulin is a hormone made by the pancreas. Insulin helps convert sugar and starches in food into energy to sustain life. There are two types of diabetes: type 1 and type 2. Type 1 diabetes is most often diagnosed in children and adolescents, and results from the body's inability to make insulin. Type 2 diabetes, which is sometimes referred to as adult-onset diabetes, is the most common form of diabetes. It is usually seen in adults and is most often associated with an inability to use the insulin made by the pancreas. Obesity is a risk factor for developing type 2 diabetes. In recent years, rates of type 2 diabetes have increased along with the rising rates of obesity.

Magnesium plays an important role in carbohydrate metabolism. It may influence the release and activity of insulin, the hormone that helps control blood glucose (sugar) levels. Low blood levels of magnesium (hypomagnesemia) are frequently seen in individuals with type 2 diabetes. Hypomagnesemia may worsen insulin resistance, a condition that often precedes diabetes, or may be a consequence of insulin resistance. Individuals with insulin resistance do not use insulin efficiently and require greater amounts of insulin to maintain blood sugar within normal levels. The kidneys possibly lose their ability to retain magnesium during periods of severe hyperglycemia (significantly elevated blood glucose). The increased loss of magnesium in urine may then result in lower blood levels of magnesium. In older adults, correcting magnesium depletion may improve insulin response and action.

The Nurses' Health Study (NHS) and the Health Professionals' Follow-up Study (HFS) follow more than 170,000 health professionals through questionnaires the participants complete every 2 years. Diet was first evaluated in 1980 in the NHS and in 1986 in the HFS, and dietary assessments have been completed every 2 to 4 years since. Information on the use of dietary supplements, including multivitamins, is also collected. As part of these studies, over 127,000 participants (85,060 women and 42,872 men) with no history of diabetes, cardiovascular disease, or cancer at baseline were followed to examine risk factors for developing type 2 diabetes. Women were followed for 18 years; men were followed for 12 years. Over time, the risk for developing type 2 diabetes was greater in men and women with a lower magnesium intake. This study supports the dietary recommendation to increase consumption of major food sources of magnesium, such as whole grains, nuts, and green leafy vegetables.

The Iowa Women's Health Study has followed a group of older women since 1986. Researchers from this study examined the association between women's risk of developing type 2 diabetes and intake of carbohydrates, dietary fiber, and dietary magnesium. Dietary intake was estimated by a food frequency questionnaire, and incidence of diabetes throughout 6 years of follow-up was determined by asking participants if they had been diagnosed by a doctor as having diabetes. Based on baseline dietary intake assessment only, researchers' findings suggested that a greater intake of whole grains, dietary fiber, and magnesium decreased the risk of developing diabetes in older women.

The Women's Health Study was originally designed to evaluate the benefits versus risks of low-dose aspirin and vitamin E supplementation in the primary prevention of cardiovascular disease and cancer in women 45 years of age and older. In an examination of almost 40,000 women participating in this study, researchers also examined the association between magnesium intake and incidence of type 2 diabetes over an average of 6 years. Among women who were overweight, the risk of developing type 2 diabetes was significantly greater among those with lower magnesium intake. This study also supports the dietary recommendation to increase consumption of major food sources of magnesium, such as whole grains, nuts, and green leafy vegetables.

On the other hand, the Atherosclerosis Risk in Communities (ARIC) study did not find any association between dietary magnesium intake and the risk for type 2 diabetes. During 6 years of follow-up, ARIC researchers examined the risk for type 2 diabetes in over 12,000 middle-aged adults without diabetes at baseline examination. In this study, there was no association between dietary magnesium intake and incidence of type 2 diabetes in either black or white participants. It can be confusing to read about studies that examine the same issue but have different results. Before reaching a conclusion on a health issue, scientists conduct and evaluate many studies. Over time, they determine when results are consistent enough to suggest a conclusion. They want to be sure they are providing correct recommendations to the public.

Several clinical studies have examined the potential benefit of supplemental magnesium on control of type 2 diabetes. In one such study, 63 subjects with below normal serum magnesium levels received either 2.5 grams of oral magnesium chloride daily "in liquid form" (providing 300 mg elemental magnesium per day) or a placebo. At the end of the 16-week study period, those who received the magnesium supplement had higher blood levels of magnesium and improved control of diabetes, as suggested by lower hemoglobin A1C levels, than those who received a placebo. Hemoglobin A1C is a test that measures overall control of blood glucose over the previous 2 to 3 months, and is considered by many doctors to be the single most important blood test for diabetics.

In another study, 128 patients with poorly controlled type 2 diabetes were randomized to receive a placebo or a supplement with either 500 mg or 1000 mg of magnesium oxide (MgO) for 30 days. All patients were also treated with diet or diet plus oral medication to control blood glucose levels. Magnesium levels increased in the group receiving 1000 mg magnesium oxide per day (equal to 600 mg elemental magnesium per day) but did not significantly change in the placebo group or the group receiving 500 mg of magnesium oxide per day (equal to 300 mg elemental magnesium per day). However, neither level of magnesium supplementation significantly improved blood glucose control.

These studies provide intriguing results but also suggest that additional research is needed to better explain the association between blood magnesium levels, dietary magnesium intake, and type 2 diabetes. In 1999, the American Diabetes Association (ADA) issued nutrition recommendations for diabetics stating that "routine evaluation of blood magnesium level is recommended only in patients at high risk for magnesium deficiency. Levels of magnesium should be [replaced] only if hypomagnesemia can be demonstrated."

Magnesium and cardiovascular disease: Magnesium metabolism is very important to insulin sensitivity and blood pressure regulation, and magnesium deficiency is common in individuals with diabetes. The observed associations between magnesium metabolism, diabetes, and high blood pressure increase the likelihood that magnesium metabolism may influence cardiovascular disease.

Some observational surveys have associated higher blood levels of magnesium with lower risk of coronary heart disease. In addition, some dietary surveys have suggested that a higher magnesium intake may reduce the risk of having a stroke. There is also evidence that low body stores of magnesium increase the risk of abnormal heart rhythms, which may increase the risk of complications after a heart attack. These studies suggest that consuming recommended amounts of magnesium may be beneficial to the cardiovascular system. They have also prompted interest in clinical trials to determine the effect of magnesium supplements on cardiovascular disease.

Several small studies suggest that magnesium supplementation may improve clinical outcomes in individuals with coronary disease. In one of these studies, the effect of magnesium supplementation on exercise tolerance (the ability to walk on a treadmill or ride a bicycle), chest pain caused by exercise, and quality of life was examined in 187 patients. Patients received either a placebo or a supplement providing 365 milligrams of magnesium citrate twice daily for 6 months. At the end of the study period researchers found that magnesium therapy significantly increased magnesium levels. Patients receiving magnesium had a 14 percent improvement in exercise duration as compared to no change in the placebo group. Those receiving magnesium were also less likely to experience chest pain caused by exercise.

In another study, 50 men and women with stable coronary disease were randomized to receive either a placebo or a magnesium supplement that provided 342 mg magnesium oxide twice daily. After 6 months, those who received the oral magnesium supplement were found to have improved exercise tolerance.

In a third study, researchers examined whether magnesium supplementation would add to the anti-thrombotic (anti-clotting) effects of aspirin in 42 coronary patients. For 3 months, each patient received either a placebo or a supplement with 400 mg of magnesium oxide two to three times daily. After a 4-week break without any treatment,

treatment groups were reversed so that each person in the study then received the alternate treatment for 3 months. Researchers found that supplemental magnesium did provide an additional anti-thrombotic effect.

These studies are encouraging, but involved small numbers. Additional studies are needed to better understand the complex relationships between magnesium intake, indicators of magnesium status, and heart disease. Doctors can evaluate magnesium status when above-mentioned medical problems occur, and determine the need for magnesium supplementation.

Magnesium and osteoporosis: Bone health is supported by many factors, most notably calcium and vitamin D. However, some evidence suggests that magnesium deficiency may be an additional risk factor for postmenopausal osteoporosis. This may be due to the fact that magnesium deficiency alters calcium metabolism and the hormones that regulate calcium. Several human studies have suggested that magnesium supplementation may improve bone mineral density. In a study of older adults, a greater magnesium intake maintained bone mineral density to a greater degree than a lower magnesium intake. Diets that provide recommended levels of magnesium are beneficial for bone health, but further investigation on the role of magnesium in bone metabolism and osteoporosis is needed.

Chapter 28

Omega-3 Fatty Acid Supplements

Chapter Contents

Section 28.1—Fish Oils 176

Section 28.2—Flaxseed and Flaxseed Oils 190

Section 28.1

Fish Oils

Background

Dietary sources of omega-3 fatty acids include fish oil and certain plant/nut oils. Fish oil contains both docosahexaenoic acid (DHA) and eicosapentaenoic acid (EPA), while some nuts (English walnuts) and vegetable oils (canola, soybean, flaxseed/linseed, olive) contain alpha-linolenic acid (ALA).

There is evidence from multiple studies supporting intake of recommended amounts of DHA and EPA in the form of dietary fish or fish oil supplements lowers triglycerides, reduces the risk of death, heart attack, dangerous abnormal heart rhythms, and strokes in people with known cardiovascular disease, slows the buildup of atherosclerotic plaques ("hardening of the arteries"), and lowers blood pressure slightly. However, high doses may have harmful effects, such as an increased risk of bleeding. Although similar benefits are proposed for alpha-linolenic acid, scientific evidence is less compelling, and beneficial effects may be less pronounced.

Some species of fish carry a higher risk of environmental contamination, such as with methylmercury.

Synonyms

Alpha-linolenic acid (ALA, C18:3n-3), cod liver oil, coldwater fish, docosahexaenoic acid (DHA, C22:6n-3), eicosapentaenoic acid (EPA, C20:5n-3), fish oil fatty acids, fish body oil, fish extract, fish liver oil, halibut oil, long chain polyunsaturated fatty acids, mackerel oil, marine oil, menhaden oil, n-3 fatty acids, n-3 polyunsaturated fatty acids, omega fatty acids, omega-3 oils, polyunsaturated fatty acids (PUFA), salmon oil, shark liver oil, w-3 fatty acids.

Note: Should not be confused with omega-6 fatty acids.

Evidence

These uses have been tested in humans or animals. Safety and effectiveness have not always been proven. Some of these conditions are potentially serious, and should be evaluated by a qualified healthcare provider. Key to grades—A (Strong scientific evidence for this use); B (Good scientific evidence for this use); C (Unclear scientific evidence for this use); D (Fair scientific evidence against this use); F (Strong scientific evidence against this use).

Uses Based on Scientific Evidence

High Blood Pressure

Multiple human trials report small reductions in blood pressure with intake of omega-3 fatty acid. DHA may have greater benefits than EPA. However, high intakes of omega-3 fatty acids per day may be necessary to obtain clinically relevant effects, and at this dose level, there is an increased risk of bleeding. Therefore, a qualified healthcare provider should be consulted prior to starting treatment with supplements. Grade: A.

Hypertriglyceridemia (Fish Oil/EPA plus DHA)

There is strong scientific evidence from human trials that omega-3 fatty acids from fish or fish oil supplements (EPA + DHA) significantly reduce blood triglyceride levels. Benefits appear to be dose-dependent. Fish oil supplements also appear to cause small improvements in high-density lipoprotein ("good cholesterol"); however, increases (worsening) in low-density lipoprotein levels (LDL/"bad cholesterol") are also observed. It is not clear if alpha-linolenic acid significantly affects triglyceride levels, and there is conflicting evidence in this area. The American Heart Association has published recommendations for EPA + DHA. Because of the risk of bleeding from omega-3 fatty acids, a qualified healthcare provider should be consulted prior to starting treatment with supplements. There is growing evidence that reducing C-reactive protein (CRP) is beneficial toward favorable cardiovascular outcomes, although additional research is pending in this area. The data on fish oils and CRP levels is mixed. Grade: A.

Secondary Cardiovascular Disease Prevention (Fish Oil/ EPA plus DHA)

Several well-conducted randomized controlled trials report that in people with a history of heart attack, regular consumption of oily fish or fish oil/omega-3 supplements reduces the risk of non-fatal heart attack, fatal heart attack, sudden death, and all-cause mortality (death due to any cause). Most patients in these studies were also using conventional heart drugs, suggesting that the benefits of fish oils may add to the effects of other therapies. Grade: A.

Primary Cardiovascular Disease Prevention (Fish Intake)

Several large studies of populations ("epidemiologic" studies) report a significantly lower rate of death from heart disease in men and women who regularly eat fish. Other epidemiologic research reports no such benefits. It is not clear if reported benefits only occur in certain groups of people, such as those at risk of developing heart disease. Overall, the evidence suggests benefits of regular consumption of fish oil. However, well-designed randomized controlled trials which classify people by their risk of developing heart disease are necessary before a firm conclusion can be drawn. Grade: B.

Protection from Cyclosporine Toxicity in Organ Transplant Patients

There are multiple studies of heart transplant and kidney transplant patients taking cyclosporine (Neoral®), who were administered fish oil supplements. The majority of trials report improvements in kidney function, and less high blood pressure compared to patients not taking fish oil. Although several recent studies report no benefits on kidney function, the weight of scientific evidence favors the beneficial effects of fish oil. Grade: B.

Rheumatoid Arthritis (Fish Oil)

Multiple randomized controlled trials report improvements in morning stiffness and joint tenderness with the regular intake of fish oil supplements for up to 3 months. Benefits have been reported as additive with anti-inflammatory medications such as NSAIDs (like ibuprofen or aspirin). However, because of weaknesses in study designs and reporting, better research is necessary before a strong favorable recommendation can be made. Effects beyond three months of treatment have not been well evaluated. Grade: B.

Angina Pectoris

Preliminary studies report reductions in angina associated with fish oil intake. Better research is necessary before a firm conclusion can be drawn. Grade: C.

Asthma

Several studies in this area do not provide enough reliable evidence to form a clear conclusion, with some studies reporting no effects, and others finding benefits. Because most studies have been small without clear descriptions of design or results, the results cannot be considered conclusive. Grade: C.

Atherosclerosis

Some research reports that regular intake of fish or fish oil supplements reduces the risk of developing atherosclerotic plaques in the arteries of the heart, while other research reports no effects. Additional evidence is necessary before a firm conclusion can be drawn in this area. Grade: C.

Bipolar Disorder

Several studies in this area do not provide enough reliable evidence to form a clear conclusion. Grade: C.

Cancer Prevention

Several population (epidemiologic) studies report that dietary omega-3 fatty acids or fish oil may reduce the risk of developing breast, colon, or prostate cancer. Randomized controlled trials are necessary before a clear conclusion can be drawn. Grade: C.

Cardiac Arrhythmias (Abnormal Heart Rhythms)

There is promising evidence that omega-3 fatty acids may decrease the risk of cardiac arrhythmias. This is one proposed mechanism behind the reduced number of heart attacks in people who regularly ingest fish oil or EPA + DHA. Additional research is needed in this area specifically before a firm conclusion can be reached. Grade: C.

Colon Cancer

Omega-3 fatty acids are commonly taken by cancer patients. Although preliminary studies report that growth of colon cancer cells may be reduced by taking fish oil, effects on survival or remission have not been measured adequately. Grade: C.

Crohn's Disease

It has been suggested that effects of omega-3 fatty acids on inflammation may be beneficial in patients with Crohn's disease when added to standard therapy, and several studies have been conducted in this area. Results are conflicting, and no clear conclusion can be drawn at this time. Grade: C.

Cystic Fibrosis

A small amount of research in this area does not provide enough reliable evidence to form a clear conclusion. Grade: C.

Dementia

Well-designed clinical trials are needed before omega-3 fatty acids can be recommended for the prevention of cognitive impairment or dementia. Grade: C.

Depression

Several studies on the use of omega 3 fatty acids in depression, including positive results in postpartum depression, do not provide enough reliable evidence to form a clear conclusion or replace standard treatments. However, based on one recent study, omega-3 fatty acids may have therapeutic benefits in childhood depression. Promising initial evidence requires confirmation with larger, well-designed trials. Grade: C.

Dysmenorrhea (Painful Menstruation)

There is preliminary evidence suggesting possible benefits of fish oil/omega-3 fatty acids in patients with dysmenorrhea. Additional research is necessary before a firm conclusion can be reached. Grade: C.

Eczema

Several studies of EPA for eczema do not provide enough reliable evidence to form a clear conclusion. Grade: C.

IgA Nephropathy

There are conflicting results from several trials in this area. Grade: C.

Infant Eye/Brain Development

Well-designed research is necessary before a clear conclusion can be reached. Grade: C.

Lupus Erythematosus

There is not enough reliable evidence to form a clear conclusion in this area. Grade: C.

Nephrotic Syndrome

There is not enough reliable evidence to form a clear conclusion in this area. Grade: C.

Preeclampsia

Several studies of fish oil do not provide enough reliable evidence to form a clear conclusion in this area. Grade: C.

Prevention of Graft Failure after Heart Bypass Surgery

There is limited study of the use of fish oils in patients after undergoing coronary artery bypass grafting (CABG). Additional evidence is necessary before a firm conclusion can be drawn in this area. Grade: C.

Prevention of Restenosis after Coronary Angioplasty (PTCA)

Several randomized controlled trials have evaluated whether omega-3 fatty acid intake reduces blockage of arteries in the heart following balloon angioplasty (percutaneous transluminal coronary angioplasty/PTCA). The evidence in this area remains inconclusive. Grade: C.

Primary Cardiovascular Disease Prevention (Alpha-Linolenic Acid [ALA])

Additional research is necessary before a conclusion can be drawn in this area. Grade: C.

Psoriasis

Several studies in this area do not provide enough reliable evidence to form a clear conclusion. Grade: C.

Schizophrenia

There is promising preliminary evidence from several randomized controlled trials in this area. Additional research is necessary before a firm conclusion can be reached. Grade: C.

Secondary Cardiovascular Disease Prevention (Alpha-Linolenic Acid [ALA])

Several randomized controlled trials have examined the effects of alpha-linolenic acid in people with a history of heart attack. Although some studies suggest benefits, others do not. Additional research is necessary before a conclusion can be drawn in this area. Grade: C.

Stroke Prevention

Several large studies of populations ("epidemiologic" studies) have examined the effects of omega-3 fatty acid intake on stroke risk. Some studies suggest benefits, while others do not. Effects are likely on ischemic or thrombotic stroke risk, and very large intakes of omega-3 fatty acids ("Eskimo" amounts) may actually increase the risk of hemorrhagic (bleeding) stroke. At this time, it is unclear if there are benefits in people with or without a history of stroke, or if effects of fish oil are comparable to other treatment strategies. Grade: C.

Ulcerative Colitis

It has been suggested that effects of omega-3 fatty acids on inflammation may be beneficial in patients with ulcerative colitis when added to standard therapy, and several studies have been conducted in this area. Better research is necessary before a clear conclusion can be drawn. Grade: C.

Appetite/Weight Loss in Cancer Patients

There is preliminary evidence that fish oil supplementation does not improve appetite or prevent weight loss in cancer patients. Further study is warranted. Grade: D.

Diabetes

The available scientific evidence suggests that there are no significant long-term effects of fish oil in patients with diabetes. Most studies in this area are not well designed. Grade: D.

Hypercholesterolemia

Although fish oil is able to reduce triglycerides, beneficial effects on blood cholesterol levels have not been demonstrated. Fish oil supplements appear to cause small improvements in high-density lipoprotein ("good cholesterol"); however, increases (worsening) in low-density lipoprotein levels ("bad cholesterol") are also observed. Fish oil does not appear to affect C-reactive protein (CRP) levels. Grade: D.

Transplant Rejection Prevention (Kidney and Heart)

There are multiple studies of heart transplant and kidney transplant patients taking cyclosporine (Neoral®), who were administered fish oil supplements. The majority of trials report improvements in kidney function (glomerular filtration rate, serum creatinine), and less hypertension (high blood pressure) compared to patients not taking fish oil. However, several recent studies report no benefits on kidney function, and no changes have been found in rates of rejection or graft survival. Grade D.

Uses Based on Tradition or Theory

The below uses are based on tradition or scientific theories. They often have not been thoroughly tested in humans, and safety and effectiveness have not always been proven. Some of these conditions are potentially serious, and should be evaluated by a qualified healthcare provider: Acute myocardial infarction (heart attack), acute respiratory distress syndrome (ARDS), age related macular degeneration, aggressive behavior, agoraphobia, AIDS [acquired immunodeficiency syndrome], allergies, Alzheimer's disease, anticoagulation, antiphospholipid syndrome, attention deficit hyperactivity disorder (ADHD), anthracycline-induced cardiac toxicity, bacterial infections, psychological disorders (borderline personality disorder), breast cysts, breast tenderness, chronic fatigue syndrome (postviral fatigue syndrome), chronic obstructive pulmonary disease, cirrhosis, common cold, congestive heart failure, critical illness, deficiency (omega-3 fatty acid), dermatomyositis, diabetic nephropathy, diabetic neuropathy, dyslexia, dyspraxia, endocrine disorders (glycogen storage diseases), exercise performance enhancement, fibromyalgia, gallstones, gingivitis, glaucoma, glomerulonephritis, gout, hay fever, headache, hepatorenal syndrome, hypoxia, ichthyosis (skin disorder), immunosuppression, inflammatory conditions (Behçet's syndrome), joint problems (cartilage repair), kidney disease prevention, kidney stones, leprosy, leukemia, malaria, male infertility, mastalgia (breast pain), memory enhancement, menopausal symptoms, menstrual cramps, methotrexate toxicity, multiple sclerosis, myopathy, nephritis (autoimmune), neuropathy, night vision enhancement, obesity, osteoarthritis, osteoporosis, otitis media (ear infection), panic disorder, peripheral vascular disease, pregnancy nutritional supplement, premature birth prevention, premenstrual syndrome, prostate cancer prevention, protection from isotretinoin drug toxicity, Raynaud's phenomenon, Refsum's syndrome, retinitis pigmentosa, Reye's syndrome, seizure disorder, Sjögren's syndrome, suicide prevention, systemic lupus erythematosus, tardive dyskinesia, tennis elbow, ulcerative colitis, urolithiasis (bladder stones), vision enhancement, weight loss.

Dosing

The below doses are based on scientific research, publications, traditional use, or expert opinion. Many herbs and supplements have not been thoroughly tested, and safety and effectiveness may not be proven. Brands may be made differently, with variable ingredients, even within the same brand. The below doses may not apply to all products. You should read product labels, and discuss doses with a qualified healthcare provider before starting therapy.

Adults (18 years and older): Average dietary intake of omega-3/omega-6 fatty acids—Average Americans consume approximately 1.6 grams of omega-3 fatty acids each day, of which about 1.4 grams (~90%) comes from alpha-linolenic acid, and only 0.1–0.2 grams (~10%) from EPA and DHA. In Western diets, people consume roughly 10 times more omega-6 fatty acids than omega-3 fatty acids. These large amounts of omega-6 fatty acids come from the common use of vegetable oils containing linoleic acid (for example: corn oil, evening primrose oil, pumpkin oil, safflower oil, sesame oil, soybean oil, sunflower oil, walnut oil, wheat germ oil). Because omega-6 and omega-3 fatty acids compete with each other to be converted to active metabolites in the body, benefits can be reached either by decreasing intake of omega-6 fatty acids, or by increasing omega-3 fatty acids.

Recommended daily intake of omega-3 fatty acids (healthy adults)—For healthy adults with no history of heart disease, the American Heart Association recommends eating fish at least two times per week. In particular, fatty fish are recommended, such as anchovies, bluefish, carp, catfish, halibut, herring, lake trout, mackerel, pompano, salmon, striped sea bass, tuna (albacore), and whitefish. It is also recommended to consume plant-derived sources of alpha-linolenic acid, such as tofu/soybeans, walnuts, flaxseed oil, and canola oil. The World Health Organization and governmental health agencies of several countries recommend consuming 0.3–0.5 grams of daily EPA + DHA and 0.8–1.1 grams of daily alpha-linolenic acid. A doctor and pharmacist should be consulted for dosing for other conditions.

Children (younger than 18 years): Omega-3 fatty acids are used in some infant formulas, although effective doses are not clearly established. Ingestion of fresh fish should be limited in young children due to the presence of potentially harmful environmental contaminants. Fish oil capsules should not be used in children except under the direction of a physician.

Safety

The U.S. Food and Drug Administration does not strictly regulate herbs and supplements. There is no guarantee of strength, purity or safety of products, and effects may vary. You should always read product labels. If you have a medical condition, or are taking other drugs, herbs, or supplements, you should speak with a qualified healthcare provider before starting a new therapy. Consult a healthcare provider immediately if you experience side effects.

Allergies

People with allergy or hypersensitivity to fish should avoid fish oil or omega-3 fatty acid products derived from fish. Skin rash has been reported rarely. People with allergy or hypersensitivity to nuts should avoid alpha linolenic acid or omega-3 fatty acid products that are derived from the types of nuts to which they react.

Side Effects and Warnings

The U.S. Food and Drug Administration classifies intake of up to 3 grams per day of omega-3 fatty acids from fish as GRAS (Generally Regarded as Safe). Caution may be warranted, however, in diabetic patients due to potential (albeit unlikely) increases in blood sugar levels, patients at risk of bleeding, or in those with high levels of low-density lipoprotein (LDL). Fish meat may contain methylmercury and caution is warranted in young children and pregnant/breastfeeding women.

Omega-3 fatty acids may increase the risk of bleeding, although there is little evidence of significant bleeding risk at lower doses. Very large intakes of fish oil/omega-3 fatty acids ("Eskimo" amounts) may increase the risk of hemorrhagic (bleeding) stroke. High doses have also been associated with nosebleed and blood in the urine. Fish oils appear to decrease platelet aggregation and prolong bleeding time, increase fibrinolysis (breaking down of blood clots), and may reduce von Willebrand factor.

Potentially harmful contaminants such as dioxins, methylmercury, and polychlorinated biphenyls (PCBs) are found in some species of fish. Methylmercury accumulates in fish meat more than in fish oil, and fish oil supplements appear to contain almost no mercury. Therefore, safety concerns apply to eating fish but likely not to ingesting fish oil supplements. Heavy metals are most harmful in young children and pregnant/nursing women.

Gastrointestinal upset is common with the use of fish oil supplements. Diarrhea may also occur, with potentially severe diarrhea at very high doses. There are also reports of increased burping, acid reflux/heartburn/indigestion, abdominal bloating, and abdominal pain. Fishy aftertaste is a common effect. Gastrointestinal side effects can be minimized if fish oils are taken with meals and if doses are started low and gradually increased.

Multiple human trials report small reductions in blood pressure with intake of omega-3 fatty acids. Reductions of 2–5 mmHg have been observed, and effects appear to be dose-responsive (higher doses have greater effects). DHA may have greater effects than EPA. Caution is warranted in patients with low blood pressure or in those taking blood-pressure lowering medications.

Although slight increases in fasting blood glucose levels have been noted in patients with type 2 ("adult onset") diabetes, the available scientific evidence suggests that there are no significant long-term effects of fish oil in patients with diabetes, including no changes in hemoglobin A1C levels. Limited reports in the 1980s of increased insulin needs in diabetic patients taking long-term fish oils may be related to other dietary changes or weight gain.

Fish oil taken for many months may cause a deficiency of vitamin E, and therefore vitamin E is added to many commercial fish oil products. As a result, regular use of vitamin E-enriched products may lead to elevated levels of this fat-soluble vitamin. Fish liver oil contains the fat-soluble vitamins A and D, and therefore fish liver oil products (such as cod liver oil) may increase the risk of vitamin A or D toxicity.

Increases (worsening) in low-density lipoprotein levels ("bad cholesterol") by 5–10% are observed with intake of omega-3 fatty acids. Effects are dose-dependent.

Mild elevations in liver function tests (alanine aminotransferase) have been reported rarely.

Skin rashes have been reported rarely.

There are rare reports of mania in patients with bipolar disorder or major depression. Restlessness and formication (the sensation of ants crawling on the skin) have also been reported.

Pregnancy and Breastfeeding

Potentially harmful contaminants such as dioxins, methylmercury, and polychlorinated biphenyls (PCBs) are found in some species of fish, and may be harmful in pregnant/nursing women. Methylmercury accumulates in fish meat more than in fish oil, and fish oil supplements appear to contain almost no mercury. Therefore, these safety concerns apply to eating fish but likely not to ingesting fish oil supplements. However, unrefined fish oil preparations may contain pesticides.

It is not known if omega-3 fatty acid supplementation of women during pregnancy or breastfeeding is beneficial to infants. It has been suggested that high intake of omega-3 fatty acids during pregnancy, particularly DHA, may increase birth weight and gestational length. However, higher doses may not be advisable due to the potential risk of bleeding. Fatty acids are added to some infant formulas.

Interactions

Most herbs and supplements have not been thoroughly tested for interactions with other herbs, supplements, drugs, or foods. The interactions listed in the following text are based on reports in scientific publications, laboratory experiments, or traditional use. You should always read product labels. If you have a medical condition, or are taking other drugs, herbs, or supplements, you should speak with a qualified healthcare provider before starting a new therapy.

Interactions with Drugs

In theory, omega-3 fatty acids may increase the risk of bleeding when taken with drugs that increase the risk of bleeding. Some examples include aspirin, anticoagulants ("blood thinners") such as warfarin (Coumadin®) or heparin, anti-platelet drugs such as clopidogrel (Plavix®), and non-steroidal anti-inflammatory drugs such as ibuprofen (Motrin®, Advil®) or naproxen (Naprosyn®, Aleve®).

Based on human studies, omega-3 fatty acids may lower blood pressure and add to the effects of drugs that may also affect blood pressure.

Fish oil supplements may lower blood sugar levels a small amount. Caution is advised when using medications that may also lower blood sugar. Patients taking drugs for diabetes by mouth or insulin should be monitored closely by a qualified healthcare provider. Medication adjustments may be necessary.

Omega-3 fatty acids lower triglyceride levels, but can actually increase (worsen) low-density lipoprotein (LDL/"bad cholesterol") levels by a small amount. Therefore, omega-3 fatty acids may add to the triglyceride-lowering effects of agents like niacin/nicotinic acid, fibrates such as gemfibrozil (Lopid®), or resins such as cholestyramine (Questran®). However, omega-3 fatty acids may work against the LDL-lowering properties of "statin" drugs like atorvastatin (Lipitor®) and lovastatin (Mevacor®).

Interactions with Herbs and Dietary Supplements

In theory, omega-3 fatty acids may increase the risk of bleeding when taken with herbs and supplements that are believed to increase the risk of bleeding. Multiple cases of bleeding have been reported with the use of *Ginkgo biloba*, and fewer cases with garlic and saw palmetto. Numerous other agents may theoretically increase the risk of bleeding, although this has not been proven in most cases.

Based on human studies, omega-3 fatty acids may lower blood pressure, and theoretically may add to the effects of agents that may also affect blood pressure.

Fish oil supplements may lower blood sugar levels a small amount. Caution is advised when using herbs or supplements that may also lower blood sugar. Blood glucose levels may require monitoring, and doses may need adjustment.

Omega-3 fatty acids lower triglyceride levels, but can actually increase (worsen) low-density lipoprotein (LDL/"bad cholesterol") levels by a small amount. Therefore, omega-3 fatty acids may add to the triglyceride-lowering effects of agents like niacin/nicotinic acid, but may work against the potential LDL-lowering properties of agents like barley, garlic, guggul, psyllium, soy, or sweet almond.

Fish oil taken for many months may cause a deficiency of vitamin E, and therefore vitamin E is added to many commercial fish oil products. As a result, regular use of vitamin E-enriched products may lead to elevated levels of this fat-soluble vitamin. Fish liver oil contains the fat-soluble vitamins A and D, and therefore fish liver oil products (such as cod liver oil) may increase the risk of vitamin A or D toxicity. Since fat-soluble vitamins can build up in the body and cause toxicity, patients taking multiple vitamins regularly or in high doses should discuss this risk with their healthcare practitioners.

Methodology

This information is based on a professional level monograph edited and peer-reviewed by contributors to the Natural Standard Research Collaboration (www.naturalstandard.com).

Selected References

1. Berbert AA, Kondo CR, Almendra CL, et al. Supplementation of fish oil and olive oil in patients with rheumatoid arthritis. *Nutrition* 2005;21(2):131–136.

2. Bittiner SB, Tucker WF, Cartwright I, et al. A double-blind, randomised, placebo-controlled trial of fish oil in psoriasis. *Lancet* 2-20-1988;1(8582):378–380.

3. Bjorneboe A, Smith AK, Bjorneboe GE, et al. Effect of dietary supplementation with n-3 fatty acids on clinical manifestations of psoriasis. *Br J Dermatol* 1988;118(1):77–83.

4. Brouwer IA, Zock PL, Camm AJ, et al. Effect of fish oil on ventricular tachyarrhythmia and death in patients with implantable cardioverter defibrillators: the Study on Omega-3 Fatty Acids and Ventricular Arrhythmia (SOFA) randomized trial. *JAMA*. 2006 Jun 14;295(22):2613–9.

5. Burns CP, Halabi S, Clamon G, et al. Phase II study of high-dose fish oil capsules for patients with cancer-related cachexia. *Cancer* 7-15-2004;101(2):370–378.

6. Chan JK, McDonald BE, Gerrard JM, et al. Effect of dietary alpha-linolenic acid and its ratio to linoleic acid on platelet and plasma fatty acids and thrombogenesis. *Lipids* 1993;28(9):811–817.

7. Dry J, Vincent D. Effect of a fish oil diet on asthma: results of a 1-year double-blind study. *Int Arch Allergy Appl Immunol*. 1991;95(2–3):156–157.

8. Duffy EM, Meenagh GK, McMillan SA, et al. The clinical effect of dietary supplementation with omega-3 fish oils and/or copper in systemic lupus erythematosus. *J Rheumatol*. 2004;31(8):1551–1556.

9. Erkkila AT, Lichtenstein AH, Mozaffarian D, et al. Fish intake is associated with a reduced progression of coronary artery atherosclerosis in postmenopausal women with coronary artery disease. *Am J Clin Nutr*. 2004;80(3):626–632.

10. Fenton WS, Dickerson F, Boronow J, et al. A placebo-controlled trial of omega-3 Fatty Acid (ethyl eicosapentaenoic Acid) supplementation for residual symptoms and cognitive impairment in schizophrenia. *Am J Psychiatry* 2001;158(12):2071–2074.

11. Lim WS, Gammack JK, Van Niekerk J, et al. Omega 3 fatty acid for the prevention of dementia. *Cochrane Database Syst Rev*. 2006 Jan 25;(1):CD005379.

12. Mostad IL, Bjerve KS, Bjorgaas MR, et al. Effects of n-3 fatty acids in subjects with type 2 diabetes: reduction of insulin sensitivity and time-dependent alteration from carbohydrate to fat oxidation. *Am J Clin Nutr*. 2006 Sep;84(3):540–50.

13. Olsen SF, Secher NJ, Tabor A, et al. Randomised clinical trials of fish oil supplementation in high risk pregnancies. Fish Oil Trials In Pregnancy (FOTIP) Team. *BJOG*. 2000;107(3):382–395.

14. Stoll AL, Severus WE, Freeman MP, et al. Omega 3 fatty acids in bipolar disorder: a preliminary double-blind, placebo-controlled trial. *Arch Gen. Psychiatry* 1999;56(5):407–412.

15. Su KP, Huang SY, Chiu CC, et al. Omega-3 fatty acids in major depressive disorder. A preliminary double-blind, placebo-controlled trial. *Eur. Neuropsychopharmacol.* 2003;13(4):267–271.

Section 28.2

Flaxseed and Flaxseed Oils

Excerpted from "Flaxseed and Flaxseed Oil," by the National Center for Complementary and Alternative Medicine (NCCAM, nccam.nih.gov), part of the National Institutes of Health, April 2008.

Flaxseed is the seed of the flax plant, which is believed to have originated in Egypt. It grows throughout Canada and the northwestern United States. Flaxseed oil comes from flaxseeds. Common names for flaxseed are flaxseed and linseed. The Latin name for flaxseed is *Linum usitatissimum*.

What Flaxseed Is Used For

- Flaxseed is most commonly used as a laxative.

- Flaxseed is also used for hot flashes and breast pain.

- Flaxseed oil is used for different conditions than flaxseed, including arthritis.

- Both flaxseed and flaxseed oil have been used for high cholesterol levels and in an effort to prevent cancer.

How Flaxseed Is Used

Whole or crushed flaxseed can be mixed with water or juice and taken by mouth. Flaxseed is also available in powder form. Flaxseed oil is available in liquid and capsule form. Flaxseed contains lignans (phytoestrogens, or plant estrogens), while flaxseed oil preparations lack lignans.

What the Science Says

- Flaxseed contains soluble fiber, like that found in oat bran, and is an effective laxative.

- Studies of flaxseed preparations to lower cholesterol levels report mixed results.

- Some studies suggest that alpha-linolenic acid (a substance found in flaxseed and flaxseed oil) may benefit people with heart disease. But not enough reliable data are available to determine whether flaxseed is effective for heart conditions.

- Study results are mixed on whether flaxseed decreases hot flashes.

- NCCAM is funding studies on flaxseed. Recent studies have looked at the effects of flaxseed on high cholesterol levels, as well as its possible role in preventing conditions such as heart disease and osteoporosis.

Side Effects and Cautions

- Flaxseed and flaxseed oil supplements seem to be well tolerated. Few side effects have been reported.

- Flaxseed, like any supplemental fiber source, should be taken with plenty of water; otherwise, it could worsen constipation or, in rare cases, even cause intestinal blockage.

- The fiber in flaxseed may lower the body's ability to absorb medications that are taken by mouth. Flaxseed should not be taken at the same time as any conventional oral medications or other dietary supplements.

- Tell your health care providers about any complementary and alternative practices you use. Give them a full picture of what you do to manage your health. This will help ensure coordinated and safe care.

Chapter 29

Selenium

What is selenium?

Selenium is a trace mineral that is essential to good health but re-quired only in small amounts. Selenium is incorporated into proteins to make selenoproteins, which are important antioxidant enzymes. The antioxidant properties of selenoproteins help prevent cellular damage from free radicals. Free radicals are natural by-products of oxygen me-tabolism that may contribute to the development of chronic diseases such as cancer and heart disease. Other selenoproteins help regulate thyroid function and play a role in the immune system.

What are some current issues and controversies about selenium?

Selenium and cancer: Observational studies indicate that death from cancer, including lung, colorectal, and prostate cancers, is lower among people with higher blood levels or intake of selenium. In addi-tion, the incidence of nonmelanoma skin cancer is significantly higher in areas of the United States with low soil selenium content. The effect of selenium supplementation on the recurrence of different types of skin cancers was studied in seven dermatology clinics in the United States from 1983 through the early 1990s. Taking a daily supplement containing 200 mcg of selenium did not affect recurrence of skin cancer,

Excerpted from text by the Office of Dietary Supplements (ODS, ods.od.nih.gov), part of the National Institutes of Health, November 12, 2009.

but significantly reduced the occurrence and death from total cancers. The incidence of prostate cancer, colorectal cancer, and lung cancer was notably lower in the group given selenium supplements.

Research suggests that selenium affects cancer risk in two ways. As an antioxidant, selenium can help protect the body from damaging effects of free radicals. Selenium may also prevent or slow tumor growth. Certain breakdown products of selenium are believed to prevent tumor growth by enhancing immune cell activity and suppressing development of blood vessels to the tumor.

However, not all studies have shown a relationship between selenium status and cancer. In 1982, over 60,000 participants of the Nurse's Health Study with no history of cancer submitted toenail clippings for selenium analysis. Toenails are thought to reflect selenium status over the previous year. After three and a half years of data collection, researchers compared toenail selenium levels of nurses with and without cancer. Those nurses with higher levels of selenium in their toenails did not have a reduced risk of cancer.

Two long-term studies, the SU.VI.MAX study in France and the Selenium and Vitamin E Cancer Prevention Trial (SELECT) in the United States and Canada, investigated whether selenium combined with at least one other dietary supplement could reduce the risk of prostate cancer in men.

The SU.VI.MAX study examined the effects of a supplement package containing moderate doses of vitamins E and C, beta-carotene, zinc, and selenium (100 mcg/day) versus placebo on the risk of chronic diseases such as cancer and cardiovascular disease. Among the 5,141 men enrolled, those randomized to the supplements who began the study with a normal (<3 ng/ml) PSA (prostate specific antigen) level at baseline had their risk of prostate cancer reduced by half. Among the men whose PSA levels were elevated at baseline, however, use of the supplements was associated with an increased incidence of prostate cancer of borderline statistical significance compared to placebo.

The Selenium and Vitamin E Cancer Prevention Trial (SELECT) was a very large randomized clinical trial begun in 2001 specifically designed to determine whether 7–12 years of daily supplementation with selenium (200 mcg), with or without synthetic vitamin E (400 IU), reduces the number of new prostate cancers in healthy men (PSA less than or equal to 4 ng/ml at baseline). The trial, which had enrolled >35,000 men, was discontinued in October 2008 when an analysis found that the supplements, taken alone or together for an average of 5.5 years, did not prevent prostate cancer. Study staff members will continue to monitor participants' health for an additional 3 years.

Selenium and heart disease: Some population surveys have suggested an association between lower antioxidant intake and a greater incidence of heart disease. Evidence also suggests that oxidative stress from free radicals, which are natural by-products of oxygen metabolism, may promote heart disease. For example, it is the oxidized form of low-density lipoproteins (LDL, often called "bad" cholesterol) that promotes plaque build-up in coronary arteries. Selenium is one of a group of antioxidants that may help limit the oxidation of LDL cholesterol and thereby help to prevent coronary artery disease. Currently there is insufficient evidence available to recommend selenium supplements for the prevention of coronary heart disease.

Selenium and arthritis: Surveys indicate that individuals with rheumatoid arthritis, a chronic disease that causes pain, stiffness, swelling, and loss of function in joints, have reduced selenium levels in their blood. In addition, some individuals with arthritis have a low selenium intake.

The body's immune system naturally makes free radicals that can help destroy invading organisms and damaged tissue, but that can also harm healthy tissue. Selenium, as an antioxidant, may help to relieve symptoms of arthritis by controlling levels of free radicals. Current findings are considered preliminary, and further research is needed before selenium supplements can be recommended for individuals with arthritis.

Selenium and HIV: HIV/AIDS [human immunodeficiency virus/acquired immunodeficiency syndrome] malabsorption can deplete levels of many nutrients, including selenium. Selenium deficiency is associated with decreased immune cell counts, increased disease progression, and high risk of death in the HIV/AIDS population. HIV/AIDS gradually destroys the immune system, and oxidative stress may contribute to further damage of immune cells. Antioxidant nutrients such as selenium help protect cells from oxidative stress, thus potentially slowing progression of the disease. Selenium also may be needed for the replication of the HIV virus, which could further deplete levels of selenium.

An examination of 125 HIV-positive men and women linked selenium deficiency with a higher rate of death from HIV. In a small study of 24 children with HIV who were observed for five years, those with low selenium levels died at a younger age, which may indicate faster disease progression. Results of research studies have led experts to suggest that selenium status may be a significant predictor of survival for those infected with HIV.

Researchers continue to investigate the relationship between selenium and HIV/AIDS, including the effect of selenium levels on disease progression and mortality. There is insufficient evidence to routinely recommend selenium supplements for individuals with HIV/AIDS, but physicians may prescribe such supplements as part of an overall treatment plan. It is also important for HIV-positive individuals to consume recommended amounts of selenium in their diet.

Chapter 30

Bone and Joint Health Supplements

Chapter Contents

Section 30.1—Calcium Supplements and Bone Health..................198

Section 30.2—Glucosamine/Chondroitin Supplements..................201
and Joint Health

197

Section 30.1

Calcium Supplements and Bone Health

From "Calcium Supplements: What to Look for," by the National Institute of Arthritis and Musculoskeletal and Skin Diseases (NIAMS, niams.nih.gov), part of the National Institutes of Health, May 2009.

Calcium is essential for many functions in the body, including the following:

- Regulating the heartbeat
- Conducting nerve impulses
- Stimulating hormone secretions
- Clotting blood
- Building and maintaining healthy bones

Calcium is a mineral found in many foods. Getting enough of this nutrient is important because the human body cannot make it. Even after you are fully grown, adequate calcium intake is important because the body loses calcium every day through the skin, nails, hair, and sweat, as well as through urine and feces. This lost calcium must be replaced daily through the diet. Otherwise, the body takes calcium from the bones to perform other functions, which makes the bones weaker and more likely to break over time.

Experts recommend that adults get 1,000 to 1,200 mg (milligrams) of calcium each day. Although food is the best source of calcium, most Americans do not get enough of it from food sources. Calcium-fortified foods (such as orange juice, bread, cereals, and many others on grocery shelves) and calcium supplements can fill the gap by ensuring that you meet your daily calcium requirement.

What to Look for in a Calcium Supplement

Calcium exists in nature only in combination with other substances. These substances are called compounds. Several different calcium compounds are used in supplements, including the following:

- Calcium carbonate
- Calcium phosphate
- Calcium citrate

These compounds contain different amounts of elemental calcium, which is the actual amount of calcium in the supplement. Read the label carefully to determine how much elemental calcium is in the supplement and how many doses or pills to take.

Calcium supplements are available without a prescription in a wide range of preparations and strengths, which can make selecting one a confusing experience. Many people ask which calcium supplement they should take. The "best" supplement is the one that meets your needs. Ask yourself these questions:

- How well does my body tolerate this kind of supplement? Does it cause any side effects (such as gas or constipation)? If so, you may want to try a different type or brand.

- Is this kind of supplement convenient? Can I remember to take it as often as recommended each day?

- Is the cost of this supplement within my budget?

- Is it widely available? Can I buy it at a store near me?

Other Important Things to Consider

Purity: Choose calcium supplements with familiar brand names. Look for labels that state "purified" or have the USP (United States Pharmacopeia) symbol. Avoid supplements made from unrefined oyster shell, bone meal, or dolomite that don't have the USP symbol because they may contain high levels of lead or other toxic metals.

Absorbability: The body easily absorbs most brand-name calcium products. If you aren't sure about your product, you can find out how well it dissolves by placing it in a small amount of warm water for 30 minutes and stirring it occasionally. If it hasn't dissolved within this time, it probably will not dissolve in your stomach. Chewable and liquid calcium supplements dissolve well because they are broken down before they enter the stomach.

The body best absorbs calcium, whether from food or supplements, when it's taken several times a day in amounts of not more than 500 mg, but taking it all at once is better than not taking it at all. Calcium carbonate is absorbed best when taken with food. Calcium citrate can be taken anytime.

Tolerance: Some calcium supplements may cause side effects, such as gas or constipation, for some people. If simple measures (such as increasing your intake of fluids and high-fiber foods) do not solve the problem, you should try another form of calcium. Also, it is important to increase the dose of your supplement gradually: take just 500 mg a day for a week, and then slowly add more calcium. Do not take more than the recommended amount of calcium without your doctor's approval.

Calcium interactions: It's important to talk with a doctor or pharmacist about possible interactions between calcium supplements and your over-the-counter and prescription medications. For example, calcium supplements may reduce the absorption of the antibiotic tetracycline. Calcium also interferes with iron absorption. So you should not take a calcium supplement at the same time as an iron supplement—unless the calcium supplement is calcium citrate or the iron supplement is taken with vitamin C. Any medications that need to be taken on an empty stomach should not be taken with calcium supplements.

Combination Products

Calcium supplements are available in a bewildering array of combinations with vitamins and other minerals. Calcium supplements often come in combination with vitamin D, which is necessary for the absorption of calcium. However, calcium and vitamin D do not need to be taken together or in the same preparation to be absorbed by the body. Minerals such as magnesium and phosphorus also are important but usually are obtained through food or multivitamins. Most experts recommend that nutrients come from a balanced diet, with multivitamins used to supplement dietary deficiencies.

Getting enough calcium—whether through your diet or with the help of supplements—will help to protect the health of your bones. However, this is only one of the steps you need to take for bone health. Exercise, a healthy lifestyle, and, for some people, medication are also important.

Section 30.2

Glucosamine/Chondroitin Supplements and Joint Health

Excerpted from "Dietary Supplements Glucosamine and/or Chondroitin Fare No Better than Placebo in Slowing Structural Damage of Knee Osteoarthritis," by the National Institutes of Health (NIH, www.nih.gov), September 29, 2008.

The dietary supplements glucosamine and chondroitin sulfate, together or alone, appeared to fare no better than placebo in slowing loss of cartilage in osteoarthritis of the knee, researchers from the Glucosamine/chondroitin Arthritis Intervention Trial (GAIT) team report in the October issue of *Arthritis & Rheumatism*.[1] Interpreting the study results is complicated, however, because participants taking placebo had a smaller loss of cartilage, or joint space width, than predicted. Loss of cartilage, the slippery material that cushions the joints, is a hallmark of osteoarthritis and its loss is typically measured as a reduction in joint space width—the distance between the ends of bones in a joint as seen on an x-ray.

"While these results are of interest, we cannot draw definitive conclusions about the utility of glucosamine or chondroitin in reducing joint space width loss, in part because the placebo group fared better than anticipated based on prior research results," said Josephine P. Briggs, MD, director of the National Center for Complementary and Alternative Medicine, at the National Institutes of Health (NIH), one of the study's funders. "The results of the study provide interesting insights for future research."

The NIH-supported study was led by University of Utah School of Medicine's Allen D. Sawitzke, MD, and Daniel O. Clegg, MD. This study was an ancillary, or additional, trial conducted by the GAIT team with a subset of participants from the original GAIT study. The original GAIT study sought to determine whether these dietary supplements could treat the pain of knee osteoarthritis and found that overall the combination of glucosamine plus chondroitin sulfate did not provide significant relief from osteoarthritis pain among all participants. However, a smaller subgroup of study participants with moderate-to-severe pain showed significant relief with the combined supplements. These results were reported in 2006.[2]

To study whether the dietary supplements could diminish the structural damage of osteoarthritis, interested GAIT patients were offered the opportunity to continue their original study treatment in the ancillary trial for an additional 18 months, for a total of 2 years. The randomly assigned study treatments were 500 milligrams glucosamine hydrochloride three times daily, sodium chondroitin sulfate 400 milligrams three times daily, the combination of glucosamine plus chondroitin sulfate, placebo, or celecoxib 200 milligrams daily. The research team enrolled 572 GAIT participants for the ancillary study. Participants entering the ancillary study had x-ray evidence of moderate (grade 2) or severe (grade 3) knee osteoarthritis in one or both knees using a scale that measures osteoarthritis severity called the Kellgren-Lawrence scale. At the end of the ancillary study, the team had gathered data on 581 knees.

"At 2 years, no treatment showed what we determined to be a clinically important reduction in joint space width loss," said Dr. Sawitzke, associate professor of medicine and lead investigator for the ancillary study. "While we found a trend toward improvement among those with milder, Kellgren-Lawrence grade 2 osteoarthritis of the knee in those taking glucosamine alone, we were not able to draw any definitive conclusions."

The joint space width in the knee, or knees, of the patients was measured with a specific x-ray protocol on entering the ancillary study and at 1 and 2 years to determine any loss in joint width. The x-ray technique required images of the knees be taken in a standardized, weight-bearing position.

The GAIT researchers expected patients in the placebo group to have a joint space width loss of approximately 0.4 millimeters over 2 years, based on results of previously published large studies. The study team hypothesized that a loss of 0.2 millimeters or less would show a slowed rate of cartilage loss. The final results, adjusted for baseline joint space width, gender, and other factors, showed the following:

- The glucosamine alone group had the least average joint space width loss of 0.013 millimeters.

- The chondroitin alone group had an average loss of 0.107 millimeters.

- The glucosamine plus chondroitin group had an average loss of 0.194 millimeters.

- The celecoxib group had an average loss of 0.111 millimeters.

- The placebo group had an average loss of 0.166 millimeters.

In addition to measuring average loss of joint space width, the study also measured the percentage of participants with progression (worsening) of their osteoarthritis—defined as a joint space width loss of more than 0.48 millimeters over the 2 years. Overall, those with grade 2 (moderate) knee osteoarthritis were least likely to have progression of osteoarthritis compared to those with more severe disease. Approximately 24 percent of participants taking the combination of glucosamine plus chondroitin sulfate showed disease progression, which was similar to placebo, but greater than either glucosamine or chondroitin sulfate alone. The researchers theorize that this may reflect interference in absorption of the two supplements when taken together.

"Research continues to reveal that osteoarthritis, the most common form of arthritis, appears to be the result of an array of factors including age, gender, genetics, obesity, and joint injuries," said Stephen I. Katz, MD, director of the National Institute of Arthritis and Musculoskeletal and Skin Diseases, co-funder of the study. "Because osteoarthritis affects an estimated 27 million Americans, we are seeking ways to not only treat pain, but also address the structural effects of the condition."

The researchers note that the study has limitations, such as a greater-than-expected variability in measurement of joint space width loss and a less-than-expected loss of joint space width in the placebo group. However, the team also notes that not only was the study designed to investigate whether glucosamine and chondroitin sulfate, either together or alone, may have an effect on structural damage, it was also designed to test the method of measuring joint space width loss and learning more about the natural progression of osteoarthritis.

"Despite the ancillary study's limitations, it has provided us with new insights on osteoarthritis progression, the techniques to use to more reliably measure loss of joint space width, the possible effects of these dietary supplements, and the characteristics of osteoarthritis patients that may best respond, all of which will assist investigators in future studies," said Dr. Clegg, professor of medicine and chief of rheumatology and principal investigator for GAIT.

References

1. Sawitzke AD, Shi H, Finco MF, et al. The Effect of Glucosamine and/or Chondroitin Sulfate on the Progression of Knee Osteoarthritis: A Report from the Glucosamine/Chondroitin Arthritis Intervention Trial. *Arthritis & Rheumatism,* 2008; 58(10):3183–3191.

2. Clegg D, Reda DJ, Harris CL, et al. Glucosamine, Chondroitin Sulfate, and the Two in Combination for Painful Knee Osteoarthritis. *New England Journal of Medicine,* 2006;354:795–808.

Chapter 31

Immune System
Support Supplements

Chapter Contents

Section 31.1—Echinacea... 206
Section 31.2—Zinc.. 208

Section 31.1

Echinacea

Excerpted from text by the National Center for Complementary and
Alternative Medicine (NCCAM, nccam.nih.gov), part of the National
Institutes of Health, March 2008.

This text provides basic information about the herb echinacea.
There are nine known species of echinacea, all of which are native to
the United States and southern Canada. The most commonly used,
Echinacea purpurea, is believed to be the most potent. Common names
include echinacea, purple coneflower, coneflower, and American coneflower. Latin names include *Echinacea purpurea, Echinacea angustifolia,* and *Echinacea pallida.*

What Echinacea Is Used For

- Echinacea has traditionally been used to treat or prevent colds,
  flu, and other infections.

- Echinacea is believed to stimulate the immune system to help
  fight infections.

- Less commonly, echinacea has been used for wounds and skin
  problems, such as acne or boils.

How Echinacea Is Used

The aboveground parts of the plant and roots of echinacea are used
fresh or dried to make teas, squeezed (expressed) juice, extracts, or
preparations for external use.

What the Science Says

- Study results are mixed on whether echinacea effectively treats
  colds or flu. For example, two NCCAM-funded studies did not
  find a benefit from echinacea, either as *Echinacea purpurea*
  fresh-pressed juice for treating colds in children, or as an unrefined mixture of *Echinacea angustifolia* root and *Echinacea*

purpurea root and herb in adults. However, other studies have shown that echinacea may be beneficial in treating upper respiratory infections.

- Most studies to date indicate that echinacea does not appear to prevent colds or other infections.

- NCCAM is continuing to support the study of echinacea for the treatment of upper respiratory infections. NCCAM is also studying echinacea for its potential effects on the immune system.

Side Effects and Cautions

- When taken by mouth, echinacea usually does not cause side effects. However, some people experience allergic reactions, including rashes, increased asthma, and anaphylaxis (a life-threatening allergic reaction). In clinical trials, gastrointestinal side effects were most common.

- People are more likely to experience allergic reactions to echinacea if they are allergic to related plants in the daisy family, which includes ragweed, chrysanthemums, marigolds, and daisies. Also, people with asthma or atopy (a genetic tendency toward allergic reactions) may be more likely to have an allergic reaction when taking echinacea.

- Tell your health care providers about any complementary and alternative practices you use. Give them a full picture of what you do to manage your health. This will help ensure coordinated and safe care.

Section 31.2

Zinc

Excerpted from "Zinc," by the Office of Dietary Supplements (ODS, ods.od.nih.gov), part of the National Institutes of Health, June 30, 2009.

Zinc is an essential mineral that is naturally present in some foods, added to others, and available as a dietary supplement. Zinc is also found in many cold lozenges and some over-the-counter drugs sold as cold remedies.

Zinc is involved in numerous aspects of cellular metabolism. It is required for the catalytic activity of approximately 100 enzymes and it plays a role in immune function, protein synthesis, wound healing, DNA [deoxyribonucleic acid] synthesis, and cell division. Zinc also supports normal growth and development during pregnancy, childhood, and adolescence and is required for proper sense of taste and smell. A daily intake of zinc is required to maintain a steady state because the body has no specialized zinc storage system.

Immune Function

Severe zinc deficiency depresses immune function, and even mild to moderate degrees of zinc deficiency can impair macrophage and neutrophil functions, natural killer cell activity, and complement activity. The body requires zinc to develop and activate T-lymphocytes. Individuals with low zinc levels have shown reduced lymphocyte proliferation response to mitogens and other adverse alterations in immunity that can be corrected by zinc supplementation. These alterations in immune function might explain why low zinc status has been associated with increased susceptibility to pneumonia and other infections in children in developing countries and the elderly.

Wound Healing

Zinc helps maintain the integrity of skin and mucosal membranes. Patients with chronic leg ulcers have abnormal zinc metabolism and low serum zinc levels, and clinicians frequently treat skin ulcers with zinc supplements. The authors of a systematic review concluded that zinc sulfate might be effective for treating leg ulcers in some patients who have low serum zinc levels. However, research has not shown that the general use of zinc sulfate in patients with chronic leg ulcers or arterial or venous ulcers is effective.

Diarrhea

Acute diarrhea is associated with high rates of mortality among children in developing countries. Zinc deficiency causes alterations in immune response that probably contribute to increased susceptibility to infections, such as those that cause diarrhea, especially in children.

Studies show that poor, malnourished children in India, Africa, South America, and Southeast Asia experience shorter courses of infectious diarrhea after taking zinc supplements. The children in these studies received 4–40 mg of zinc a day in the form of zinc acetate, zinc gluconate, or zinc sulfate.

In addition, results from a pooled analysis of randomized controlled trials of zinc supplementation in developing countries suggest that zinc helps reduce the duration and severity of diarrhea in zinc-deficient or otherwise malnourished children. Similar findings were reported in a meta-analysis published in 2008 and a 2007 review of zinc supplementation for preventing and treating diarrhea. The effects of zinc supplementation on diarrhea in children with adequate zinc status, such as most children in the United States, are not clear.

The World Health Organization and UNICEF [United Nations Children's Fund] now recommend short-term zinc supplementation (20 mg of zinc per day, or 10 mg for infants under 6 months, for 10–14 days) to treat acute childhood diarrhea.

The Common Cold

The effect of zinc treatment on the severity or duration of cold symptoms is controversial. Researchers have hypothesized that zinc directly inhibits rhinovirus binding and replication in the nasal mucosa and suppresses inflammation. However, no data are available to support this hypothesis.

In a randomized, double-blind, placebo-controlled clinical trial, 50 subjects (within 24 hours of developing the common cold) took a zinc acetate lozenge (13.3 mg zinc) or placebo every 2–3 wakeful hours. Compared with placebo, the zinc lozenges significantly reduced the duration of cold symptoms (cough, nasal discharge, and muscle aches).

Complementary and Alternative Medicine Sourcebook, Fourth Edition

In another clinical trial involving 273 participants with experimentally induced colds, zinc gluconate lozenges (providing 13.3 mg zinc) significantly reduced the duration of illness compared with placebo but had no effect on symptom severity. However, treatment with zinc acetate lozenges (providing 5 or 11.5 mg zinc) had no effect on either cold duration or severity. Neither zinc gluconate nor zinc acetate lozenges affected the duration or severity of cold symptoms in 281 subjects with natural (not experimentally induced) colds in another trial.

In 77 participants with natural colds, a combination of zinc gluconate nasal spray and zinc orotate lozenges (37 mg zinc every 2–3 wakeful hours) was also found to have no effect on the number of asymptomatic patients after 7 days of treatment.

In September of 2007, Caruso and colleagues published a structured review of the effects of zinc lozenges, nasal sprays, and nasal gels on the common cold. Of the 14 randomized, placebo-controlled studies included, 7 (5 using zinc lozenges, 2 using a nasal gel) showed that the zinc treatment had a beneficial effect and 7 (5 using zinc lozenges, 1 using a nasal spray, and 1 using lozenges and a nasal spray) showed no effect. A Cochrane review of the effects of zinc lozenges on cold symptoms also reported inconclusive findings, although the author of another review concluded that zinc can reduce the duration and severity of cold symptoms.

The available data are therefore inconclusive regarding the use of zinc lozenges, nasal gels, and sprays to treat the common cold.

As previously noted, the safety of intranasal zinc has been called into question because of numerous reports of anosmia (loss of smell), in some cases long-lasting or permanent, from the use of zinc-containing nasal gels or sprays.

Age-Related Macular Degeneration

Researchers have suggested that both zinc and antioxidants delay the progression of age-related macular degeneration (AMD) and vision loss, possibly by preventing cellular damage in the retina. In a population-based cohort study in the Netherlands, high dietary intake of zinc as well as beta carotene, vitamin C, and vitamin E was associated with reduced risk of AMD in elderly subjects. However, the authors of a systematic review and meta-analysis published in 2007 concluded that zinc is not effective for the primary prevention of early AMD, although zinc might reduce the risk of progression to advanced AMD.

The Age-Related Eye Disease Study (AREDS), a large, randomized, placebo-controlled, clinical trial (n = 3,597), evaluated the effect of high doses of selected antioxidants (500 mg vitamin C, 400 IU vitamin E, and 15 mg beta-carotene) with or without zinc (80 mg as zinc oxide) on the development of advanced AMD in older individuals with varying degrees of AMD. Participants also received 2 mg copper to prevent the copper deficiency associated with high zinc intakes. After an average follow-up period of 6.3 years, supplementation with antioxidants plus zinc (but not antioxidants alone) significantly reduced the risk of developing advanced AMD and reduced visual acuity loss. Zinc supplementation alone significantly reduced the risk of developing advanced AMD in subjects at higher risk but not in the total study population. Visual acuity loss was not significantly affected by zinc supplementation alone.

Two other small clinical trials evaluated the effects of supplementation with 200 mg zinc sulfate (providing 45 mg zinc) for 2 years in subjects with drusen or macular degeneration. Zinc supplementation significantly reduced visual acuity loss in one of the studies but had no effect in the other.

A Cochrane review concluded that the evidence supporting the use of antioxidant vitamins and zinc for AMD comes primarily from the AREDS study. Further research is required before public health recommendations can be made, but individuals who have or are developing AMD might wish to talk to their physician about using dietary supplements.

Chapter 32

Mood and Brain Health Supplements

Chapter Contents

Section 32.1—Ginkgo Biloba 214

Section 32.2—St. John's Wort 216

Section 32.1

Ginkgo Biloba

Excerpted from "Ginkgo," by the National Center for Complementary
and Alternative Medicine (NCCAM, nccam.nih.gov), part of the National
Institutes of Health, November 2008.

This text provides basic information about the herb ginkgo. The
ginkgo tree is one of the oldest types of trees in the world. Ginkgo
seeds have been used in traditional Chinese medicine for thousands
of years, and cooked seeds are occasionally eaten. Common names
include ginkgo, *Ginkgo biloba,* fossil tree, maidenhair tree, Japanese
silver apricot, baiguo, bai guo ye, kew tree, and yinhsing (yin-hsing).
The Latin name is *Ginkgo biloba.*

What Ginkgo Biloba Is Used For

- Ginkgo leaf extract has been used to treat a variety of ailments
  and conditions, including asthma, bronchitis, fatigue, and tinnitus (ringing or roaring sounds in the ears).

- Today, people use ginkgo leaf extracts hoping to improve memory; to treat or help prevent Alzheimer disease and other types of
  dementia; to decrease intermittent claudication (leg pain caused
  by narrowing arteries); and to treat sexual dysfunction, multiple
  sclerosis, tinnitus, and other health conditions.

How Ginkgo Biloba Is Used

Extracts are usually taken from the ginkgo leaf and are used to
make tablets, capsules, or teas. Occasionally, ginkgo extracts are used
in skin products.

What the Science Says

- Numerous studies of ginkgo have been done for a variety of conditions. Some promising results have been seen for intermittent claudication, but larger, well-designed research studies are needed.

- An NCCAM-funded study of the well-characterized ginkgo product, EGb-761, found it ineffective in lowering the overall incidence of dementia and Alzheimer disease in the elderly. Further analysis of the same data also found ginkgo to be ineffective in slowing cognitive decline. In this clinical trial, known as the Ginkgo Evaluation of Memory study, researchers recruited more than 3,000 volunteers age 75 and over who took 240 mg of ginkgo daily. Participants were followed for an average of approximately 6 years.

- Some smaller studies for memory enhancement have had promising results, but a trial sponsored by the National Institute on Aging of more than 200 healthy adults over age 60 found that ginkgo taken for 6 weeks did not improve memory.

- Other NCCAM-funded research includes studies on ginkgo for asthma, symptoms of multiple sclerosis, vascular function (intermittent claudication), cognitive decline, sexual dysfunction due to antidepressants, and insulin resistance. NCCAM is also looking at potential interactions between ginkgo and prescription drugs.

Side Effects and Cautions

- Side effects of ginkgo may include headache, nausea, gastrointestinal upset, diarrhea, dizziness, or allergic skin reactions. More severe allergic reactions have occasionally been reported.

- There are some data to suggest that ginkgo can increase bleeding risk, so people who take anticoagulant drugs, have bleeding disorders, or have scheduled surgery or dental procedures should use caution and talk to a health care provider if using ginkgo.

- Uncooked ginkgo seeds contain a chemical known as ginkgotoxin, which can cause seizures. Consuming large quantities of seeds over time can cause death. Ginkgo leaf and ginkgo leaf extracts appear to contain little ginkgotoxin.

- Tell your health care providers about any complementary and alternative practices you use. Give them a full picture of what you do to manage your health. This will help ensure coordinated and safe care.

Section 32.2

St. John's Wort

Excerpted from "St. John's Wort," by the National Center for Complementary and Alternative Medicine (NCCAM, nccam.nih.gov), part of the National Institutes of Health, March 2008.

This text provides basic information about the herb St. John's wort. St. John's wort is a plant with yellow flowers whose medicinal uses were first recorded in ancient Greece. The name St. John's wort apparently refers to John the Baptist, as the plant blooms around the time of the feast of St. John the Baptist in late June. Common names include St. John's wort, hypericum, Klamath weed, and goat weed. The Latin name for St. John's wort is *Hypericum perforatum*.

What St. John's Wort Is Used For

- St. John's wort has been used for centuries to treat mental disorders and nerve pain.

- St. John's wort has also been used as a sedative and a treatment for malaria, as well as a balm for wounds, burns, and insect bites.

- Today, St. John's wort is used by some for depression, anxiety, and/or sleep disorders.

How St. John's Wort Is Used

The flowering tops of St. John's wort are used to prepare teas and tablets containing concentrated extracts.

What the Science Says

- There is some scientific evidence that St. John's wort is useful for treating mild to moderate depression. However, two large studies, one sponsored by NCCAM, showed that the herb was no more effective than placebo in treating major depression of moderate severity.

- NCCAM is studying the use of St. John's wort in a wider spectrum of mood disorders, including minor depression.

Side Effects and Cautions

St. John's wort may cause increased sensitivity to sunlight. Other side effects can include anxiety, dry mouth, dizziness, gastrointestinal symptoms, fatigue, headache, or sexual dysfunction.

Research shows that St. John's wort interacts with some drugs. The herb affects the way the body processes or breaks down many drugs; in some cases, it may speed or slow a drug's breakdown. Drugs that can be affected include the following:

- Antidepressants

- Birth control pills

- Cyclosporine, which prevents the body from rejecting transplanted organs

- Digoxin, which strengthens heart muscle contractions

- Indinavir and possibly other drugs used to control HIV [human immunodeficiency virus] infection

- Irinotecan and possibly other drugs used to treat cancer

- Warfarin and related anticoagulants

When combined with certain antidepressants, St. John's wort may increase side effects such as nausea, anxiety, headache, and confusion.

St. John's wort is not a proven therapy for depression. If depression is not adequately treated, it can become severe. Anyone who may have depression should see a health care provider. There are effective proven therapies available.

Tell your health care providers about any complementary and alternative practices you use. Give them a full picture of what you do to manage your health. This will help ensure coordinated and safe care.

Chapter 33

Probiotics: Supplements for Gastrointestinal Health

Probiotics are live microorganisms (in most cases, bacteria) that are similar to beneficial microorganisms found in the human gut. They are also called friendly bacteria or good bacteria. Probiotics are available to consumers mainly in the form of dietary supplements and foods. They can be used as complementary and alternative medicine (CAM).

What Probiotics Are

Experts have debated how to define probiotics. One widely used definition, developed by the World Health Organization and the Food and Agriculture Organization of the United Nations, is that probiotics are "live microorganisms, which, when administered in adequate amounts, confer a health benefit on the host." (Microorganisms are tiny living organisms—such as bacteria, viruses, and yeasts—that can be seen only under a microscope.)

Probiotics are not the same thing as prebiotics—nondigestible food ingredients that selectively stimulate the growth and/or activity of beneficial microorganisms already in people's colons. When probiotics and prebiotics are mixed together, they form a synbiotic.

Probiotics are available in foods and dietary supplements (for example, capsules, tablets, and powders) and in some other forms as well. Examples of foods containing probiotics are yogurt, fermented

Excerpted from "An Introduction to Probiotics," by the National Center for Complementary and Alternative Medicine (NCCAM, nccam.nih.gov), part of the National Institutes of Health, August 1, 2008.

and unfermented milk, miso, tempeh, and some juices and soy beverages. In probiotic foods and supplements, the bacteria may have been present originally or added during preparation.

Most probiotics are bacteria similar to those naturally found in people's guts, especially in those of breastfed infants (who have natural protection against many diseases). Most often, the bacteria come from two groups, *Lactobacillus* or *Bifidobacterium*. Within each group, there are different species (for example, *Lactobacillus acidophilus* and *Bifidobacterium bifidus*), and within each species, different strains (or varieties). A few common probiotics, such as *Saccharomyces boulardii,* are yeasts, which are different from bacteria.

Some probiotic foods date back to ancient times, such as fermented foods and cultured milk products. Interest in probiotics in general has been growing; Americans' spending on probiotic supplements, for example, nearly tripled from 1994 to 2003.

Uses for Health Purposes

There are several reasons that people are interested in probiotics for health purposes.

First, the world is full of microorganisms (including bacteria), and so are people's bodies—in and on the skin, in the gut, and in other orifices. Friendly bacteria are vital to proper development of the immune system, to protection against microorganisms that could cause disease, and to the digestion and absorption of food and nutrients. Each person's mix of bacteria varies. Interactions between a person and the microorganisms in his body, and among the microorganisms themselves, can be crucial to the person's health and well-being.

This bacterial balancing act can be thrown off in two major ways:

1. It can be thrown off by antibiotics, when they kill friendly bacteria in the gut along with unfriendly bacteria. Some people use probiotics to try to offset side effects from antibiotics like gas, cramping, or diarrhea. Similarly, some use them to ease symptoms of lactose intolerance—a condition in which the gut lacks the enzyme needed to digest significant amounts of the major sugar in milk, and which also causes gastrointestinal symptoms.

2. "Unfriendly" microorganisms such as disease-causing bacteria, yeasts, fungi, and parasites can also upset the balance. Researchers are exploring whether probiotics could halt these unfriendly agents in the first place and/or suppress their growth and activity in conditions like the following:

- Infectious diarrhea

- Irritable bowel syndrome

- Inflammatory bowel disease (e.g., ulcerative colitis and Crohn disease)

- Infection with *Helicobacter pylori* (*H. pylori*), a bacterium that causes most ulcers and many types of chronic stomach inflammation

- Tooth decay and periodontal disease

- Vaginal infections

- Stomach and respiratory infections that children acquire in daycare

- Skin infections

Another part of the interest in probiotics stems from the fact there are cells in the digestive tract connected with the immune system. One theory is that if you alter the microorganisms in a person's intestinal tract (as by introducing probiotic bacteria), you can affect the immune system's defenses.

What the Science Says

Scientific understanding of probiotics and their potential for preventing and treating health conditions is at an early stage, but moving ahead. In November 2005, a conference that was cofunded by the National Center for Complementary and Alternative Medicine (NCCAM) and convened by the American Society for Microbiology explored this topic.

According to the conference report, some uses of probiotics for which there is some encouraging evidence from the study of specific probiotic formulations are as follows:

- To treat diarrhea (this is the strongest area of evidence, especially for diarrhea from rotavirus)

- To prevent and treat infections of the urinary tract or female genital tract

- To treat irritable bowel syndrome

- To reduce recurrence of bladder cancer

- To shorten how long an intestinal infection lasts that is caused by a bacterium called *Clostridium difficile*

- To prevent and treat pouchitis (a condition that can follow surgery to remove the colon)

- To prevent and manage atopic dermatitis (eczema) in children

The conference panel also noted that in studies of probiotics as cures, any beneficial effect was usually low; a strong placebo effect often occurs; and more research (especially in the form of large, carefully designed clinical trials) is needed in order to draw firmer conclusions.

Some other areas of interest to researchers on probiotics include the following:

- An area of interest is what is going on at the molecular level with the bacteria themselves and how they may interact with the body (such as the gut and its bacteria) to prevent and treat diseases. Advances in technology and medicine are making it possible to study these areas much better than in the past.

- Issues of quality are also of interest. For example, what happens when probiotic bacteria are treated or are added to foods—is their ability to survive, grow, and have a therapeutic effect altered?

- Scientists want to understand the best ways to administer probiotics for therapeutic purposes, as well as the best doses and schedules.

- Scientists want to understand probiotics' potential to help with the problem of antibiotic-resistant bacteria in the gut.

- Another area of interest is whether they can prevent unfriendly bacteria from getting through the skin or mucous membranes and traveling through the body (e.g., which can happen with burns, shock, trauma, or suppressed immunity).

Side Effects and Risks

Some live microorganisms have a long history of use as probiotics without causing illness in people. Probiotics' safety has not been thoroughly studied scientifically, however. More information is especially needed on how safe they are for young children, elderly people, and people with compromised immune systems.

Probiotics' side effects, if they occur, tend to be mild and digestive (such as gas or bloating). More serious effects have been seen in some people. Probiotics might theoretically cause infections that need to be treated with antibiotics, especially in people with underlying health conditions. They could also cause unhealthy metabolic activities, too much stimulation of the immune system, or gene transfer (insertion of genetic material into a cell).

Probiotic products taken by mouth as a dietary supplement are manufactured and regulated as foods, not drugs.

Some Other Points to Consider

- If you are thinking about using a probiotic product as CAM, consult your health care provider first. No CAM therapy should be used in place of conventional medical care or to delay seeking that care.

- Effects from one species or strain of probiotics do not necessarily hold true for others, or even for different preparations of the same species or strain.

- If you use a probiotic product and experience an effect that concerns you, contact your health care provider.

Chapter 34

Sports and Energy Supplements

Chapter Contents

Section 34.1—Sports Supplements 226

Section 34.2—Energy Drinks 231

Section 34.1

Sports Supplements

If you're a competitive athlete or a fitness buff, improving your sports performance is probably on your mind. Lots of people wonder if taking sports supplements could offer fast, effective results without so much hard work. But do sports supplements really work? And are they safe?

What Are Sports Supplements?

Sports supplements (also called ergogenic aids) are products used to enhance athletic performance that may include vitamins, minerals, amino acids, herbs, or botanicals (plants)—or any concentration, extract, or combination of these. These products are generally available over the counter without a prescription.

Sports supplements are considered a dietary supplement. Dietary supplements do not require U.S. Food and Drug Administration (FDA) approval before they come on the market. Supplement manufacturers do have to follow the FDA's current good manufacturing practices to ensure quality and safety of their product, though. And the FDA is responsible for taking action if a product is found to be unsafe after it has gone on the market.

Critics of the supplement industry point out cases where manufacturers haven't done a good job of following standards. They also mention instances where the FDA hasn't enforced regulations. Both of these can mean that supplements contain variable amounts of ingredients or even ingredients not listed on the label.

Some over-the-counter medicines and prescription medications, including anabolic steroids, are used to enhance performance but they are not considered supplements. Although medications are FDA approved, using medicines—even over-the-counter ones—in ways other than their intended purpose puts the user at risk of serious side effects.

For example, teen athletes who use medications like human growth hormone (hGH) that haven't been prescribed for them may have problems with development and hormone levels.

Lots of sports organizations have developed policies on sports supplements. The National Football League (NFL), the National Collegiate Athletic Association (NCAA), and the International Olympic Committee (IOC) have banned the use of steroids, ephedra, and androstenedione by their athletes, and competitors who use them face fines, ineligibility, and suspension from their sports.

The National Federation of State High School Associations (NFHS) strongly recommends that student athletes consult with their doctor before taking any supplement.

Common Supplements and How They Affect the Body

Whether you hear about sports supplements from your teammates in the locker room or the sales clerk at your local vitamin store, chances are you're not getting the whole story about how supplements work, if they are really effective, and the risks you take by using them.

Androstenedione and DHEA

Androstenedione (also known as andro) and dehydroepiandrosterone (also known as DHEA) are prohormones or "natural steroids" that can be broken down into testosterone. When researchers studied these prohormones in adult athletes, DHEA and andro did not increase muscle size, improve strength, or enhance performance.

The side effects of these "natural" steroid supplements like DHEA and andro aren't well known. But experts believe that, when taken in large doses, they cause effects similar to stronger anabolic steroids.

What is known is that andro and DHEA can cause hormone imbalances in people who use them. Both may have the same effects as taking anabolic steroids and may lead to dangerous side effects like testicular cancer, infertility, stroke, and an increased risk of heart disease. As with anabolic steroids, teens who use andro while they are still growing may not reach their full adult height. Natural steroid supplements can also cause breast development and shrinking of testicles in guys.

Creatine

Creatine is already manufactured by the body in the liver, kidneys, and pancreas. It also occurs naturally in foods such as meat and fish. Creatine supplements are available over the counter, and teens make up a large portion of the supplement's users.

People who take creatine usually take it to improve strength, but the long-term and short-term effects of creatine use haven't been studied in teens and kids. Research in adults found that creatine is most effective for athletes doing intermittent high-intensity exercise with short recovery intervals, such as sprinting and power lifting. However, researchers found no effect on athletic performance in nearly a third of athletes studied. Creatine has not been found to increase endurance or improve aerobic performance.

The most common side effects of creatine supplements include weight gain, diarrhea, abdominal pain, and muscle cramps. People with kidney problems should not use creatine because it may affect kidney function. The American College of Sports Medicine recommends that people younger than 18 years old do not use creatine. If you are considering using creatine, talk with your doctor about the risks and benefits, as well as appropriate dosing.

Fat Burners

Fat burners (sometimes known as thermogenics) were often made with an herb called ephedra, also known as ephedrine or ma huang, which acts as a stimulant and increases metabolism. Some athletes use fat burners to lose weight or to increase energy—but ephedra-based products can be one of the most dangerous supplements. Evidence has shown that it can cause heart problems, stroke, and occasionally even death.

Because athletes and others have died using this supplement, ephedra has been taken off the market. Since the ban, "ephedra-free" products have emerged, but they often contain ingredients with ephedra-like properties, including bitter orange or country mallow. Similar to ephedra, these supplements can cause high blood pressure, heart attack, stroke, and seizures.

Many of these products also contain caffeine, along with other caffeine sources (such as yerba mate and guarana). This combination may lead to restlessness, anxiety, racing heart, irregular heart beat, and increases the chance of having a life-threatening side effect.

Will Supplements Make Me a Better Athlete?

Sports supplements haven't been tested on teens and kids. But studies on adults show that the claims of many supplements are weak at best. Most won't make you any stronger, and none will make you any faster or more skillful.

Many factors go into your abilities as an athlete—including your diet, how much sleep you get, genetics and heredity, and your training program. But the fact is that using sports supplements may put you at risk for serious health conditions. So instead of turning to supplements to improve your performance, concentrate on nutrition and follow a weight-training and aerobic-conditioning program.

Tips for Dealing with Athletic Pressure and Competition

Advertisements for sports supplements often use persuasive before and after pictures that make it look easy to get a muscular, toned body. But the goal of supplement advertisers is to make money by selling more supplements, and many claims may be misleading. Teens and kids may seem like an easy sell on supplements because they may feel dissatisfied or uncomfortable with their still-developing bodies, and many supplement companies try to convince teens that supplements are an easy solution.

Don't waste your money on expensive and dangerous supplements. Instead, try these tips for getting better game:

- **Make downtime a priority.** Studies show that teens need more than 8 hours of sleep a night, and sleep is important for athletes. Organize time for sleep into your schedule by doing as much homework as possible on the weekend or consider cutting back on after-school job hours during your sports season.

- **Try to relax.** Your school, work, and sports schedules may have you sprinting from one activity to the next, but taking a few minutes to relax can be helpful. Meditating or visualizing your success during the next game may improve your performance; sitting quietly and focusing on your breathing can give you a brief break and prepare you for your next activity.

- **Choose good eats.** Fried, fatty, or sugary foods will interfere with your performance. Instead, focus on eating foods such as lean meats, whole grains, vegetables, fruits, and low-fat dairy products. Celebrating with the team at the local pizza place after a big game is fine once in a while. But for most meals and snacks, choose healthy foods to keep your weight in a healthy range and your performance at its best.

- **Eat often.** Sometimes people skip breakfast or have an early lunch, then try to play a late afternoon game. Not getting enough food to fuel an activity can quickly wear you out—and even place you at risk for injury or muscle fatigue. Be sure to eat lunch on practice and game days. If you feel hungry before the game, pack easy-to-carry, healthy snacks in your bag, such as fruit, trail mix, or string cheese. It's important to eat well after a workout.

- **Avoid harmful substances.** Smoking will diminish your lung capacity and your ability to breathe, alcohol can make you sluggish and tired, and can impair your hand-eye coordination and reduce your alertness. And you can kiss your team good-bye if you get caught using drugs or alcohol—many schools have a no-tolerance policy for harmful substances.

- **Train harder and smarter.** If you get out of breath easily during your basketball game and you want to increase your endurance, work on improving your cardiovascular conditioning. If you think more leg strength will help you excel on the soccer field, consider weight training to increase your muscle strength. Before changing your program, though, get advice from your doctor.

- **Consult a professional.** If you're concerned about your weight or whether your diet is helping your performance, talk to your doctor or a registered dietitian who can evaluate your nutrition and steer you in the right direction. Coaches can help too. And if you're still convinced that supplements will help you, talk to your doctor or a sports medicine specialist. The doc will be able to offer alternatives to supplements based on your body and sport.

Section 34.2

Energy Drinks

Excerpted from "Energy Drinks: Power Boosts or Empty Boasts?" by the Substance Abuse and Mental Health Services Administration (SAMHSA, family.samhsa.gov), part of the U.S. Department of Health and Human Services, April 30, 2007.

Slick packaging, edgy themes, exotic ingredients, and special formulas are all part of the hype about energy drinks. A growing number of beverages promise quick energy as well as performance and nutritional benefits to athletes, students, partygoers—anyone who wants a pick-me-up. Yet, claims about these products often are inflated while health risks such as dehydration, overstimulation, and the double danger of combining energy drinks with alcohol receive little attention.

Do you know what your child drinks between meals and when he works out or plays sports? Make sure both of you understand which ingredients energy drinks contain and the effects they produce.

Looking for a Liquid Lift

The energy drink market is hot. With names that suggest extreme power, a growing number of beverages are aimed at anyone who wants to improve athletic performance, study late, dance all night, or just counter a mid-afternoon slump.

These products are sold with claims that include boosting energy, raising alertness, lowering reaction time, improving concentration, speeding up metabolism, increasing stamina, and enhancing nutrition. Perhaps the most powerful energy drink is named after an illegal drug. Although this product does not contain the drug, it promises a high followed by a long-lasting energy buzz.

What's behind these claims? Although the makers of energy drinks tout mixtures of vitamins, minerals, and tropical extracts, the main ingredient is caffeine. The difference between the caffeine in energy drinks and other beverages is the amount—they have at least as much caffeine as coffee and much more than soft drinks.

Caffeine Concerns

Caffeine perks up the central nervous system and provides the lift that energy drinks are all about. The central nervous system, which includes the brain and the spinal cord, is the main "processing center" that controls all of the body's organs and systems.

However, the high levels of caffeine in energy drinks can cause problems. Because caffeine can send you to the bathroom more often, it can dehydrate your body—meaning that you do not have as much water and fluids as you should—when you are also sweating during exercise.

Caffeine also can speed up a person's heart and raise blood pressure. The amount of caffeine in energy drinks is not good for children. Caffeine may cause a child to become agitated, irritable, or nervous. In addition, caffeine is a concern for pregnant women as well as the children they carry. The Food and Drug Administration advises pregnant women to use caffeine in moderation.

How much caffeine is too much? It depends—the effects of caffeine vary from one person to another according to traits such as age, size, and health. For most people, three 8-ounce cups of coffee per day is considered a moderate amount of caffeine.

Mixing energy drinks with alcohol poses a special risk. The stimulation from a caffeine-heavy energy drink can make a person feel less intoxicated than she really is. As a result, she may keep drinking or take a risk such as driving without realizing the danger. In addition, because caffeine dehydrates the body, alcohol becomes harder to absorb, which makes its toxic effects much more damaging to the body.

School starts early, activities and jobs create tight schedules, and nighttime often finds today's youth up late doing homework, listening to music, playing computer games, and instant messaging their friends. As a result, kids often do not get the sleep they need, leaving them more likely to reach for a caffeine jolt. In fact, the more caffeine kids consume, the less sleep they get. So, work with your child to adjust his schedule so he has enough time for sleep and offer him noncaffeinated drinks such as juice, milk, and water after dinner.

What's in the Mix?

Other energy drink ingredients add to the possible problems. Guarana, or guarine, is a caffeine-like substance. Taurine is an amino acid that the body produces naturally, but exactly how it works or how much is too much is not known. Vitamins, minerals, and herbs added to energy drinks are not risky by themselves, but they could upset one's nutritional balance and could cause a bad reaction to medication.

Finally, energy drinks contain carbohydrates—carbs for short—that we need to fuel long exercise sessions. However, energy drinks provide more carbs than most people need for exercise. The result—excess calories—is just what we are trying to avoid or burn off. And because carbs make it harder for the body to absorb fluids, they can cause dehydration, especially in hot weather.

Choosing Wisely

While an energy drink every so often will not be a problem for most people, make sure that your child knows the real deal about these products. Talk with him about situations in which sports drinks could have unexpected effects. Remind him that many other products or just plain water can give him the lift he is looking for, often at a much lower cost than an energy drink. Making careful choices when he wants to kick it up a notch will pay off in safety and results. As a bonus, he'll end up with more money in his pocket.

Chapter 35

Supplements Used
for Weight Loss

Chapter Contents

Section 35.1— Green Tea... 236
Section 35.2—Hoodia 238

Section 35.1

Green Tea

Excerpted from text by the National Center for Complementary and Alternative Medicine (NCCAM, nccam.nih.gov), part of the National Institutes of Health, November 2008.

This text provides basic information about green tea. All types of tea (green, black, and oolong) are produced from the *Camellia sinensis* plant using different methods. Fresh leaves from the *Camellia sinensis* plant are steamed to produce green tea. Common names include green tea, Chinese tea, and Japanese tea. The Latin name for green tea is *Camellia sinensis*.

What Green Tea Is Used For

- Green tea and green tea extracts, such as its component EGCG [epigallocatechin gallate], have been used to prevent and treat a variety of cancers, including breast, stomach, and skin cancers.

- Green tea and green tea extracts have also been used for improving mental alertness, aiding in weight loss, lowering cholesterol levels, and protecting skin from sun damage.

How Green Tea Is Used

Green tea is usually brewed and drunk as a beverage. Green tea extracts can be taken in capsules and are sometimes used in skin products.

What the Science Says

- Laboratory studies suggest that green tea may help protect against or slow the growth of certain cancers, but studies in people have shown mixed results.

- Some evidence suggests that the use of green tea preparations improves mental alertness, most likely because of its caffeine content. There are not enough reliable data to determine whether green tea can aid in weight loss, lower blood cholesterol levels, or protect the skin from sun damage.

- NCCAM is supporting studies to learn more about the components in green tea and their effects on conditions such as cancer, diabetes, and heart disease.

Side Effects and Cautions

- Green tea is safe for most adults when used in moderate amounts.

- There have been some case reports of liver problems in people taking concentrated green tea extracts. This problem does not seem to be connected with green tea infusions or beverages. Although these cases are very rare and the evidence is not definitive, experts suggest that concentrated green tea extracts be taken with food, and that people should discontinue use and consult a heath care practitioner if they have a liver disorder or develop symptoms of liver trouble, such as abdominal pain, dark urine, or jaundice.

- Green tea and green tea extracts contain caffeine. Caffeine can cause insomnia, anxiety, irritability, upset stomach, nausea, diarrhea, or frequent urination in some people.

- Green tea contains small amounts of vitamin K, which can make anticoagulant drugs, such as warfarin, less effective.

- Tell your health care providers about any complementary and alternative practices you use. Give them a full picture of what you do to manage your health. This will help ensure coordinated and safe care.

Section 35.2

Hoodia

Excerpted from text by the National Center for Complementary and
Alternative Medicine (NCCAM, nccam.nih.gov), part of the National
Institutes of Health, June 2008.

This text provides basic information about the herb hoodia. Hoodia is a flowering, cactus-like plant native to the Kalahari Desert in southern Africa. Its harvest is protected by conservation laws. Common names include hoodia, Kalahari cactus, and Xhoba. The Latin name for it is *Hoodia gordonii*.

What Hoodia Is Used For

- Kalahari Bushmen have traditionally eaten hoodia stems to reduce their hunger and thirst during long hunts.

- Today, hoodia is marketed as an appetite suppressant for weight loss.

How Hoodia Is Used

Dried extracts of hoodia stems and roots are used to make capsules, powders, and chewable tablets. Hoodia can also be used in liquid extracts and teas. Hoodia products often contain other herbs or minerals, such as green tea or chromium picolinate.

What the Science Says

There is no reliable scientific evidence to support hoodia's use. No studies of the herb in people have been published.

Side Effects and Cautions

- Hoodia's safety is unknown. Its potential risks, side effects, and interactions with medicines and other supplements have not been studied.

- The quality of hoodia products varies widely. News reports suggest that some products sold as hoodia do not contain any hoodia.

- Tell your health care providers about any complementary and alternative practices you use. Give them a full picture of what you do to manage your health. This will help ensure coordinated and safe care.

Part Four

Biologically Based Therapies

Chapter 36

Biologically Based Therapies: An Overview

Definition of Scope of Field

The complementary and alternative medicine (CAM) domain of biologically based practices includes, but is not limited to, botanicals, animal-derived extracts, vitamins, minerals, fatty acids, amino acids, proteins, prebiotics and probiotics, whole diets, and functional foods.

Dietary supplements are a subset of this CAM domain. In the Dietary Supplement Health and Education Act (DSHEA) of 1994, Congress defined a dietary supplement as a product taken by mouth that contains a "dietary ingredient" intended to supplement the diet. The "dietary ingredients" in these products may include vitamins, minerals, herbs or other botanicals, amino acids, and substances such as enzymes, organ tissues, glandulars, and metabolites. Dietary supplements can also be extracts or concentrates, and they can occur in many forms, such as tablets, capsules, softgels, gelcaps, liquids, or powders.

The Food and Drug Administration (FDA) regulates dietary supplements differently than drug products (either prescription or over-the-counter). First, drugs are required to follow defined good manufacturing practices (GMPs). The FDA is developing GMPs for dietary supplements. However, until they are issued, companies must follow existing manufacturing requirements for foods. Second, drug products must

Excerpted from "Biologically Based Practices: An Overview," by the National Center for Complementary and Alternative Medicine (NCCAM, nccam.nih.gov), part of the National Institutes of Health, March 2007.

be approved by the FDA as safe and efficacious prior to marketing. In contrast, manufacturers of dietary supplements are responsible for ensuring that their products are safe. While the FDA monitors adverse effects after dietary supplement products are on the market, newly marketed dietary supplements are not subject to premarket approval or a specific postmarket surveillance period. Third, while DSHEA requires companies to substantiate claims of benefit, citation of existing literature is considered sufficient to validate such claims. Manufacturers are not required, as they are for drugs, to submit such substantiation data to the FDA; instead, it is the Federal Trade Commission that has primary responsibility for monitoring dietary supplements for truth in advertising. A 2004 Institute of Medicine (IOM) report on the safety of dietary supplements recommends a framework for cost-effective and science-based evaluation by the FDA.

History and Demographic Use of Biologically Based Practices

Dietary supplements reflect some of humankind's first attempts to improve the human condition. The personal effects of the mummified prehistoric "Ice Man" found in the Italian Alps in 1991 included medicinal herbs. By the Middle Ages, thousands of botanical products had been inventoried for their medicinal effects. Many of these, including digitalis and quinine, form the basis of modern drugs.

Interest in and use of dietary supplements have grown considerably in the past two decades. Consumers state that their primary reason for using herbal supplements is to promote overall health and wellness, but they also report using supplements to improve performance and energy, to treat and prevent illnesses (e.g., colds and flu), and to alleviate depression. According to a 2002 national survey on Americans' use of CAM, use of supplements may be more frequent among Americans who have one or more health problems, who have specific diseases such as breast cancer, who consume high amounts of alcohol, or who are obese. Supplement use differs by ethnicity and across income strata. On average, users tend to be women, older, better educated, live in one- or two-person households, have slightly higher incomes, and live in metropolitan areas.

Use of vitamin and mineral supplements, a subset of dietary supplements, by the U.S. population has been a growing trend since the 1970s. National surveys—such as the Third National Health and Nutrition Examination Survey (NHANES III, 1988–1994); NHANES, 1999–2000; and the 1987 and 1992 National Health Interview Surveys—indicate that 40 to 46 percent of Americans reported taking at least one vitamin or mineral supplement at some time within the month surveyed. Data from national surveys collected before the enactment of DSHEA in 1994, however, may not reflect current supplement consumption patterns.

In 2002, sales of dietary supplements increased to an estimated $18.7 billion per year, with herbs/botanical supplements accounting for an estimated $4.3 billion in sales. Consumers consider the proposed benefits of herbal supplements less believable than those of vitamins and minerals. From 2001 to 2003, sales of herbs experienced negative growth. This was attributed to consumers' withering confidence and confusion. Within the herbal category, however, formulas led single herbs in sales; products became increasingly condition-specific; and sales of women's products actually increased by approximately 25 percent.

In contrast to dietary supplements, functional foods are components of the usual diet that may have biologically active components (e.g., polyphenols, phytoestrogens, fish oils, carotenoids) that may provide health benefits beyond basic nutrition. Examples of functional foods include soy, nuts, chocolate, and cranberries. These foods' bioactive constituents are appearing with increasing frequency as ingredients in dietary supplements. Functional foods are marketed directly to consumers. Sales increased from $11.3 billion in 1995 to about $16.2 billion in 1999. Unlike dietary supplements, functional foods may claim specific health benefits. The Nutrition Labeling and Education Act (NLEA) of 1990 delineates the permissible labeling of these foods for health claims.

Whole diet therapy has become an accepted practice for some health conditions. However, the popularity of unproven diets, especially for the treatment of obesity, has risen to a new level as the prevalence of obesity and metabolic syndrome among Americans has increased and traditional exercise and diet "prescriptions" have failed. Popular diets today include the Atkins, Zone, and Ornish diets, Sugar Busters, and others. The range of macronutrient distributions of these popular diets is very wide. The proliferation of diet books is phenomenal. Recently, food producers and restaurants have been targeting their marketing messages to reflect commercially successful low-carbohydrate diets.

Public need for information about dietary supplements, functional foods, and selected strict dietary regimens has driven research on the effectiveness and safety of these interventions and the dissemination of research findings.

Scope of the Research

Range of Studies

Research on dietary supplements spans the spectrum of basic to clinical research and includes ethnobotanical investigations, analytical research, and method development/validation, as well as bioavailability, pharmacokinetic, and pharmacodynamic studies. However, the basic and preclinical research is better delineated for supplements composed of single chemical constituents (e.g., vitamins and minerals) than for the more complex products (e.g., botanical extracts). There is an abundance of clinical research for all types of dietary supplements. Most of this research involves small phase II studies.

The literature on functional foods is vast and growing; it includes clinical trials, animal studies, experimental in vitro laboratory studies, and epidemiological studies. Much of the current evidence for functional foods is preliminary or not based on well-designed trials. However, the foundational evidence gained through other types of investigations is significant for some functional foods and their "health-promoting" constituents. The strongest evidence for effectiveness is that developed in accordance with the NLEA guidelines for preapproved health claims (e.g., oat bran or psyllium).

An important gap in knowledge concerns the role of diet composition in energy balance. Popular diets low in carbohydrates have been purported to enhance weight loss. Shorter-term clinical studies show equivocal results. In addition, mechanisms by which popular diets affect energy balance, if at all, are not well understood. Although numerous animal studies assessing the impact of diet composition on appetite and body weight have been conducted, these studies have been limited by availability and use of well-defined and standardized diets. The research on weight loss is more abundant than that on weight maintenance.

Primary Challenges

Many clinical studies of dietary supplements are flawed because of inadequate sample size, poor design, limited preliminary dosing data, lack of blinding even when feasible, and/or failure to incorporate objective or standardized outcome instruments. In addition, the lack of reliable data on the absorption, disposition, metabolism, and excretion of these entities in living systems has complicated the selection of products to be used in clinical trials. This is more problematic for complex preparations (e.g., botanicals) than for products composed of single chemical moieties (e.g., zinc).

The lack of consistent and reliable botanical products represents a formidable challenge both in clinical trials and in basic research. Most have not been sufficiently characterized or standardized for the conduct of clinical trials capable of adequately demonstrating safety or efficacy, or predicting that similarly prepared products would also be safe and effective in wider public use. Consequently, obtaining sufficient quantities of well-characterized products for evaluation in clinical trials would be advantageous. Several issues regarding the choice of clinical trial material require special attention, for example:

- Influences of climate and soil
- Use of different parts of the plants
- Use of different cultivars and species
- Optimal growing, harvesting, and storage conditions
- Use of the whole extract or a specific fraction
- Method of extraction
- Chemical standardization of the product
- Bioavailability of the formulation
- Dose and length of administration

Some nonbotanical dietary supplements, such as vitamins, carnitine, glucosamine, and melatonin, are single chemical entities. Botanicals, however, are complex mixtures. Their putative active ingredients may be identified, but are rarely known for certain. Usually, there is more than one of these ingredients, often dozens. When active compounds are unknown, it is necessary to identify marker or reference compounds, even though they may be unrelated to biological effects. Qualitative and quantitative determinations of the active and marker compounds, as well as the presence of product contaminants, can be assessed by capillary electrophoresis, gas chromatography, liquid chromatography-mass spectrometry, gas chromatography-mass spectrometry, high-performance liquid chromatography, and liquid chromatography-multidimensional nuclear magnetic resonance. Fingerprinting techniques can map out the spectrum of compounds in a plant extract. New applications of older techniques and new analytical methods continue to be developed and validated. However, there remains a paucity of analytical tools that are precise, accurate, specific, and robust. Steps are currently being taken to apply molecular tools, such as DNA fingerprinting, to verify species in products, while transient expression systems, and microarray and proteomic analyses, are beginning to be used to define the cellular and biological activities of dietary supplements.

Particular attention should be paid to the issues of complex botanicals and clinical dosing. Quality control of complex botanicals is difficult, but must be accomplished, because it is not ethical to administer an unknown product to patients. The use of a suboptimal dose that is safe but ineffective does not serve the larger goals of NCCAM, the CAM community, or public health. Although the trial would indicate only that the tested dose of the intervention was ineffective, the public might conclude that all doses of the intervention are ineffective, and patients would be denied a possible benefit from the intervention. Overdosing, on the other hand, might produce unnecessary adverse effects. Phase I/II studies should be conducted first to determine the safety of various doses, and the optimal dose should then be tested in a phase III trial. As a result, maximum benefit would be seen in the trial; also, any negative result would be definitive.

To a great extent, the difference between a dietary supplement and a drug lies in the use of the agent, not in the nature of the agent itself. If an herb, vitamin, mineral, or amino acid is used to resolve a nutritional deficiency or to improve or sustain the structure or function of the body, the agent is considered a dietary supplement. If the agent is used to diagnose, prevent, treat, or cure a disease, the agent is considered a drug. This distinction is key when the FDA determines whether proposed research on a product requires an investigational new drug (IND) exemption. If the proposed investigation of a lawfully marketed botanical dietary supplement is to study its effects on diseases (i.e., to cure, treat, mitigate, prevent, or diagnose a disease and its associated symptoms), then the supplement is more likely to be subject to IND requirements. The FDA has worked with NCCAM to provide direction to investigators and created a Botanical Review Team to ensure consistent interpretation of the document *Guidance for Industry—Botanical Drug Products*.

Similarly, little attention has been paid to the quality of probiotics. Quality issues for probiotic supplements may include the following:

- Viability of bacteria in the product

- Types and titer of bacteria in the product

- Stability of different strains under different storage conditions and in different product formats

- Enteric protection of the product

Therefore, for optimal studies, documentation of the type of bacteria (genus and species), potency (number of viable bacteria per dose), purity (presence of contaminating or ineffective microorganisms), and disintegration properties must be provided for any strain to be considered for use as a probiotic product. Speciation of the bacteria must be established by means of the most current, valid methodology.

Many of the challenges identified for research on dietary supplements, including issues of composition and characterization, are applicable to research on functional foods and whole diets. In addition, challenges of popular diet research include adherence to the protocol for longer-term studies, inability to blind participants to intervention assignment, and efficacy versus effectiveness.

Summary of the Major Threads of Evidence

Over the past few decades, thousands of studies of various dietary supplements have been performed. To date, however, no single supplement has been proven effective in a compelling way. Nevertheless, there are several supplements for which early studies yielded positive, or at least encouraging, data. Good sources of information on some of them can be found at the Natural Medicines Comprehensive Database and a number of National Institutes of Health (NIH) websites. The NIH Office of Dietary Supplements (ODS) annually publishes a bibliography of resources on significant advances in dietary supplement research. Finally, the ClinicalTrials.gov database lists all NIH-supported clinical studies of dietary supplements that are actively accruing patients.

For a few dietary supplements, data have been deemed sufficient to warrant large-scale trials. For example, multicenter trials have concluded or are in progress on ginkgo (*Ginkgo biloba*) for prevention of dementia, glucosamine hydrochloride and chondroitin sulfate for osteoarthritis of the knee, saw palmetto (*Serenoa repens*)/African plum (*Prunus africana*) for benign prostatic hypertrophy, vitamin E/selenium for prevention of prostate cancer, shark cartilage for lung cancer, and St. John's wort (*Hypericum perforatum*) for major and minor depression. The results of one of the depression studies showed that St. John's wort is no more effective for treating major depression of moderate severity than placebo. Other studies of this herb, including its possible value in treatment of minor depression, are under way.

Reviews of the data regarding some dietary supplements have been conducted, including some by the members of the Cochrane Collaboration. The Agency for Healthcare Research and Quality has produced a number of evidence-based reviews of dietary supplements, including garlic, antioxidants, milk thistle, omega-3 fatty acids, ephedra, and S-adenosyl-L-methionine (SAMe). The following are examples of findings from some of these reviews:

- Analysis of the literature shows generally disappointing results for the efficacy of antioxidant supplementation (vitamins C and E, and coenzyme Q10) to prevent or treat cancer. Because this finding contrasts with the benefits reported from observational studies, additional research is needed to understand why these two sources of evidence disagree.

- Similarly, the literature on the roles of the antioxidants vitamins C and E and coenzyme Q10 for cardiovascular disease also shows discordance between observational and experimental data. Therefore, the thrust of new research into antioxidants and cardiovascular disease should be randomized trials.

- The clinical efficacy of milk thistle to improve liver function is not clearly established. Interpretation of the evidence is hampered by poor study methods or poor quality of reporting in publications. Possible benefit has been shown most frequently, but not consistently, for improvement in aminotransferase levels. Liver function tests are overwhelmingly the most common outcome measure studied. Available evidence is not sufficient to suggest whether milk thistle is more effective for some liver diseases than others. Available evidence does suggest that milk thistle is associated with few, and generally minor, adverse effects. Despite substantial in vitro and animal research, the mechanism of action of milk thistle is not well defined and may be multifactorial.

- The review of SAMe for the treatment of depression, osteoarthritis, and liver disease identified a number of promising areas for future research. For example, it would be helpful to conduct (1) additional review studies, studies elucidating the pharmacology of SAMe, and clinical trials; (2) studies that would lead to a better understanding of the risk-benefit ratio of SAMe compared to that of conventional therapy; (3) good dose-escalation studies using the oral formulation of SAMe for depression, osteoarthritis, or liver disease; and (4) larger clinical trials once the efficacy of the most effective oral dose of SAMe has been demonstrated.

- Two high-quality randomized controlled trials provide good evidence that cranberry juice may decrease the number of symptomatic urinary tract infections in women over a 12-month period. It

250

is not clear if it is effective in other groups. The fact that a large number of women dropped out of these studies indicates that cranberry juice may not be acceptable over long periods of time. Finally, the optimal dosage or method of administration of cranberry products (e.g., juice or tablets) is not clear.

There has been some study of other popular dietary supplements. For example, valerian is an herb often consumed as a tea for improved sleep, and melatonin is a pineal hormone touted for the same purpose. Small studies suggest that these two supplements may relieve insomnia, and there may be little harm in a trial course of either one. Echinacea has long been taken to treat or prevent colds; other supplements currently used for colds include zinc lozenges and high doses of vitamin C. As yet, only moderate-sized studies have been conducted with echinacea or zinc, and their outcomes have been conflicting. Large trials of high doses of oral vitamin C showed little, if any, benefit in preventing or treating the common cold.

Because of widespread use, often for centuries, and because the products are "natural," many people assume dietary supplements to be inert or at least innocuous. Yet, recent studies show clearly that interactions between these products and drugs do occur. For example, the active ingredients in ginkgo extract are reported to have antioxidant properties and to inhibit platelet aggregation. Several cases have been reported of increased bleeding associated with ginkgo's use with drugs that have anticoagulant or antiplatelet effects. St. John's wort induces a broad range of enzymes that metabolize drugs and transport them out of the body. It has been shown to interact with a number of drugs that serve as substrates for the cytochrome P450 CYP3A enzymes responsible for metabolism of approximately 60 percent of current pharmaceutical agents. Other dietary supplements shown to potentiate or interfere with prescription drugs include garlic, glucosamine, ginseng (Panax), saw palmetto, soy, valerian, and yohimbe.

In addition to interacting with other agents, some herbal supplements can be toxic. Misidentification, contamination, and adulteration may contribute to some of the toxicities. But other toxicities may result from the products themselves. For example, in 2001, extracts of kava were associated with fulminant liver failure. More recently, the FDA banned the sale of ephedra after it was shown to be associated with an increased risk of adverse events.

The FDA lists warnings and safety information on dietary supplements (e.g., androstenedione, aristolochic acid, comfrey, kava, and PC SPES) as they become available.

Chapter 37

Apitherapy

What is apitherapy?

As a technique, it is the medical use of the products of the honeybee hive often used with essential oils.

As a philosophy, it is a form of harmony between the individual and the environment.

As a medical principle, it is primarily the cultivation of health and its re-establishment when sickness interferes.

What products are used in apitherapy?

They are: honey, pollen, propolis, royal jelly, and bee venom. These products can be used individually. More frequently, several of those are used together.

Essential oils, already present in honey and propolis, are often used in conjunction with the products of the hive.

What kinds of conditions are treated with apitherapy?

Currently the most popular and well-known uses of honeybee venom in the United States are for people suffering from MS [multiple sclerosis] and many forms of arthritis. Now, the only condition that has actual scientific data supporting the use of apitherapy for treatment is post-herpetic neuralgia. There were several articles written

"Frequently Asked Questions about Apitherapy," © 2009 American Apitherapy Association (www.apitherapy.org). Reprinted with permission.

in the first half of the 1900s about using bee venom in the treatment of osteoarthritis and rheumatoid arthritis and there is some ongoing research now looking at its effect in multiple sclerosis. Anecdotal reports suggest that it might have some usefulness in the treatment of infectious, autoimmune, cardiovascular, pulmonary, gastrointestinal, neuropathic pain, and other chronic pain conditions.

How are MS and arthritis treated?

Bee venom, in synergy with other bee products, is the major therapeutic agent. Live bee stings or a commercially available venom extract which can be injected by doctors are used in conjunction with one or more of the products of the bee hive mentioned above.

Where can I find someone who can help me with apitherapy?

The American Apitherapy Society (AAS) has information on its database of practitioners and of people ready to give information and assistance. This information is available to society members.

Who practices apitherapy?

Practitioners include physicians, nurses, acupuncturists, and naturopaths, as well as interested laypersons including bee keepers who can provide persons who want bee venom therapy with bees and instruct them how to treat themselves.

Is apitherapy covered by insurance?

No, however, many AAS members practitioners do not charge for the procedure but some do charge for their time. A donation to AAS is appreciated to support the dissemination of information about and education about apitherapy. The amount of the donation can vary and can be discussed with the practitioner. Joining the AAS is another way to support the organization and you get an informative and entertaining newsletter quarterly as part of the membership.

Is apitherapy a recognized therapy in the United States?

No official body in the United States has sanctioned apitherapy as a recognized treatment modality. Bee venom has been approved by the FDA [U.S. Food and Drug Administration] for desensitization purposes only. Apitherapy is considered, from both the legal and medical viewpoint, an experimental approach.

What about bee sting allergy?

Contrary to popular belief allergy to honeybee sting is relatively rare: About seven in 1,000 persons are allergic. Of this proportion only a small percentage risks anaphylactic shock. Nevertheless bee venom treatment is always to be preceded by a test of sensitivity. A sensitive person can be d-sensitized to bee venom, thus allowing apitherapy to proceed. AAS recommends that anyone that uses or administers bee venom have readily available an epinephrine kit to be used in case of anaphylactic response and know how to use it. Many people erroneously consider swelling after a sting to be an allergic reaction. Swelling is a normal response of the body as are localized redness, swelling, and itching.

Chapter 38

Aromatherapy and Essential Oils

What is aromatherapy?

Aromatherapy is the use of essential oils from plants to support and balance the mind, body, and spirit. It is used by patients with cancer mainly as a form of supportive care that may improve quality of life and reduce stress and anxiety. Aromatherapy may be combined with other complementary treatments like massage therapy and acupuncture, as well as with standard treatments.

Essential oils (also known as volatile oils) are the basic materials of aromatherapy. They are made from fragrant essences found in many plants. These essences are made in special plant cells, often under the surface of leaves, bark, or peel, using energy from the sun and elements from the air, soil, and water. If the plant material is crushed, the essence and its unique fragrance are released.

When essences are extracted from plants in natural ways, they become essential oils. They may be distilled with steam and/or water, or mechanically pressed. Oils that are made with chemical processes are not considered true essential oils.

There are many essential oils used in aromatherapy, including Roman chamomile, geranium, lavender, tea tree, lemon, cedarwood, and bergamot. Each type of essential oil has a different chemical structure that affects how it smells, how it is absorbed, and how it is used by

PDQ® Cancer Information Summary. National Cancer Institute; Bethesda, MD. Aromatherapy and Essential Oils (PDQ®): CAM—Patient. Updated 01/2010. Available at http://cancer.gov. Accessed January 13, 2009.

the body. Even varieties of plants within the same species may have chemical structures different from each other because they are grown or harvested in different ways or locations.

Essential oils are very concentrated. For example, it takes about 220 pounds of lavender flowers to make about 1 pound of essential oil. Essential oils are very volatile, evaporating quickly when they come in contact with air.

What is the history of the discovery and use of aromatherapy as a complementary and alternative treatment for cancer?

Fragrant plants have been used in healing practices for thousands of years across many cultures, including ancient China, India, and Egypt. Ways to extract essential oils from plants were first discovered during the Middle Ages.

The history of modern aromatherapy began in the early 20th century, when French chemist Rene Gattefosse coined the term "aromatherapie" and studied the effects of essential oils on many kinds of diseases. In the 1980s and 1990s, aromatherapy was rediscovered in Western countries as interest in complementary and alternative medicine (CAM) began to grow.

What is the theory behind the claim that aromatherapy is useful in treating cancer?

Aromatherapy is generally not suggested as a treatment for cancer, but as a form of supportive care to manage symptoms of cancer or side effects of cancer treatment. There are different theories about how aromatherapy and essential oils work. One theory is that smell receptors in the nose may respond to the smells of essential oils by sending chemical messages along nerve pathways to the brain's limbic system, which affects moods and emotions. Imaging studies in humans help show the effects of smells on the limbic system and its emotional pathways. Another theory suggests that because essential oils are extracted from whole aromatic plants, they have a life force or vitality that can affect the body in unique ways.

How is aromatherapy administered?

Aromatherapy is most often used in one of two ways:

- **Inhalation (taking into the body by breathing):** This can be done by using a diffuser or placing drops of essential oils near the patient.

- **Topical treatment (applied to the surface of the body), usually in a diluted form:** This can be done by massaging with essential oils diluted in a carrier oil, or by using essential oils in bath water, lotions, or dressings.

Aromatherapy is rarely taken by mouth.

There are some essential oils commonly chosen to treat specific conditions. However, the types of oils used and the ways they are combined may vary, depending on the experience and training of the aromatherapist. This lack of standard methods has led to conflicting research on the effects of aromatherapy.

Have any preclinical (laboratory or animal) studies been conducted using aromatherapy?

Many studies of essential oils have found that they have antibacterial effects when applied to the skin. In addition, studies in rats have shown that different essential oils can be calming or energizing. When rats were exposed to certain fragrances under stressful conditions, their behavior and immune responses were improved.

One study showed that after essential oils were inhaled, markers of the fragrance compounds were found in the bloodstream, suggesting that aromatherapy affects the body directly like a drug, rather than indirectly through the central nervous system.

Have any clinical trials (research studies with people) of aromatherapy been conducted?

Clinical trials of aromatherapy have mainly studied its use in the treatment of stress, anxiety, and other health-related conditions in seriously ill patients. Several clinical trials of aromatherapy in patients with cancer have been published with mixed results.

A few early studies have shown that aromatherapy may improve quality of life in patients with cancer. Some patients receiving aromatherapy have reported improvement in symptoms such as nausea or pain, and have lower blood pressure, pulse, and respiratory rates.

A small study of tea tree oil as a topical treatment to clear antibiotic -resistant MRSA [methicillin-resistant *Staphylococcus aureus*] bacteria from the skin of hospital patients found that it was as effective as the standard treatment. No studies in scientific or medical literature discuss aromatherapy as a treatment for cancer.

Have any side effects or risks been reported from aromatherapy?

Safety testing on essential oils shows very few bad side effects or risks when they are used as directed. Some essential oils have been approved as ingredients in food and are classified as GRAS (generally recognized as safe) by the U.S. Food and Drug Administration, within specific limits. Eating large amounts of essential oils is not recommended.

Allergic reactions and skin irritation may occur in aromatherapists or in patients, especially when essential oils are in contact with the skin for long periods of time. Sun sensitivity may develop when citrus or other oils are applied to the skin before sun exposure.

Lavender and tea tree oils have been found to have some hormone-like effects. They have effects similar to estrogen (female sex hormone) and also block or decrease the effect of androgens (male sex hormones). Applying lavender and tea tree oils to the skin over a long period of time has been linked to breast enlargement in boys who have not yet reached puberty. It is not known if the use of lavender and tea tree oils is safe for women who have a high risk for breast cancer that is estrogen-receptive.

Is aromatherapy approved by the U.S. Food and Drug Administration (FDA) for use as a cancer treatment in the United States?

Aromatherapy products do not need approval by the Food and Drug Administration because no specific claims are made for the treatment of cancer or other diseases.

Aromatherapy is not regulated by state law, and there is no licensing required to practice aromatherapy in the United States. Professionals often combine aromatherapy training with another field in which they are licensed, for example, massage therapy, registered nursing, acupuncture, or naturopathy.

The National Association for Holistic Aromatherapy (www.naha. org) and the Alliance of International Aromatherapists (www.alliance-aromatherapists.org) are two organizations that have national educational standards for aromatherapists. The National Association for Holistic Aromatherapy (NAHA) plans to have a standard aromatherapy certification in the United States. At this time, there are 19 schools that offer certificate programs approved by NAHA. National exams in aromatherapy are held twice a year.

The Canadian Federation of Aromatherapists (www.cfacanada.com) certifies aromatherapists in Canada. See the International Federation of Aromatherapists website (www.ifaroma.org) for a list of international aromatherapy programs.

Chapter 39

Diet-Based Therapies

Chapter Contents

Section 39.1—Detoxification Diets 264

Section 39.2—Fasting 267

Section 39.3—Gerson Therapy 269

Section 39.4—Macrobiotics 273

Section 39.5—Veganism 275

Section 39.6—Vegetarianism 279

Section 39.1

Detoxification Diets

What Is a Detox Diet?

The name sounds reassuring—everyone knows that anything toxic
is bad for you. Plus these diets encourage you to eat natural foods and
involve lots of water and veggies—all stuff you know is good for you.
You hear about celebrities going on detox diets, and people who go into
drug or alcohol rehabs are said to be detoxing. So shouldn't a detox
diet be a good bet?

Not really. Like many other fad diets, detox diets can have harmful
side effects, especially for teens.

A toxin is a chemical or poison that is known to have harmful effects
on the body. Toxins can come from food or water, from chemicals used
to grow or prepare food, and even from the air that we breathe. Our
bodies process those toxins through organs like the liver and kidneys
and eliminate them in the form of sweat, urine, and feces.

Although detox diet theories have not been proven scientifically, the
people who support them believe that toxins don't always leave our
bodies properly during the elimination of waste. Instead, they think
toxins hang around in our digestive, lymph, and gastrointestinal systems as well as in our skin and hair causing problems like tiredness,
headaches, and nausea.

The basic idea behind detox diets is to temporarily give up certain
kinds of foods that are thought to contain toxins. The idea is to purify
and purge the body of all the "bad" stuff. But the truth is, the human
body is designed to purify itself.

Detox diets vary. Most involve some version of a fast: that is, giving
up food for a couple of days and then gradually reintroducing certain
foods into the diet. Many of these diets also encourage people to have
colonic irrigation or enemas to "clean out" the colon. (An enema flushes

out the rectum and colon using water.) Others recommend that you take special teas or supplements to help the "purification" process.

There are lots of claims about what a detox diet can do, from preventing and curing disease to giving people more energy or focus. Of course, eating a diet lower in fat and higher in fiber can help many people feel healthier. But people who support detox diets claim that this is because of the elimination of toxins. There's no scientific proof that these diets help rid the body of toxins faster or that the elimination of toxins will make you a healthier, more energetic person.

What Should You Watch out For?

Detox diets are supposedly to help "clean out the system" but many people think they will lose weight if they try these diets. Here's the truth:

Detox diets are not recommended for teens. Normal teenagers need lots of nutritional goodies; like enough calories and protein to support rapid growth and development. So diets that involve fasting and severe restriction of food are not a good idea. For teens who are involved in sports and physical activities that require ample food, fasting does not provide enough fuel to support these activities. For these reasons, detox diets can be especially risky for teenagers.

Detox diets aren't for people with health conditions. They're not recommended for people with diabetes, heart disease, or other chronic medical conditions. Detox diets should be avoided if you are pregnant or have an eating disorder.

Detox diets can be addicting. That's because there's a certain feeling that comes from going without food or having an enema— almost like the high other people get from nicotine or alcohol. This can become a dangerous addiction that leads to health problems, including serious eating disorders, heart problems, and even death.

Detox supplements can have side effects. Many of the supplements used during detox diets are actually laxatives, which are designed to make people go to the bathroom more often, and that can get messy. Laxative supplements are never a good idea because they can cause dehydration, mineral imbalances, and problems with the digestive system.

Detox diets don't help people lose fat. Finally, people who fast for several days may drop pounds, but most of it will be water and some of it may be muscle. Most people regain the weight they lost soon after completing the program.

Detox diets are for short-term purposes only. In addition to causing other health problems, fasting for long periods can slow down a person's metabolism, making it harder to keep the weight off or to lose weight later.

Eat Right and Your Body Does the Rest

Of course, it's a great idea to eat lots of fruits and veggies, get lots of fiber, and drink water. But you also need to make sure you're getting all of the nutrients you need from other foods, including protein (from sources such as lean meats, eggs, beans, or peas) and calcium (from foods like low-fat or fat-free milk or yogurt). You definitely shouldn't start a detox diet or stop eating from any major food group without talking to your doctor or a registered dietitian.

The human body is designed to purify itself. Your liver and kidneys will do the job they're supposed to do if you eat a healthy diet that includes fiber, fruits, veggies, and plenty of water. If you're feeling tired or run down, or if you're concerned that you're overweight, talk with a doctor who can help you determine the cause and recommend ways to address the problem.

Section 39.2

Fasting

This treatment modality is used in place of conventional therapies to treat cancer. Seek advice from a qualified physician before replacing standard cancer therapy with fasting and juice therapies.

What do fasting and juice therapies involve?

Fasting, or voluntarily abstaining from food, and juice therapy, the consumption of certain fruit and vegetable juices instead of food, are believed by supporters to cleanse and detoxify the body internally. Fasting has long been practiced around the world as a part of religious beliefs to purify the soul. Only recently has fasting been thought to purify the physical body.

How are fasting and juice therapies thought to treat cancer?

Proponents believe that fasting or just consuming certain juices aids the body in cleansing itself of toxins and impurities. The immune system is believed by its supporters to work better, heal the body, and get rid of poisons when the body's physiologic systems have a chance to rest. Juice can also provide nutrients and calories if a patient is unable to keep solid food down.

What has been proven about the benefit of fasting and juice therapies?

The American Cancer Society does not believe that detoxification by fasting is based on scientific fact, nor does it cure cancer. While short-term fasting does aid weight loss in the severely obese, there is no evidence that it can rid the body of toxins or aid in treatment of disease. The mainstream medical community states the denying the body of necessary nutrients and calories actually weakens the immune system, resulting in the deterioration, not improvement, of health. Patients with advanced cancer are encouraged to avoid fasting. While not a magic cure-all, juice can serve as a valuable nutritional supplement for cancer patients. Juice does not contain fiber, fat, and protein and these need to be ingested as well to maintain energy and reach optimum health.

What is the potential risk or harm of fasting and juice therapies?

Fasting and juice therapies can cause fatigue, anemia, dizziness, and an irregular heartbeat. Supporters do not believe these are harmful symptoms. In fact, they view them as indicators of movement towards well-being and mental sharpness. Certain medical conditions such as diabetes can be aggravated by the ingestion of juices. Acidic citrus and tomato juices can irritate the stomach of sensitive patients.

How much do fasting and juice therapies cost?

Eating nothing or just juice is sure to cut back on one's grocery bill. Most treatments are self-help remedies and are performed at home. Occasionally, a physician might oversee the patient to ensure no additional health problems develop as a result of the therapy.

For Additional Information

American Association of Naturopathic Physicians
8201 Greensboro Drive, Suite 300
McLean, VA 22102
Phone: 877-969-2267
Website: www.naturopathic.org

Section 39.3

Gerson Therapy

PDQ® Cancer Information Summary. National Cancer Institute; Bethesda, MD. Gerson Therapy (PDQ®): CAM—Patient. Updated 06/2009. Available at http://cancer.gov. Accessed December 10, 2009.

What is the Gerson therapy?

The Gerson therapy has been used by some people to treat cancer and other diseases. It is based on the role of minerals, enzymes, and other dietary factors. There are three key parts to the therapy:

- **Diet:** Organic fruits, vegetables, and whole grains to give the body plenty of vitamins, minerals, enzymes, and other nutrients. The fruits and vegetables are low in sodium (salt) and high in potassium.

- **Supplementation:** The addition of certain substances to the diet to help correct cell metabolism (the chemical changes that take place in a cell to make energy and basic materials needed for the body's life processes).

- **Detoxification:** Treatments, including enemas, to remove toxic (harmful) substances from the body.

What is the history of the discovery and use of the Gerson therapy as a complementary or alternative treatment for cancer?

The Gerson therapy was named after Dr. Max B. Gerson (1881–1959), who first used it to treat his migraine headaches. In the 1930s, Dr. Gerson's therapy became known to the public as a treatment for a type of tuberculosis (TB). The Gerson therapy was later used to treat other conditions, including cancer.

What is the theory behind the claim that the Gerson therapy is useful in treating cancer?

The Gerson therapy is based on the idea that cancer develops when there are changes in cell metabolism because of the buildup of toxic substances in the body. Dr. Gerson said the disease process makes more toxins

269

and the liver becomes overworked. According to Dr. Gerson, people with cancer also have too much sodium and too little potassium in the cells in their bodies, which causes tissue damage and weakened organs.

The goal of the Gerson therapy is to restore the body to health by repairing the liver and returning the metabolism to its normal state. According to Dr. Gerson, this can be done by removing toxins from the body and building up the immune system with diet and supplements. The enemas are said to widen the bile ducts of the liver so toxins can be released. According to Dr. Gerson, the liver is further overworked as the treatment regimen breaks down cancer cells and rids the body of toxins. Pancreatic enzymes are given to decrease the demands on the weakened liver and pancreas to make enzymes for digestion. An organic diet and nutritional supplements are used to boost the immune system and support the body as the regimen cleans the body of toxins. Foods low in sodium and high in potassium are said to help correct the tissue damage caused by having too much sodium in the cells.

How is the Gerson therapy administered?

The Gerson therapy requires that the many details of its treatment plan be followed exactly. Some key parts of the regimen include the following:

- A person must drink 13 glasses of juice a day. The juice must be freshly made from organic fruits and vegetables and be taken once every hour.

- A person must eat vegetarian meals of organically grown fruits, vegetables, and whole grains.

- A person must take a number of supplements, including the following:

  - Potassium

  - Lugol's Solution (potassium iodide, iodine, and water)

  - Coenzyme Q10 injected with vitamin B_{12} (The original regimen used crude liver extract instead of coenzyme Q10.)

  - Vitamins A, C, and B_3 (niacin)

  - Flaxseed oil

  - Pancreatic enzymes

  - Pepsin (a stomach enzyme)

- A person must take coffee or chamomile enemas regularly to remove toxins from the body.

- A person must prepare food without salt, spices, or oils, and without using aluminum cookware or utensils.

Have any preclinical (laboratory or animal) studies been conducted using the Gerson therapy?

No results of laboratory or animal studies have been published in scientific journals.

Have any clinical trials (research studies with people) of the Gerson therapy been conducted?

Most of the published information on the use of the Gerson therapy reports on retrospective studies (reviews of past cases). Dr. Gerson published case histories (detailed reports of the diagnosis, treatment, and follow-up of individual patients) of 50 of his patients. He treated several different types of cancer in his practice. The reports include Dr. Gerson's notes, with some X-rays of the patients over time. The follow-up was contact with patients by mail or phone and included anecdotal reports (incomplete descriptions of the medical and treatment histories of one or more patients).

In 1947 and 1959, the National Cancer Institute (NCI) reviewed the cases of a total of 60 patients treated by Dr. Gerson. The NCI found that the available information did not prove the regimen had benefit.

The following studies of the Gerson therapy were published:

- In 1983–1984, a retrospective study of 38 patients treated with the Gerson therapy was done. Medical records were not available to the authors of the study; information came from patient interviews. These case reviews did not provide information that supports the usefulness of the Gerson therapy for treating cancer.

- In 1990, a study of a diet regimen similar to the Gerson therapy was done in Austria. The patients received standard treatment along with the special diet. The authors of the study reported that the diet appeared to help patients live longer than usual and have fewer side effects. The authors said it needed further study.

- In 1995, the Gerson Research Organization did a retrospective study of their melanoma patients who were treated with the Gerson therapy. The study reported that patients who had stage

271

III or stage IV melanoma lived longer than usual for patients with these stages of melanoma. There have been no clinical trials that support the findings of this retrospective study.

- A case review of six patients with metastatic cancer who used the Gerson therapy reported that the regimen helped patients in some ways, both physically and psychologically. Based on these results, the reviewers recommended that clinical trials of the Gerson therapy be conducted.

Have any side effects or risks been reported from use of the Gerson therapy?

Reports of three deaths that may be related to coffee enemas have been published. Taking too many enemas of any kind can cause changes in normal blood chemistry, chemicals that occur naturally in the body and keep the muscles, heart, and other organs working properly.

Is the Gerson therapy approved by the U.S. Food and Drug Administration (FDA) for use as a cancer treatment in the United States?

The Gerson therapy has not been approved by the FDA for use as a treatment for cancer or any other disease.

For most cancer patients, nutrition guidelines include eating a well-balanced diet with plenty of fruits, vegetables, and whole-grain products. However, general guidelines such as these may have to be changed to meet the specific needs of an individual patient. Patients should talk with their health care providers about an appropriate diet to follow. Information about diet during cancer treatment is also available from the Cancer Information Service (800-4-CANCER [TTY: 800-332-8615]).

Section 39.4

Macrobiotics

This treatment modality is thought to promote wellness and optimize overall health. Macrobiotics should be used with, not in place of, standard cancer therapy.

What does macrobiotics therapy involve?

Macrobiotics therapy is a combination of diet, spiritual, and social philosophy and a way of healthful living. The macrobiotics philosophy combines elements of Buddhism with dietary principles based on simplicity and avoidance of "toxic" animal products. Although a relatively new therapy, macrobiotics teaches that it is necessary to maintain balance and harmony between two antagonistic but complementary forces, Yin and Yang, a traditional Chinese medicine concept. The diet, originally termed the "Zen macrobiotic diet," was very restrictive and has since been modified by other practitioners in the macrobiotic movement. The diet consists mainly of whole grains, vegetables, and beans with the occasional use of fish and some fruits. Foods not allowed in the diet include coffee, dairy products, eggs, sugar, meats, and processed foods. The macrobiotics diet also requires special methods of food preparation such as using only pots, pans, and utensils made of certain materials. There is not a single diet for everyone, but rather a diet "principle" that considers different climates, ages, sex, level of activity, and changing personal needs.

How is macrobiotics thought to promote wellness and optimize overall health?

Traditional Chinese medicine believes that imbalances of Yin and Yang lead to illness. Therefore, macrobiotics attempts to rebalance Yin and Yang and regain health through diet and a change in lifestyle and life philosophy. The macrobiotics diet can lower fat and cholesterol and, like other fat-reducing diets, may help prevent some cancers that appear to be related to higher fat intake, such as colon cancer. This fat-free diet can also lower blood pressure and reduce the chance of heart disease. Other aspects of the macrobiotics therapy may promote a reduction in stress.

What has been proven about the benefit of macrobiotics?

According to the University of Texas MD Anderson Cancer Center, peer-reviewed research concerning the ability of the macrobiotics diet to cure cancer is currently limited. After an extensive search only three human studies on macrobiotics applicable to cancer were found. None demonstrated beyond a reasonable doubt that macrobiotics therapy should be viewed as a curative therapy. Macrobiotics is a "lifestyle" approach that can help prevent cancer, promote wellness, and optimize health.

What is the potential risk or harm of macrobiotics therapy?

A nutrient, vitamin, and calorie restrictive diet can be dangerous for frail cancer patients. The most serious effects occur when the diet is deficient in calories, vitamin D, vitamin B_{12}, protein, and iron. Increased caloric needs to fight illness and recover from treatment may not be met with the macrobiotics diet, which is high in bulk and low in fat. Children on the macrobiotics diet tend to have growth and nutrient deficiencies.

How much does macrobiotics therapy cost?

The cost of consuming a macrobiotics diet is probably comparable to consumption of a typical American diet when all factors are taken into consideration. Higher costs for macrobiotics include the initial setup of a macrobiotics kitchen and special foods. However, eating a macrobiotic diet can decrease costs because of the elimination of meat and poultry and the tendency to dine outside the home.

Section 39.5

Veganism

What Is a Vegan?

Vegetarians do not eat meat, fish, or poultry. Vegans, in addition to
being vegetarian, do not use other animal products and by-products
such as eggs, dairy products, honey, leather, fur, silk, wool, and cosmetics and soaps derived from animal products.

Why Veganism?

People choose to be vegan for health, environmental, and/or ethical
reasons. For example, some vegans feel that one promotes the meat
industry by consuming eggs and dairy products. That is, once dairy
cows or egg laying chickens are too old to be productive, they are often
sold as meat. Some people avoid these items because of conditions associated with their production.

Many vegans chose this lifestyle in order to promote a more humane
and caring world. They know they are not perfect, but believe they have
a responsibility to try to do their best, while not being judgmental of
others.

Common Vegan Foods

[Common vegan foods include]: Oatmeal, stir-fried vegetables, cereal, toast, orange juice, peanut butter on whole wheat bread, frozen
fruit desserts, lentil soup, salad bar items like chickpeas and three
bean salad, dates, apples, macaroni, fruit smoothies, popcorn, spaghetti,
vegetarian baked beans, guacamole, chili.

Vegans also eat: Tofu lasagna, homemade pancakes without eggs,
hummus, eggless cookies, soy ice cream, tempeh, corn chowder, soy
yogurt, rice pudding, fava beans, banana muffins, spinach pies, oat nut
burgers, seitan, corn fritters, French toast made with soy milk, soy hot
dogs, vegetable burgers, pumpkin casserole, scrambled tofu, falafel.

When Eating Out

Try these foods: Pizza without cheese, Chinese moo shu vegetables, Indian curries and dahl, eggplant dishes without the cheese, bean tacos without the lard and cheese (available from Taco Bell and other Mexican restaurants), Middle Eastern hummus and tabouli, Ethiopian injera (flat bread) and lentil stew, Thai vegetable curries.

Egg and Dairy Replacers

As a binder substitute for each egg:

- 1/4 cup (2 ounces) soft tofu blended with the liquid ingredients of the recipe

- 1 small banana, mashed

- 1/4 cup applesauce

- 2 tablespoons cornstarch or arrowroot starch

- Ener-G Egg Replacer or another commercial mix found in health food stores.

Dairy substitutes:

- Soy milk, rice milk, potato milk, nut milk, or water (in some recipes) may be used.

- Buttermilk can be replaced with soured soy or rice milk. For each cup of buttermilk, use 1 cup soy milk plus 1 tablespoon of vinegar.

- Soy cheese available in health food stores. (Be aware that many soy cheeses contain casein, which is a dairy product.)

- Crumbled tofu can be substituted for cottage cheese or ricotta cheese in lasagna and similar dishes.

- Several brands of nondairy cream cheese are available in supermarkets and kosher stores.

Vegan Nutrition

The key to a nutritionally sound vegan diet is variety. A healthy and varied vegan diet includes fruits, vegetables, plenty of leafy greens, whole grain products, nuts, seeds, and legumes.

Protein

It is very easy for a vegan diet to meet the recommendations for protein as long as calorie intake is adequate. Strict protein planning or combining is not necessary. The key is to eat a varied diet.

Sources of protein: Almost all foods except for alcohol, sugar, and fats provide some protein. Vegan sources include: lentils, chickpeas, tofu, peas, peanut butter, soy milk, almonds, spinach, rice, whole wheat bread, potatoes, broccoli, and kale.

For example, if part of a day's menu included the following foods, you would meet the Recommended Dietary Allowance (RDA) for protein for an adult male:

- 1 cup oatmeal
- 1 cup soy milk
- 2 slices whole wheat bread
- 1 bagel
- 2 Tablespoons peanut butter
- 1 cup vegetarian baked beans
- 5 ounces tofu
- 2 tablespoons almonds
- 1 cup broccoli
- 1 cup brown rice

Fat

Vegan diets are free of cholesterol and are generally low in saturated fat. Thus eating a vegan diet makes it easy to conform to recommendations given to reduce the risk of major chronic diseases such as heart disease and cancer. High-fat foods, which should be used sparingly, include oils, margarine, nuts, nut butters, seed butters, avocado, and coconut.

Vitamin D

Vitamin D is not found in the vegan diet but can be made by humans following exposure to sunlight. At least 10 to 15 minutes of summer sun on hands and face two to three times a week is recommended for adults so that vitamin D production can occur. Food sources of vitamin D include vitamin D-fortified orange juice and vitamin D-fortified soy milk and rice milk.

Calcium

Calcium, needed for strong bones, is found in dark green leafy vegetables, tofu made with calcium sulfate, calcium-fortified soy milk and orange juice, and many other foods commonly eaten by vegans. Although lower animal protein intake may reduce calcium losses, there is currently not enough evidence to suggest that vegans have lower calcium needs. Vegans should eat foods that are high in calcium and/or use a calcium supplement.

Other good sources of calcium include: okra, turnip greens, soybeans, tempeh, almond butter, broccoli, bok choy, calcium-fortified soy yogurt.

The recommended intake for calcium for adults 19 through 50 years is 1,000 milligrams/day.

Note: It appears that oxalic acid, which is found in spinach, rhubarb, chard, and beet greens, binds with calcium and reduces calcium absorption. Calcium is well absorbed from other dark green vegetables.

Zinc

Vegan diets can provide zinc at levels close to or even higher than the RDA. Zinc is found in grains, legumes, and nuts.

Iron

Dried beans and dark green leafy vegetables are especially good sources of iron, better on a per calorie basis than meat. Iron absorption is increased markedly by eating foods containing vitamin C along with foods containing iron.

Sources of iron: Soybeans, lentils, blackstrap molasses, kidney beans, chickpeas, black-eyed peas, Swiss chard, tempeh, black beans, prune juice, beet greens, tahini, peas, bulghur, bok choy, raisins, watermelon, millet, kale.

Omega-3 Fatty Acids

In order to maximize production of DHA and EPA ([docosahexaenoic acid and eicosapentaenoic acid] omega-3 fatty acids), vegans should include good sources of alpha-linolenic acid in their diet such as flaxseed, flaxseed oil, canola oil, tofu, soybeans, and walnuts.

Vitamin B_{12}

The requirement for vitamin B_{12} is very low but it is an essential nutrient. It is especially important for pregnant and lactating women, infants, and children to have reliable sources of vitamin B_{12} in their diets. Non-animal sources include cereals, soy milk, rice milk, and meat analogues that have been fortified with vitamin B_{12}. Also, around 2 teaspoons of Red Star nutritional yeast T6635, often labeled as Vegetarian Support Formula, supplies the adult RDA.

Read labels carefully or contact companies since fortification levels can change. Vitamin B_{12} supplements are another option. There are supplements which do not contain animal products. Claims of a high vitamin B_{12} content in fermented soy foods (miso and tempeh) and for sea vegetables and Spirulina are unfounded. Unless fortified, no plant food contains significant amounts of active vitamin B_{12}.

Section 39.6

Vegetarianism

"Vegetarianism," October 2008, reprinted with permission from www.kidshealth.org. Copyright © 2008 The Nemours Foundation. This information was provided by KidsHealth, one of the largest resources online for medically reviewed health information written for parents, kids, and teens. For more articles like this one, visit www.KidsHealth.org, or www.TeensHealth.org.

Vegetarianism is a popular choice for many individuals and families. But parents may wonder if kids can safely follow a vegetarian diet and still get all necessary nutrients. Most dietary and medical experts agree that a well-planned vegetarian diet can actually be a very healthy way to eat.

But special care must be taken when serving kids and teens a vegetarian diet, especially if it doesn't include dairy and egg products. And as with any diet, you'll need to understand that the nutritional needs of kids change as they grow.

Types of Vegetarian Diets

Before your child or family switches to a vegetarian diet, it's important to note that all vegetarian diets are not alike. Major vegetarian categories include:

- **Ovo-vegetarian:** Eats eggs; no meat

- **Lacto-ovo vegetarian:** Eats dairy and egg products; no meat

- **Lacto-vegetarian:** Eats dairy products; no eggs or meat

- **Vegan:** Eats only food from plant sources

And many other people are semi-vegetarians who have eliminated red meat, but may eat poultry or fish.

The Choice of Vegetarianism

Kids or families may follow a vegetarian diet for a variety of reasons. Younger vegetarians are usually part of a family that eats vegetarian meals for health, cultural, or other reasons. Older kids may decide to become vegetarians because of concern for animals, the environment, or their own health.

In most cases, you shouldn't be alarmed if your child chooses vegetarianism. Discuss what it means and how to implement it, ensuring your child makes healthy and nutritious food choices.

Nutrition for All Ages

Your doctor or a registered dietitian can help you plan and monitor a healthy vegetarian diet. Parents should give their kids a variety of foods that provide enough calories and nutrients to enable them to grow normally.

A well-planned vegetarian diet can meet kids' nutritional needs and has some health benefits. For example, a diet rich in fruits and veggies will be high in fiber and low in fat, factors known to improve cardiovascular health by reducing blood cholesterol and maintaining a healthy weight. However, kids and teens on a vegetarian diet may need to be careful that they get an adequate amount of certain vitamins and minerals.

Here are nutrients that vegetarians should get and some of their best food sources:

- **Vitamin B_{12}:** Dairy products, eggs, and vitamin-fortified products, such as cereals, breads, and soy and rice drinks, and nutritional yeast

- **Vitamin D:** Milk, vitamin D-fortified orange juice, and other vitamin D-fortified products

- **Calcium:** Dairy products, dark green leafy vegetables, broccoli, dried beans, and calcium-fortified products, including orange juice, soy and rice drinks, and cereals

- **Protein:** Dairy products, eggs, tofu and other soy products, dried beans, and nuts

- **Iron:** Eggs, dried beans, dried fruits, whole grains, leafy green vegetables, and iron-fortified cereals and bread

- **Zinc:** Wheat germ, nuts, fortified cereal, dried beans, and pumpkin seeds

Depending on the type of vegetarian diet chosen, kids may miss out on some of these important nutrients if the diet isn't monitored by the parents. The less restrictive the vegetarian diet, the easier it will be for your child to get enough of the necessary nutrients. In some cases, fortified foods or supplements can help meet nutritional needs.

Vegetarian Infants

The main sources of protein and nutrients for infants are breast milk and formula (soy formula for vegan infants), especially in the first 6 months of life. Breastfed infant vegans should receive a source of vitamin B_{12}, if the mother's diet isn't supplemented, and breastfed infants and infants drinking less than 32 ounces (1 liter) of formula should get vitamin D supplements.

Guidelines for the introduction of solid foods are the same for vegetarian and nonvegetarian infants. Breastfed infants 6 months and older should receive iron from complementary foods, such as iron-fortified infant cereal.

Once an infant is introduced to solids, protein-rich vegetarian foods can include pureed tofu, cottage cheese, yogurt or soy yogurt, and pureed and strained legumes (legumes include beans, peas, chickpeas, and lentils).

Vegetarian Toddlers

Toddlers are already a challenge when it comes to eating. As they come off of breast milk or formula, kids are at risk for nutritional deficiencies. After the age of 1, strict vegan diets may not offer growing toddlers enough essential vitamins and minerals, such as vitamin D, vitamin B_{12}, iron, calcium, and zinc. So it's important to serve fortified cereals and nutrient-dense foods. Vitamin supplementation is recommended for young children whose diets may not provide adequate nutrients.

Toddlers are typically picky about which foods they'll eat and, as a result, some may not get enough calories from a vegetarian diet to thrive. For vegan toddlers, the amount of vegetables needed for proper nutrition and calories may be too bulky for their tiny stomachs. During the picky toddler stage, it's important for vegetarian parents to make sure their young child eats enough calories. You can get enough fat and calories in a vegan child's diet, but you have to plan carefully.

Older Vegetarian Kids and Teens

Preteens and teens often voice their independence through the foods they choose to eat. One strong statement is the decision to stop eating meat. This is common among teens, who may decide to embrace vegetarianism in support of animal rights, for health reasons, or because friends are doing it.

If it's done right, a meat-free diet can actually be a good choice for adolescents, especially considering that vegetarians often eat more of the foods that most teens don't get enough of—fruits and vegetables.

A vegetarian diet that includes dairy products and eggs (lacto-ovo) is the best choice for growing teens. A more strict vegetarian diet may fail to meet a teen's need for certain nutrients, such as iron, zinc, calcium, and vitamins D and B_{12}. If you're concerned that your child is not getting enough of these important nutrients, talk to your doctor, who may recommend a vitamin and mineral supplement.

The good news for young vegetarians—and their parents—is that many schools are offering vegetarian fare, including salad bars and other healthy vegetarian choices. Schools publish lists of upcoming lunch menus; be sure to scan them to see if your child will have a vegetarian choice. If not, you can pack lunch. That old standby—a peanut butter and jelly sandwich—is a great fast vegetarian lunch.

If your vegetarian preteen or teen would rather make his or her own school lunch or opts to buy lunch, keep in mind that your child's idea of a healthy vegetarian meal may be much different from yours (e.g., french fries and a soda). Talk to your child about the importance of eating right, especially when following a vegetarian diet.

Also be wary if your child has self-imposed a very restrictive diet. A teen with an eating disorder may drastically reduce calories or cut out all fat or carbohydrates and call it "vegetarianism" because it's considered socially acceptable and healthy.

Even if preteens or teens are approaching vegetarianism in a healthy way, it's still important for them to understand which nutrients might be missing in their diet. To support your child's dietary decision and promote awareness of the kinds of foods your preteen or teen should be eating, consider having the whole family eat a vegetarian meal at least one night a week.

A Healthy Lifestyle

A vegetarian diet can be a healthy choice for all kids, as long as it's properly planned.

The principles of planning a vegetarian diet are the same as planning any healthy diet—provide a variety of foods and include foods from all of the food groups. A balanced diet will provide the right combinations to meet nutritional needs. But be aware of potential nutrient deficiencies in your child's diet and figure out how you'll account for them. With a little exploration, you may find more vegetarian options than you realized.

If you aren't sure your child is getting all necessary nutrients or if you have any questions about vegetarian diets, check in with your family doctor, pediatrician, or a registered dietitian.

Chapter 40

Oxygen Therapy

Overview

Hyperbaric oxygen therapy (HBOT) is the inhalation of 100 percent oxygen inside a hyperbaric chamber that is pressurized to greater than 1 atmosphere (atm). HBOT causes both mechanical and physiologic effects by inducing a state of increased pressure and hyperoxia.

HBOT is typically administered at 1 to 3 atm. While the duration of an HBOT session is typically 90 to 120 minutes, the duration, frequency, and cumulative number of sessions have not been standardized. HBOT is administered in two primary ways, using a monoplace chamber or a multiplace chamber. The monoplace chamber is the less-costly option for initial setup and operation but provides less opportunity for patient interaction while in the chamber. Multiplace chambers allow medical personnel to work in the chamber and care for acute patients to some extent. The entire multiplace chamber is pressurized, so medical personnel may require a controlled decompression, depending on how long they were exposed to the hyperbaric air environment.

The purpose of this text is to provide a guide to the strengths and limitations of the evidence about the use of HBOT to treat patients who have brain injury, cerebral palsy, and stroke. Brain injury can be caused by an external physical force (also known as traumatic brain injury, or TBI);

Excerpted from "Hyperbaric Oxygen Therapy for Brain Injury, Cerebral Palsy, and Stroke." Summary, Evidence Report/Technology Assessment: Number 85. AHRQ Publication Number 03-E049, September 2003. Agency for Healthcare Research and Quality, Rockville, MD. http://www.ahrq.gov/clinic/epcsums/hypoxsum .htm. Reviewed by David A. Cooke, MD, FACP, January 23, 2010.

rapid acceleration or deceleration of the head; bleeding within or around the brain; lack of sufficient oxygen to the brain; or toxic substances passing through the blood-brain barrier. Brain injury results in temporary or permanent impairment of cognitive, emotional, and/or physical functioning. Cerebral palsy refers to a motor deficit that usually manifests itself by 2 years of age and is secondary to an abnormality of at least the part of the brain that relates to motor function. Stroke refers to a sudden interruption of the blood supply to the brain, usually caused by a blocked artery or a ruptured blood vessel, leading to an interruption of homeostasis of cells, and symptoms such as loss of speech and loss of motor function.

While these conditions have different etiologies, prognostic factors, and outcomes, they also have important similarities. Each condition represents a broad spectrum, from barely perceptible or mild disabilities to devastating ones. All three are characterized by acute and chronic phases and by changes over time in the type and degree of disability. Another similarity is that the outcome of conventional treatment is often unsatisfactory. For brain injury in particular, there is a strong sense that conventional treatment has made little impact on outcomes.

Predicting the outcome of brain injury, cerebral palsy, and stroke is difficult. Prognostic instruments, such as the Glasgow Coma Scale (GCS) for brain injury, are not precise enough to reliably predict an individual patient's mortality and long-term functional status. Various prognostic criteria for the cerebral palsy patient's function have been developed over the years. For example, if a patient is not sitting independently when placed by age 2, then one can predict with approximately 95 percent confidence that he/she never will be able to walk. However, it is not possible to predict precisely when an individual patient is likely to acquire a particular ability, such as smiling, recognizing other individuals, or saying or understanding a new word.

Mortality and morbidity from a stroke are related to older age, history of myocardial infarction, cardiac arrhythmias, diabetes mellitus, and the number of stroke deficits. Functional recovery is dependent on numerous variables, including age, neurologic deficit, comorbidities, psychosocial factors, educational level, vocational status, and characteristics of the stroke survivor's environment.

Reporting the Evidence

This text addresses the following questions:

- Does HBOT improve mortality and morbidity in patients who have traumatic brain injury or nontraumatic brain injury, such as anoxic ischemic encephalopathy?

- Does HBOT improve functional outcomes in patients who have cerebral palsy? (Examples of improved functional outcomes are decreased spasticity, improved speech, increased alertness, increased cognitive abilities, and improved visual functioning.)

- Does HBOT improve mortality and morbidity in patients who have suffered a stroke?

- What are the adverse effects of using HBOT in these conditions?

Findings

Brain Injury

- For traumatic brain injury, one randomized trial provided fair evidence that HBOT might reduce mortality or the duration of coma in severely injured TBI (traumatic brain injuries) patients. However, in this trial, HBOT also increased the chance of a poor functional outcome. A second fair quality randomized trial found no difference in mortality or morbidity overall, but a significant reduction in mortality in one subgroup. Therefore, they provide insufficient evidence to determine whether the benefits of HBOT outweigh the potential harms.

- The quality of the controlled trials was fair, meaning that deficiencies in the design add to uncertainty about the validity of results.

- Due to flaws in design or small size, the observational studies of HBOT in TBI do not establish a clear, consistent relationship between physiologic changes after HBOT sessions and measures of clinical improvement.

- The evidence for use of HBOT in other types of brain injury is inconclusive. No good- or fair-quality studies were found.

Cerebral Palsy

- There is insufficient evidence to determine whether the use of HBOT improves functional outcomes in children with cerebral palsy. The results of the only truly randomized trial were difficult to interpret because of the use of pressurized room air in the control group. As both groups improved, the benefit of pressurized air and of HBOT at 1.3 to 1.5 atm should both be examined in future studies.

- The only other controlled study compared HBOT treatments with 1.5 atm to delaying treatment for 6 months. As in the placebo-controlled study, significant improvements were seen, but there was not a significant difference between groups.

- Two fair-quality uncontrolled studies (one time-series, one before-after) found improvements in functional status comparable to the degree of improvement seen in both groups in the controlled trial.

- Although none of the studies adequately measured caregiver burden, study participants often noted meaningful reductions in caregiver burden as an outcome of treatment.

Stroke

- Although a large number of studies address HBOT for the treatment of stroke, the evidence is insufficient to determine whether HBOT reduces mortality in any subgroup of stroke patients because no controlled trial assessed was designed to assess mortality.

- Among controlled trials, the evidence about morbidity is conflicting. The three best-quality trials found no difference in neurological measures in patients treated with HBOT versus patients treated with pressurized room air.

- Two other controlled trials, one randomized and one nonrandomized, found that HBOT improved neurological outcomes on some measures. However, both were rated poor-quality.

- Most observational studies reported favorable, and sometimes dramatic, results, but failed to prove that these results can be attributed to HBOT. For example, one retrospective study found better mortality rates in patients who received HBOT than a comparison group of patients from a different hospital who did not. The study did not provide information on mortality rates from other causes in each hospital; this information would have made it easier to judge whether the improved survival was due to HBOT or to differences in overall quality of care at the HBOT hospital.

- The observational studies of HBOT provided insufficient evidence to establish a clear relationship between physiologic changes after HBOT sessions and measures of clinical improvement. Few studies established that patients were stable at baseline.

Adverse Events

- Evidence about the type, frequency, and severity of adverse events in actual practice is inadequate. Reporting of adverse effects was limited, and no study was designed specifically to assess adverse effects.

- The few data that are available from controlled trials and cohort studies of TBI suggest that the risk of seizure may be higher in patients with brain injuries treated with HBOT.

- No study of HBOT for brain injury, cerebral palsy, or stroke has been designed to identify the chronic neurologic complications.

- Pulmonary complications were relatively common in the trials of brain-injured patients. There are no reliable data on the incidence of aspiration in children treated for cerebral palsy with hyperbaric oxygen.

- Ear problems are a known potential adverse effect of HBOT. While ear problems were reported in brain injury, cerebral palsy, and stroke studies the incidence, severity, and effect on outcome are not clear. However, the rates reported among cerebral palsy patients were higher (up to 47 percent experiencing a problem) than reported with brain injury or stroke. However, the data in brain injury are limited by the use of prophylactic myringotomies.

Supplemental Qualitative Analysis

- Opinions about the frequency and severity of risks of HBOT vary widely.

- Several participants emphasized the importance of continued treatments to maximize results.

- Patients and caregivers value any degree of benefit from HBOT highly. An improvement that may appear small on a standard measure of motor, language, or cognitive function can have a very large impact on caregiver burden and quality of life.

Part Five

Mind-Body Medicine

Chapter 41

Mind-Body Medicine: An Overview

Mind-body medicine focuses on the interactions among the brain, mind, body, and behavior, and the powerful ways in which emotional, mental, social, spiritual, and behavioral factors can directly affect health. It regards as fundamental an approach that respects and enhances each person's capacity for self-knowledge and self-care, and it emphasizes techniques that are grounded in this approach.

Definition of Scope of Field

Mind-body medicine typically focuses on intervention strategies that are thought to promote health, such as relaxation, hypnosis, visual imagery, meditation, yoga, biofeedback, tai chi, qi gong, cognitive-behavioral therapies, group support, autogenic training, and spirituality. The field views illness as an opportunity for personal growth and transformation, and health care providers as catalysts and guides in this process.

Mind-body interventions constitute a major portion of the overall use of CAM by the public. In 2002, five relaxation techniques and imagery, biofeedback, and hypnosis, taken together, were used by more than 30 percent of the adult U.S. population. Prayer was used by more than 50 percent of the population.

Excerpted from "Mind-Body Medicine: An Overview," by the National Center for Complementary and Alternative Medicine (NCCAM, nccam.nih.gov), part of the National Institutes of Health, May 2007.

Background

The concept that the mind is important in the treatment of illness is integral to the healing approaches of traditional Chinese and Ayurvedic medicine, dating back more than 2,000 years. It was also noted by Hippocrates, who recognized the moral and spiritual aspects of healing, and believed that treatment could occur only with consideration of attitude, environmental influences, and natural remedies (ca. 400 BC). While this integrated approach was maintained in traditional healing systems in the East, developments in the Western world by the 16th and 17th centuries led to a separation of human spiritual or emotional dimensions from the physical body. This separation began with the redirection of science, during the Renaissance and Enlightenment eras, to the purpose of enhancing humankind's control over nature. Technological advances (e.g., microscopy, the stethoscope, the blood pressure cuff, and refined surgical techniques) demonstrated a cellular world that seemed far apart from the world of belief and emotion. The discovery of bacteria and, later, antibiotics further dispelled the notion of belief influencing health. Fixing or curing an illness became a matter of science (i.e., technology) and took precedence over, not a place beside, healing of the soul. As medicine separated the mind and the body, scientists of the mind (neurologists) formulated concepts, such as the unconscious, emotional impulses, and cognitive delusions, that solidified the perception that diseases of the mind were not "real," that is, not based in physiology and biochemistry.

In the 1920s, Walter Cannon's work revealed the direct relationship between stress and neuroendocrine responses in animals. Coining the phrase "fight or flight," Cannon described the primitive reflexes of sympathetic and adrenal activation in response to perceived danger and other environmental pressures (e.g., cold, heat). Hans Selye further defined the deleterious effects of stress and distress on health. At the same time, technological advances in medicine that could identify specific pathological changes, and new discoveries in pharmaceuticals, were occurring at a very rapid pace. The disease-based model, the search for a specific pathology, and the identification of external cures were paramount, even in psychiatry.

During World War II, the importance of belief reentered the web of health care. On the beaches of Anzio, morphine for the wounded soldiers was in short supply, and Henry Beecher, MD, discovered that much of the pain could be controlled by saline injections. He coined the term "placebo effect," and his subsequent research showed that up to 35 percent of a therapeutic response to any medical treatment could be the result of belief. Investigation into the placebo effect and debate about it are ongoing.

Since the 1960s, mind-body interactions have become an extensively researched field. The evidence for benefits for certain indications from biofeedback, cognitive-behavioral interventions, and hypnosis is quite good, while there is emerging evidence regarding their physiological effects.

Less research supports the use of CAM approaches like meditation and yoga. The following is a summary of relevant studies.

Mind-Body Interventions and Disease Outcomes

Over the past 20 years, mind-body medicine has provided considerable evidence that psychological factors can play a substantive role in the development and progression of coronary artery disease. There is evidence that mind-body interventions can be effective in the treatment of coronary artery disease, enhancing the effect of standard cardiac rehabilitation in reducing all-cause mortality and cardiac event recurrences for up to 2 years.

Mind-body interventions have also been applied to various types of pain. Clinical trials indicate that these interventions may be a particularly effective adjunct in the management of arthritis, with reductions in pain maintained for up to 4 years and reductions in the number of physician visits. When applied to more general acute and chronic pain management, headache, and low-back pain, mind-body interventions show some evidence of effects, although results vary based on the patient population and type of intervention studied.

Evidence from multiple studies with various types of cancer patients suggests that mind-body interventions can improve mood, quality of life, and coping, as well as ameliorate disease- and treatment-related symptoms, such as chemotherapy-induced nausea, vomiting, and pain. Some studies have suggested that mind-body interventions can alter various immune parameters, but it is unclear whether these alterations are of sufficient magnitude to have an impact on disease progression or prognosis.

Mind-Body Influences on Immunity

There is considerable evidence that emotional traits, both negative and positive, influence people's susceptibility to infection. Following systematic exposure to a respiratory virus in the laboratory, individuals who report higher levels of stress or negative moods have been shown to develop more severe illness than those who report less stress or more positive moods. Recent studies suggest that the tendency to report positive, as opposed to negative, emotions may be associated with greater resistance to objectively verified colds. These laboratory studies are supported by longitudinal studies pointing to associations between psychological or emotional traits and the incidence of respiratory infections.

Meditation and Imaging

Meditation, one of the most common mind-body interventions, is a conscious mental process that induces a set of integrated physiological changes termed the relaxation response. Functional magnetic resonance imaging (fMRI) has been used to identify and characterize the brain regions that are active during meditation. This research suggests that various parts of the brain known to be involved in attention and in the control of the autonomic nervous system are activated, providing a neurochemical and anatomical basis for the effects of meditation on various physiological activities. Recent studies involving imaging are advancing the understanding of mind-body mechanisms. For example, meditation has been shown in one study to produce significant increases in left-sided anterior brain activity, which is associated with positive emotional states. Moreover, in this same study, meditation was associated with increases in antibody titers to influenza vaccine, suggesting potential linkages among meditation, positive emotional states, localized brain responses, and improved immune function.

Physiology of Expectancy (Placebo Response)

Placebo effects are believed to be mediated by both cognitive and conditioning mechanisms. Until recently, little was known about the role of these mechanisms in different circumstances. Now, research has shown that placebo responses are mediated by conditioning when unconscious physiological functions such as hormonal secretion are involved, whereas they are mediated by expectation when conscious physiological processes such as pain and motor performance come into play, even though a conditioning procedure is carried out.

Positron emission tomography (PET) scanning of the brain is providing evidence of the release of the endogenous neurotransmitter dopamine in the brain of Parkinson disease patients in response to placebo. Evidence indicates that the placebo effect in these patients is powerful and is mediated through activation of the nigrostriatal dopamine system, the system that is damaged in Parkinson disease.

This result suggests that the placebo response involves the secretion of dopamine, which is known to be important in a number of other reinforcing and rewarding conditions, and that there may be mind-body strategies that could be used in patients with Parkinson disease in lieu of or in addition to treatment with dopamine-releasing drugs.

Stress and Wound Healing

Individual differences in wound healing have long been recognized. Clinical observation has suggested that negative mood or stress is associated with slow wound healing. Basic mind-body research is now confirming this observation. Matrix metalloproteinases (MMPs) and the tissue inhibitors of metalloproteinases (TIMPs), whose expression can be controlled by cytokines, play a role in wound healing. Using a blister chamber wound model on human forearm skin exposed to ultraviolet light, researchers have demonstrated that stress or a change in mood is sufficient to modulate MMP and TIMP expression and, presumably, wound healing. Activation of the hypothalamic-pituitary-adrenal (HPA) and sympathetic-adrenal medullary (SAM) systems can modulate levels of MMPs, providing a physiological link among mood, stress, hormones, and wound healing. This line of basic research suggests that activation of the HPA and SAM axes, even in individuals within the normal range of depressive symptoms, could alter MMP levels and change the course of wound healing in blister wounds.

Surgical Preparation

Mind-body interventions are being tested to determine whether they can help prepare patients for the stress associated with surgery. Initial randomized controlled trials—in which some patients received audiotapes with mind-body techniques (guided imagery, music, and instructions for improved outcomes) and some patients received control tapes—found that subjects receiving the mind-body intervention recovered more quickly and spent fewer days in the hospital.

Behavioral interventions have been shown to be an efficient means of reducing discomfort and adverse effects during percutaneous vascular and renal procedures. Pain increased linearly with procedure time in a control group and in a group practicing structured attention, but remained flat in a group practicing a self-hypnosis technique. The self-administration of analgesic drugs was significantly higher in the control group than in the attention and hypnosis groups. Hypnosis also improved hemodynamic stability.

Conclusion

Evidence from randomized controlled trials and, in many cases, systematic reviews of the literature, suggest the following:

- Mechanisms may exist by which the brain and central nervous system influence immune, endocrine, and autonomic functioning, which is known to have an impact on health.

- Multicomponent mind-body interventions that include some combination of stress management, coping skills training, cognitive-behavioral interventions, and relaxation therapy may be appropriate adjunctive treatments for coronary artery disease and certain pain-related disorders, such as arthritis.

- Multimodal mind-body approaches, such as cognitive-behavioral therapy, particularly when combined with an educational/informational component, can be effective adjuncts in the management of a variety of chronic conditions.

- An array of mind-body therapies (e.g., imagery, hypnosis, relaxation), when employed presurgically, may improve recovery time and reduce pain following surgical procedures.

- Neurochemical and anatomical bases may exist for some of the effects of mind-body approaches.

Mind-body approaches have potential benefits and advantages. In particular, the physical and emotional risks of using these interventions are minimal. Moreover, once tested and standardized, most mind-body interventions can be taught easily. Finally, future research focusing on basic mind-body mechanisms and individual differences in responses is likely to yield new insights that may enhance the effectiveness and individual tailoring of mind-body interventions. In the meantime, there is considerable evidence that mind-body interventions, even as they are being studied today, have positive effects on psychological functioning and quality of life, and may be particularly helpful for patients coping with chronic illness and in need of palliative care.

Chapter 42

Art Therapy

Art therapy is the therapeutic use of art making, within a professional relationship, by people who experience illness, trauma, or challenges in living, and by people who seek personal development. Through creating art and reflecting on the art products and processes, people can increase awareness of self and others; cope with symptoms, stress, and traumatic experiences; enhance cognitive abilities; and enjoy the life-affirming pleasures of making art.

Art therapists are professionals trained in both art and therapy. They are knowledgeable about human development, psychological theories, clinical practice, spiritual, multicultural, and artistic traditions, and the healing potential of art. They use art in treatment, assessment, and research, and provide consultations to allied professionals. Art therapists work with people of all ages: individuals, couples, families, groups, and communities. They provide services, individually and as part of clinical teams, in settings that include mental health, rehabilitation, medical, and forensic institutions; community outreach programs; wellness centers; schools; nursing homes; corporate structures; open studios and independent practices.

The American Art Therapy Association encourages educational, professional, and ethical standards for its members. The Art Therapy Credentials Board, Inc. (ATCB), an independent organization, grants art therapy credentials based on educational attainment.

"About Art Therapy," © 2009 American Art Therapy Association (www.american arttherapyassociation.org). Reprinted with permission.

- Registration (ATR [Registered Art Therapist]) is granted upon completion of graduate education and post-graduate supervised experience.

- Board Certification (ATR-BC) is granted to Registered Art Therapists who pass a written examination, and is maintained through continuing education.

- Some states regulate the practice of art therapy and in many states art therapists can become licensed as counselors or mental health therapists.

Defining Art Therapy

Art therapy is a mental health profession that uses the creative process of art making to improve and enhance the physical, mental, and emotional well-being of individuals of all ages. It is based on the belief that the creative process involved in artistic self-expression helps people to resolve conflicts and problems, develop interpersonal skills, manage behavior, reduce stress, increase self-esteem and self-awareness, and achieve insight.

Art therapy integrates the fields of human development, visual art (drawing, painting, sculpture, and other art forms), and the creative process with models of counseling and psychotherapy. Art therapy is used with children, adolescents, adults, older adults, groups, and families to assess and treat the following: anxiety, depression, and other mental and emotional problems and disorders; substance abuse and other addictions; family and relationship issues; abuse and domestic violence; social and emotional difficulties related to disability and illness; trauma and loss; physical, cognitive, and neurological problems; and psychosocial difficulties related to medical illness. Art therapy programs are found in a number of settings including hospitals, clinics, public and community agencies, wellness centers, educational institutions, businesses, and private practices.

Art therapists are master's level professionals who hold a degree in art therapy or a related field. Educational requirements include: theories of art therapy, counseling, and psychotherapy; ethics and standards of practice; assessment and evaluation; individual, group, and family techniques; human and creative development; multicultural issues; research methods; and practicum experiences in clinical, community, and/or other settings. Art therapists are skilled in the application of a variety of art modalities (drawing, painting, sculpture, and other media) for assessment and treatment.

Frequently Asked Questions

How did art therapy begin?

Visual expression has been used for healing throughout history, but art therapy did not emerge as a distinct profession until the 1940s. In the early 20th century, psychiatrists became interested in the artwork created by their patients with mental illness. At around the same time, educators were discovering that children's art expressions reflected developmental, emotional, and cognitive growth. By mid-century, hospitals, clinics, and rehabilitation centers increasingly began to include art therapy programs along with traditional "talk therapies," underscoring the recognition that the creative process of art making enhanced recovery, health, and wellness. As a result, the profession of art therapy grew into an effective and important method of communication, assessment, and treatment with children and adults in a variety of settings. Currently, the field of art therapy has gained attention in health-care facilities throughout the United States and within psychiatry, psychology, counseling, education, and the arts.

Where do art therapists work?

Art therapists work in a wide variety of settings, including, but not limited to, the following:

- Hospitals and clinics, both medical and psychiatric
- Outpatient mental health agencies and day treatment facilities
- Residential treatment centers
- Halfway houses
- Domestic violence and homeless shelters
- Community agencies and non-profit settings
- Sheltered workshops
- Schools, colleges, and universities
- Correctional facilities
- Elder care facilities
- Art studios
- Private practice

An art therapist may work as part of a team that includes physicians, psychologists, nurses, mental health counselors, marriage and family therapists, rehabilitation counselors, social workers, and teachers.

Together, they determine and implement a client's therapeutic goals and objectives. Other art therapists work independently and maintain private practices with children, adolescents, adults, groups, and/or families.

What are the requirements to become an art therapist?

Personal qualifications: An art therapist must have sensitivity, empathy, emotional stability, patience, interpersonal skills, insight into human behavior, and an understanding of art media. An art therapist must also be an attentive listener and a keen observer. Flexibility and a sense of humor are important in adapting to client needs and work setting.

Educational requirements: One must complete the required core curriculum as outlined in the American Art Therapy Association's Education Standards to qualify as a professional art therapist. Entry into the profession of art therapy is at the master's level. Graduate level art therapy programs include:

- master's degree in art therapy;

- master's degree with an emphasis in art therapy;

- twenty-four (24) semester units in art therapy coursework with a master's degree in a related field.

Contact the National Office for more information concerning current educational requirements and programs.
[See www.americanarttherapyassociation.org for contact information.]

Registration and Board Certification Requirements: The ATR and ATR-BC are the recognized standards for the field of art therapy, and are conferred by the Art Therapy Credentials Board (ATCB). In order to qualify as a registered art therapist (ATR), in addition to the educational requirements, an individual must complete a minimum of 1,000 direct client contact hours after graduation. One hour of supervision is required for every 10 hours of client contact.

Chapter 43

Biofeedback

What is biofeedback?

Biofeedback is a mind-body technique using electronic instruments to help individuals gain awareness and control over their body and mind. Biofeedback instruments measure muscle activity, skin temperature, electrodermal activity, respiration, heart rate, blood pressure, brain electrical activity, and brain blood flow. Biofeedback is useful in medical care, mental health treatment, physical and occupational therapy, dental care, and education.

When is biofeedback appropriate? Who should seek it and when?

Biofeedback is a useful self-help tool that can benefit almost every living human being. Biofeedback is a pathway to learning important voluntary control skills that are useful throughout life. Biofeedback enables individuals to increase bodily awareness, acquire relaxation skills, and gain control over a variety of organ systems in the body. Many persons feel encouraged and "empowered" by biofeedback. After gaining control over their body they feel more capable of gaining control over their lives.

"Biofeedback: Consumer Questions Answered," by Donald Moss, PhD, 2002. © Association for Applied Psychophysiology and Biofeedback (www.aapb.org). Reprinted with permission. The text that follows this document under the heading *"Health Reference Series* Medical Advisor's Notes and Updates" was provided to Omnigraphics, Inc. by David A. Cooke, MD, FACP, January 23, 2010. Dr. Cooke is not affiliated with the Association for Applied Psychophysiology and Biofeedback.

Anyone who is suffering from life stress and anxiety can benefit from biofeedback strategies for physical and mental relaxation. Anyone suffering from medical problems that are caused or aggravated by stress will benefit from biofeedback. In addition, individuals with many organic medical problems, such as spinal injury related motor control problems, may find that biofeedback helps them compensate for their medical condition and function better.

What are some of the most common uses for biofeedback?

Research shows that biofeedback can benefit individuals with a broad range of mental health and medical problems, including:

- alcoholism and addictions;
- anxiety;
- asthma;
- attention deficit hyperactivity disorder (ADHD);
- closed head injury;
- depression;
- diabetes mellitus;
- enuresis;
- epilepsy;
- essential hypertension;
- headache—migraine;
- headache—tension;
- incontinence (fecal and urinary);
- insomnia;
- irritable bowel syndrome;
- learning disabilities;
- motion sickness;
- neuromuscular disorders (e.g., Bell's palsy, whiplash, muscle-tendon transfers, torticollis, cerebral palsy, peripheral nerve problems, spasm);
- pain—myofascial;
- pain—rheumatoid arthritis;
- pain—temporomandibular dysfunction;

- Raynaud's syndrome and disease;
- sleep disorders;
- stroke.

How does it work and what are the benefits?

Biofeedback teaches human beings to recognize the link between their bodies and minds. The biofeedback instrument monitors one bodily system (like a muscle) and gives the individual immediate feedback when the body changes. This increases personal awareness of the bodily process, which leads to control over the body.

The first level of benefit most people encounter is improved relaxation of the entire body—reversing the effects of stress on the body.

The second level of benefit is ongoing reduction in everyday tensions and anxieties.

The third level of benefit is relief from specific medical and mental health problems. There are biofeedback treatments for the emotional disorders, attention deficit, alcoholism, and a wide range of medical problems.

The fourth level of benefit is a growing sense of personal power and confidence, a feeling that "I can learn skills which make a difference in my life."

What do people need to know about biofeedback before pursuing it? What information do they need?

It helps to learn about the idea of biofeedback, and to understand how it works, by reading a book chapter about biofeedback, such as those listed in the References portion of text. Then the individual should carefully identify a competent well-trained biofeedback professional.

What are some of the misconceptions that people have about biofeedback that need to be cleared up?

Some persons are afraid that biofeedback will do something harmful to them. Biofeedback is only a tool to enable the individual to gain control over his or her own body and mind. The instruments measure your bodily processes, and provide feedback to you. The instruments do not actively do anything *to* your body.

The second myth is that biofeedback will replace all need for medical treatment or medication. Many medical problems are complex, and a combination of traditional medical care with biofeedback is often more effective than biofeedback alone. This is true for headaches and hypertension, for instance.

How should a person select a biofeedback practitioner? What criteria should a person use in the selection process?

I recommend asking the biofeedback practitioner several questions, before committing to the treatment process:

- **Are you certified by the Biofeedback Certification Institute of America (BCIA)?** BCIA has excellent standards for the knowledge and skills a biofeedback practitioner should have. Therapists must accumulate educational credit, practical supervised experience, and pass an exam. Therapists should learn about biofeedback through college classes, approved training workshops, extensive reading, and supervised training and practice. The BCIA certification tells the patient that this therapist has done all of these things.

- **What state and national biofeedback organizations do you belong to, and what state and national conferences or biofeedback training workshops have you attended in the past two years?** Competent professionals belong to professional societies and attend meetings in order to keep their skills and knowledge current.

- **What journals and newsmagazines do you subscribe to in order to keep up with progress in biofeedback treatment?** Again, competent professionals keep their knowledge current by reading current reports.

- **Are you licensed or certified for independent practice as a health care provider in this state?** Biofeedback professionals usually are also licensed within a profession, such as medicine, psychology, nursing, or physical therapy.

Once biofeedback is used for the control of migraine headaches or some other health problem does the person need maintenance sessions of any kind, or will they need to repeat the entire treatment process again and again?

Most patients learn skills that continue to work for them for a lifetime. That is the beauty of biofeedback. Medicines for psychiatric or medical problems often work only until you stop them. Biofeedback teaches self-control skills that one can use over and over for new problems that arise in life.

Some persons periodically return for additional biofeedback sessions to brush up their skills. Dr. Joel Lubar, who developed the biofeedback treatment for ADHD, reports that most of his patients function for years with improved attention, and only occasionally come back for a short refresher course. Some problems, like migraine headache, may require extensive additional treatment at various times in life.

Is biofeedback something people can do on their own? If so, how is it best learned?

It is easier to learn biofeedback through treatment with a qualified professional. There are many related self-help skills that one can learn on one's own, such as progressive muscle relaxation, autogenic training, and meditation. Relaxation and meditation classes and workbooks are inexpensive ways to gain these skills.

There are several biofeedback systems being developed for patient self-education or for home training in between biofeedback therapy sessions. For example, the Heart Math company has a "trainer" unit that patients can use to train themselves in cardiovascular relaxation. The East 3 Company is working on a home EEG [electroencephalography] trainer, for patients to use with children with attention problems.

What is a visit to a biofeedback practitioner like? What should a person expect and should they do anything to prepare?

The treatment should begin with a clinical interview, in which the therapist learns all about the patient's life, family, work, sources of stress, coping skills, and medical and emotional problems. Biofeedback is a "holistic" mind-body therapy, meaning that biofeedback practitioners see any illness or problem as involving the whole person. So one must begin by getting to know the person who has the illness.

Next the therapist will do a biofeedback evaluation (also called a "psychophysiological stress profile"), to identify the patient's unique stress response. The interview and biofeedback evaluation are used to design the treatment.

No preparation is necessary prior to the first interview, although it helps to prepare a written timeline showing the onset and progression of one's symptoms, along with important life events in the same time period.

How many sessions are needed and generally what is the cost?

The length of treatment varies depending on the presenting problem. For most mental health problems and many medical problems eight to 12 sessions can provide excellent results. For some problems like epilepsy, alcoholism, or attention deficit, frequent and lengthy treatment is necessary: two to three sessions a week for 30–60 sessions.

Costs vary around the country, and are higher in urban areas. Half-hour training sessions can cost from $30 to $75. One-hour sessions range from $60 to $150.

Has there been any scientific research to support the use of biofeedback as a treatment method? If so, how can one find such research?

Yes, there is extensive scientific evidence proving the effectiveness of biofeedback. See the References portion of text for books and book chapters reviewing research on biofeedback treatment. AAPB also publishes a booklet summarizing the research showing that biofeedback is effective for many disorders (Shellenberger, Amar, Schneider, & Turner, 1994).

References

Lawlis, G.F. (2001). Biofeedback (pp. 196–224). In L.W. Freeman, & G.F. Lawlis (2001). *Mosby's Complementary and alternative medicine: A research based approach.* St. Louis, MO: Mosby.

Moss, D. (2001). Biofeedback. In S. Shannon (Ed.), *Handbook of complementary medicine in mental health.* San Diego, CA: Academic Press.

Moss, D., Wickramasekera, I., McGrady, A., & Davies, T. (Eds.). (2003). *Handbook of mind-body medicine in primary care: Behavioral and physiological tools.* Thousand Oaks, CA: Sage Publications.

Schwartz, M. & Associates. (2nd edition, 1995). *Biofeedback: A practitioner's guide.* NY: Guilford.

Schwartz, M., & Andrasik, F. (3rd edition, 2003). *Biofeedback: A practitioner's guide.* NY: Guilford.

Shellenberger, R., Amar, P., Schneider., P., & Turner, J. (1994). *Clinical efficacy and cost effectiveness of biofeedback therapy. Guidelines for third party reimbursement.* Wheat Ridge, Co.: Association for Applied Psychophysiology and Biofeedback.

Health Reference Series *Medical Advisor's Notes and Updates*

There is a great deal of variation in the strength and quality of the evidence supporting the use of biofeedback for the above listed disorders. While there is fairly good scientific support for some uses, the data supporting others are questionable. Additional research is needed to fairly evaluate which disorders benefit from biofeedback and to what degree.

Chapter 44

Deep Breathing Exercises

Cancer pain can be managed effectively in most patients with cancer or with a history of cancer. Although cancer pain cannot always be relieved completely, therapy can lessen pain in most patients. Pain management improves the patient's quality of life throughout all stages of the disease.

Flexibility is important in managing cancer pain. As patients vary in diagnosis, stage of disease, responses to pain and treatments, and personal likes and dislikes, management of cancer pain must be individualized. Patients, their families, and their health care providers must work together closely to manage a patient's pain effectively.

Physical and Psychosocial Interventions

Noninvasive physical and psychological methods can be used along with drugs and other treatments to manage pain during all phases of cancer treatment. The effectiveness of the pain interventions depends on the patient's participation in treatment and his or her ability to tell the health care provider which methods work best to relieve pain.

Physical Interventions

Weakness, muscle wasting, and muscle/bone pain may be treated with heat (a hot pack or heating pad); cold (flexible ice packs); massage,

Excerpted from PDQ® Cancer Information Summary. National Cancer Institute; Bethesda, MD. Pain (PDQ®): Supportive Care—Patient. Updated 02/2009. Available at http://cancer.gov. Accessed January 7, 2009.

pressure, and vibration (to improve relaxation); exercise (to strengthen weak muscles, loosen stiff joints, help restore coordination and balance, and strengthen the heart); changing the position of the patient; restricting the movement of painful areas or broken bones; stimulation; controlled low-voltage electrical stimulation; or acupuncture.

Thinking and Behavioral Interventions

Thinking and behavior interventions are also important in treating pain. These interventions help give patients a sense of control and help them develop coping skills to deal with the disease and its symptoms. Beginning these interventions early in the course of the disease is useful so that patients can learn and practice the skills while they have enough strength and energy. Several methods should be tried, and one or more should be used regularly.

- **Relaxation and imagery:** Simple relaxation techniques may be used for episodes of brief pain (for example, during cancer treatment procedures). Brief, simple techniques are suitable for periods when the patient's ability to concentrate is limited by severe pain, high anxiety, or fatigue.

- **Hypnosis:** Hypnotic techniques may be used to encourage relaxation and may be combined with other thinking/behavior methods. Hypnosis is effective in relieving pain in people who are able to concentrate and use imagery and who are willing to practice the technique.

- **Redirecting thinking:** Focusing attention on triggers other than pain or negative emotions that come with pain may involve distractions that are internal (for example, counting, praying, or saying things like "I can cope") or external (for example, music, television, talking, listening to someone read, or looking at something specific). Patients can also learn to monitor and evaluate negative thoughts and replace them with more positive thoughts and images.

- **Patient education:** Health care providers can give patients and their families information and instructions about pain and pain management and assure them that most pain can be controlled effectively. Health care providers should also discuss the major barriers that interfere with effective pain management.

- **Psychological support:** Short-term psychological therapy helps some patients. Patients who develop clinical depression or adjustment disorder may see a psychiatrist for diagnosis.

- **Support groups and religious counseling:** Support groups help many patients. Religious counseling may also help by providing spiritual care and social support.

Relaxation Exercises

The following relaxation exercises may be helpful in relieving pain.

Exercise 1: Slow Rhythmic Breathing for Relaxation*

1. Breathe in slowly and deeply, keeping your stomach and shoulders relaxed.

2. As you breathe out slowly, feel yourself beginning to relax; feel the tension leaving your body.

3. Breathe in and out slowly and regularly at a comfortable rate. Let the breath come all the way down to your stomach, as it completely relaxes.

4. To help you focus on your breathing and to breathe slowly and rhythmically: Breathe in as you say silently to yourself, "in, two, three" or each time you breathe out, say silently to yourself a word such as "peace" or "relax."

5. Do steps 1 through 4 only once or repeat steps 3 and 4 for up to 20 minutes.

6. End with a slow deep breath. As you breathe out say to yourself, "I feel alert and relaxed."

Exercise 2: Simple Touch, Massage, or Warmth for Relaxation*

Touch and massage are traditional methods of helping others relax. Some examples include the following:

- Brief touch or massage, such as hand holding or briefly touching or rubbing a person's shoulders, can help relax the patient.

- Soaking feet in a basin of warm water or wrapping the feet in a warm, wet towel can be relaxing.

- Massage (3 to 10 minutes) of the whole body or just the back, feet, or hands. If the patient is modest or cannot move or turn easily in bed, consider massage of the hands and feet.

- Use a warm lubricant. A small bowl of hand lotion may be warmed in the microwave oven or a bottle of lotion may be warmed in a sink of hot water for about 10 minutes.

- Massage for relaxation is usually done with smooth, long, slow strokes. Try several degrees of pressure along with different types of massage, such as kneading and stroking, to determine which is preferred.

Especially for the elderly person, a back rub that effectively produces relaxation may consist of no more than 3 minutes of slow, rhythmic stroking (about 60 strokes per minute) on both sides of the spine, from the crown of the head to the lower back. Continuous hand contact is maintained by starting one hand down the back as the other hand stops at the lower back and is raised. Set aside a regular time for the massage. This gives the patient something pleasant to anticipate.

*Exercise 3: Peaceful Past Experiences**

Something may have happened to you a while ago that brought you peace or comfort. You may be able to draw on that experience to bring you peace or comfort now. Think about these questions:

- Can you remember any situation, even when you were a child, when you felt calm, peaceful, secure, hopeful, or comfortable?

- Have you ever daydreamed about something peaceful? What were you thinking?

- Do you get a dreamy feeling when you listen to music? Do you have any favorite music?

- Do you have any favorite poetry that you find uplifting or reassuring?

- Have you ever been active religiously? Do you have favorite readings, hymns, or prayers? Even if you haven't heard or thought of them for many years, childhood religious experiences may still be very soothing.

Additional points: Some of the things that may comfort you, such as your favorite music or a prayer, can probably be recorded for you. Then you can listen to the tape whenever you wish. Or, if your memory is strong, you may simply close your eyes and recall the events or words.

*Exercise 4: Active Listening to Recorded Music**

1. Obtain the following:

    *   An MP3, CD, or tape player (Small, battery-operated ones are more convenient.)

    *   Earphones or a headset (Helps focus the attention better than a speaker a few feet away, and avoids disturbing others.)

    *   Music you like (Most people prefer fast, lively music, but some select relaxing music. Other options are comedy routines, sporting events, old radio shows, or stories.)

2. Mark time to the music; for example, tap out the rhythm with your finger or nod your head. This helps you concentrate on the music rather than on your discomfort.

3. Keep your eyes open and focus on a fixed spot or object. If you wish to close your eyes, picture something about the music.

4. Listen to the music at a comfortable volume. If the discomfort increases, try increasing the volume; decrease the volume when the discomfort decreases.

5. If this is not effective enough, try adding or changing one or more of the following: Massage your body in rhythm to the music; try other music; or mark time to the music in more than one manner, such as tapping your foot and finger at the same time.

Additional points: Many patients have found this technique to be helpful. It tends to be very popular, probably because the equipment is usually readily available and is a part of daily life. Other advantages are that it is easy to learn and not physically or mentally demanding. If you are very tired, you may simply listen to the music and omit marking time or focusing on a spot.

*Note: Adapted and reprinted with permission from McCaffery M, Beebe A: *Pain: Clinical Manual for Nursing Practice.* St. Louis, Mo: CV Mosby: 1989.

Chapter 45

Feng Shui

What Is It?

Feng shui is the study of how humans interact with their environment. More specifically feng shui is all about creating an atmosphere in buildings in which the people who use them can best succeed. Feng shui is based on the premise that human beings contain and are surrounded by a subtle field of electromagnetic energy known as chi in China. This can be photographed using Kirlian Photography and looks like a multi colored gas flame around any living creature. In humans the color and shape changes depending on emotional responses, so this energy can be said to contain some of a person's emotional energy.

In China this energy is called chi and chi is widely used in most traditional oriental humanistic pursuits; including acupuncture, chi gong [qigong], shiatsu, Reiki, martial arts, and feng shui. The idea in feng shui is that each building has its own atmospheric chi and that this energy will influence the chi energy field around the human body. Once a person interacts with the energy of a building he or she will begin to feel different.

How Does It Work?

The principle behind feng shui is that your own chi carries your thoughts and emotions around and through your body and that if

"Feng Shui Principles," © 2006 ChiEnergy (http://chienergy.co.uk). Reprinted with permission. For additional information about feng shui, visit http://chienergy.co.uk/freeinformation_fs.htm.

something changes your chi you will find that you feel and think differently. Each building has its own atmosphere and this energy will influence your own chi energy field. For example you will feel different standing in a large empty cathedral and sitting in a small crowded cafe.

The aim of modern feng shui is to create buildings in which people will be able to best succeed in that environment. Therefore the only question a feng shui consultant will be interested in is how will people who use the space feel whilst they are there and what kind of human feelings will best help each person succeed.

What Do You Want?

When using feng shui it is helpful to know what you want from life, what you could change about yourself to achieve it more easily and then how you can set up your home or work space so that you feel better able to make those changes. For example if you wanted to get a promotion but felt you needed to be more outgoing and expressive to achieve that you would need to set up the spaces you spent most time so that the atmosphere brought out those aspects of your character more. In this feng shui example bright colors, mirrors, plants, up lighting, and sunshine would help.

In addition to looking at the way people react with their buildings feng shui examines the relationship between buildings and their environment. The way a building is exposed to sunlight is a prime factor as the sun's solar radiation alters the atmosphere in different parts of a building. The local terrain, water, earth's magnetic field, earth energies, and nearby buildings will all contribute to defining how a new building can best harmonize with its environment and harness this to improve the internal feng shui atmosphere.

Feng Shui at Work

To give people the best opportunity to fulfill their potential it is important to look at the kind of work that is done and think through what atmosphere would encourage the kind of emotions that bring success. For example someone who is dealing with complaints will need to be patient, sensitive, diplomatic, and understanding. So here a softer feng shui work environment with pastel colors and curved forms would be ideal.

Office environments can be set up so that people feel empowered and best able to master the work required. Most important in this situation is the seating position relative to the room. Feng shui principles suggest staff would sit facing into the room in a way that he or she can

318

see the door to the office and any windows. This means most of what is happening in an office is going on in front of the person and he or she can feel protected from behind by a wall.

Pollution, EMF (Electromagnetic Fields), and Noise

Potentially toxic fumes given off by the synthetic surface materials and paints often pollute the modern office. In addition the electronic equipment, computers, fax machines, and copiers tend to emit electromagnetic fields and this makes it harder to maintain good health and concentration from a feng shui perspective. One way to combat office pollution is to fill the space with plants. Healthy plants will clean the air and reduce the influence of the electrical equipment. In addition plants have excellent properties for reducing sound.

Chapter 46

Guided Imagery and Hypnosis

Chapter Contents

Section 46.1—Guided Imagery 322

Section 46.2—Hypnosis 324

Section 46.1

Guided Imagery

"Guided Imagery," © Center for Integrative Health and Healing. Reprinted with permission. For additional information, visit www.cihh.net. The date of this document is unknown. The text that follows this document under the heading "Health Reference Series Medical Advisor's Notes and Updates" was provided to Omnigraphics, Inc. by David A. Cooke, MD, FACP, January 23, 2010. Dr. Cooke is not affiliated with the Center for Integrative Health and Healing.

Train your brain to improve your health. While that may sound funny, it's a powerful technique you can use to heal your body and even prevent the onset of disease. It's called guided imagery and it's a remarkable trend in holistic medicine.

Who can benefit?

Research has proven guided imagery to be helpful with the following and more:

- Posttraumatic stress disorder (PTSD)
- Lower blood pressure
- Reduce cholesterol
- Reduce anxiety and depression
- Speed up healing from cuts, fractures, and burns
- Enhance immune function
- Cancer patient support
- Irritable bowel syndrome (IBS)
- Reduce chronic pain and fibromyalgia
- Reduce length of hospital stay in postoperative patients
- Reduce allergic reactions

What is guided imagery?

Guided imagery is a form of deliberate daydreaming; a mixture of guided hypnosis and guided meditation. It utilizes both the power of one's imagination and suggestive words and phrases to evoke one's memory and multi-sensory fantasies for the purpose of healing or the development of a management strategy in the face of adverse situations.

A meditative styled hypnosis, guided imagery is a gentle yet powerful practice which is easy for most people to do and produces very effective results. The only prerequisite is motivation.

How does guided imagery work?

Imagery works by sending healing images straight into one's brain and nervous system by way of primitive, sensory pathways. Because the route of travel of these messages goes to the right brain (non-dominant brain) which feels, perceives, and senses as opposed to the left brain which is busy judging, deciding, and analyzing, healing imagery can be a very effective intervention tool for many diseases, stress, and traumatic conditions.

Guided imagery easily supports other ongoing therapies and also provides the patient his own powerful tool which grows more effective with continued use.

What's a guided imagery session like?

Initially, you will meet with the practitioner to discuss the personal issues you wish to overcome using guided imagery before the actual session occurs.

The 1-hour session takes place in a warm and tranquil room where you can chose between sitting in a comfortable chair or lying down on a soft massage table. The practitioner dims the lights and sits nearby.

Carefully selected music serves to enhance the imagery work by subtly falling into the background of the therapeutic session while at the same time promoting momentum for it.

The practitioner begins meditation and breath work to prepare you for a relaxed state. The first part of your session involves discovering your sacred place from which you can feel utter safety. This sacred place can be from a real or imagined memory. From this inner protective sanctuary, healing images are evoked.

With the practitioner's guidance, these powerful healing images interact with the symptom image to reduce or eliminate its effects. The second and third sessions further develop and attune these skills for continued independent use.

Health Reference Series *Medical Advisor's Notes and Updates*

Use of guided imagery for problems listed in the "Who can benefit?" section and others remains quite controversial. Different studies have produced conflicting results, some showing benefits and others no effect. Many of these conditions are difficult to measure and may naturally vary over time, so the reliability of the data is questionable. Many experts feel that the effectiveness of guided imagery is neither proven nor disproved at this point.

Section 46.2

Hypnosis

While you may think of hypnosis as something you see only in the movies or novels, hypnosis is used in real life as part of the treatment plan for people with numerous health ailments ranging from depression to gastrointestinal disorders. Based on research showing that hypnosis can help people manage—and in some cases recover from illness, hypnosis is becoming a more common part of many patients' recommended health treatment.

Definition

According to the American Psychological Association (APA)'s Division of Psychological Hypnosis, hypnosis is a procedure during which a health professional or researcher suggests while treating someone that he or she experience changes in sensations, perceptions, thoughts, or behavior. Although some hypnosis is used to make people more alert, most hypnosis includes suggestions for relaxation, calmness, and well-being. Instructions to imagine or think about pleasant experiences are also commonly included during hypnosis. People respond to hypnosis in different ways. Some describe hypnosis as a state of focused attention, in which they feel very calm and relaxed. Most people describe the experience as pleasant.

Is There Evidence That Hypnosis Works?

Yes. While there are plenty of examples in the scientific literature attesting to the usefulness of clinical hypnosis, a study published in the journal *Gut* is noteworthy. The study involved 204 people suffering from Irritable Bowel Syndrome (IBS). Treatment consisted of 12 weekly sessions of hypnosis (lasting about 1 hour each). Fifty-eight percent of the men and 75 percent of the women reported significant symptom relief immediately after finishing treatment. More than 80 percent of those who reported initial relief were still improved up to 6 years later. Fewer than 10 percent of the participants tried other treatments after hypnotherapy. (*Gut*, November 2003).

Can Everyone Be Hypnotized?

People differ in the degree to which they respond to hypnosis. A person's ability to experience hypnosis can be inhibited by fears and concerns arising from some common misconceptions. Contrary to some depictions of hypnosis in books, movies, or television, people who have been hypnotized do not lose control over their behavior. Unless amnesia has specifically been suggested, people remain aware of who they are, where they are, and remember what transpired during hypnosis. Hypnosis makes it easier for people to experience suggestions, but it does not force them to have these experiences.

Is Hypnosis Therapy?

Hypnosis is not a type of psychotherapy. It also is not a treatment in and of itself; rather, it is a procedure that can be used to facilitate other types of therapies and treatments. Clinical hypnosis should be conducted only by properly trained and credentialed health care professionals (e.g., psychologists) who also have been trained in the use of hypnosis and who are working within the limits of their professional expertise.

Practical Uses for Hypnosis

Hypnosis has been used in the treatment of pain; depression; anxiety and phobias; stress; habit disorders; gastrointestinal disorders; skin conditions; post-surgical recovery; relief from nausea and vomiting; childbirth; treatment of hemophilia; and many other conditions. However, it may not be useful for all psychological and/or medical problems or for all patients or clients. The decision to use hypnosis as an adjunct to treatment should only be made in consultation with a qualified health care provider who has been trained in the use and limitations of clinical hypnosis. In addition to its use in clinical settings, hypnosis is used in research and forensic settings. Researchers study the value of hypnosis in the treatment of physical and psychological problems and examine the impact of hypnosis on sensation, perception, learning, and memory.

Professional Hypnosis Organizations

APA Division 30, Society of Psychological Hypnosis: http://www.apa.org/divisions/div30 (Executive Committee of the American Psychological Association, Division of Psychological Hypnosis—promotes professional education and exchange of scientific information and develops standards of care).

American Board of Psychological Hypnosis (ABPH)
c/o Gary R. Elkins, PhD, ABPH
Scott & White Clinic
Department of Psychiatry
2401 South 31st Street
Temple, TX 76508
E-mail:
gelkins@swmail.sw.org

American Society of Clinical Hypnosis (ASCH)
140 North Bloomingdale Road
Bloomingdale, IL 60108-1017
Phone: 630-980-4740
Fax: 630-351-8490
E-mail:
info@asch.net
Website:
http://www.asch.net

The International Society of Hypnosis (ISH)
c/o Dr. E. Vermetten
University Medical Center Utrecht
P.O. Box 342
4000 AH TIEL
The Netherlands
Tel. + 31 344 615 427
Fax + 31 344 655 260
E-mail:
info@ish-web.org

Society for Clinical and Experimental Hypnosis (SCEH)
2201 Haeder Road, Suite 1
Pullman, WA 99163
Phone: 509-332-7555
Fax: 509-332-5907
E-mail:
sceh@pullman.com

Chapter 47

Meditation

Meditation is a mind-body practice in complementary and alternative medicine (CAM). There are many types of meditation, most of which originated in ancient religious and spiritual traditions. Generally, a person who is meditating uses certain techniques, such as a specific posture, focused attention, and an open attitude toward distractions. Meditation may be practiced for many reasons, such as to increase calmness and physical relaxation, to improve psychological balance, to cope with illness, or to enhance overall wellness.

Overview

The term meditation refers to a group of techniques, such as mantra meditation, relaxation response, mindfulness meditation, and Zen Buddhist meditation. Most meditative techniques started in Eastern religious or spiritual traditions. These techniques have been used by many different cultures throughout the world for thousands of years. Today, many people use meditation outside of its traditional religious or cultural settings, for health and wellness purposes.

In meditation, a person learns to focus attention. Some forms of meditation instruct the practitioner to become mindful of thoughts, feelings, and sensations and to observe them in a nonjudgmental way. This practice is believed to result in a state of greater calmness and

From "Meditation: An Introduction," by the National Center for Complementary and Alternative Medicine (NCCAM, nccam.nih.gov), part of the National Institutes of Health, February 2009.

physical relaxation, and psychological balance. Practicing meditation can change how a person relates to the flow of emotions and thoughts in the mind.

Most types of meditation have four elements in common:

- **A quiet location:** Meditation is usually practiced in a quiet place with as few distractions as possible. This can be particularly helpful for beginners.

- **A specific, comfortable posture:** Depending on the type being practiced, meditation can be done while sitting, lying down, standing, walking, or in other positions.

- **A focus of attention:** Focusing one's attention is usually a part of meditation. For example, the meditator may focus on a mantra (a specially chosen word or set of words), an object, or the sensations of the breath. Some forms of meditation involve paying attention to whatever is the dominant content of consciousness.

- **An open attitude:** Having an open attitude during meditation means letting distractions come and go naturally without judging them. When the attention goes to distracting or wandering thoughts, they are not suppressed; instead, the meditator gently brings attention back to the focus. In some types of meditation, the meditator learns to "observe" thoughts and emotions while meditating.

Meditation used as CAM is a type of mind-body medicine. Generally, mind-body medicine focuses on the following:

- The interactions among the brain/mind, the rest of the body, and behavior

- The ways in which emotional, mental, social, spiritual, and behavioral factors can directly affect health

Uses of Meditation for Health in the United States

A 2007 national government survey that asked about CAM use in a sample of 23,393 U.S. adults found that 9.4 percent of respondents (representing more than 20 million people) had used meditation in the past 12 months—compared with 7.6 percent of respondents (representing more than 15 million people) in a similar survey conducted in 2002. The 2007 survey also asked about CAM use in a sample of 9,417 children; 1 percent (representing 725,000 children) had used meditation in the past 12 months.

People use meditation for various health problems, such as the following:

- Anxiety
- Pain
- Depression
- Stress
- Insomnia
- Physical or emotional symptoms that may be associated with chronic illnesses (such as heart disease, HIV/AIDS [human immunodeficiency syndrome/acquired immunodeficiency syndrome], and cancer) and their treatment

Meditation is also used for overall wellness.

Examples of Meditation Practices

Mindfulness meditation and Transcendental Meditation (also known as TM) are two common forms of meditation. NCCAM-sponsored research projects are studying both of these types of meditation.

Mindfulness meditation is an essential component of Buddhism. In one common form of mindfulness meditation, the meditator is taught to bring attention to the sensation of the flow of the breath in and out of the body. The meditator learns to focus attention on what is being experienced, without reacting to or judging that experience. This is seen as helping the meditator learn to experience thoughts and emotions in normal daily life with greater balance and acceptance.

The TM technique is derived from Hindu traditions. It uses a mantra (a word, sound, or phrase repeated silently) to prevent distracting thoughts from entering the mind. The goal of TM is to achieve a state of relaxed awareness.

How Meditation Might Work

Practicing meditation has been shown to induce some changes in the body. By learning more about what goes on in the body during meditation, researchers hope to be able to identify diseases or conditions for which meditation might be useful.

Some types of meditation might work by affecting the autonomic (involuntary) nervous system. This system regulates many organs and muscles, controlling functions such as the heartbeat, sweating, breathing, and digestion. It has two major parts:

- The sympathetic nervous system helps mobilize the body for action. When a person is under stress, it produces the "fight-or-flight response": The heart rate and breathing rate go up and blood vessels narrow (restricting the flow of blood).

- The parasympathetic nervous system causes the heart rate and breathing rate to slow down, the blood vessels to dilate (improving blood flow), and digestive juices to increase.

It is thought that some types of meditation might work by reducing activity in the sympathetic nervous system and increasing activity in the parasympathetic nervous system.

In one area of research, scientists are using sophisticated tools to determine whether meditation is associated with significant changes in brain function. A number of researchers believe that these changes account for many of meditation's effects.

It is also possible that practicing meditation may work by improving the mind's ability to pay attention. Since attention is involved in performing everyday tasks and regulating mood, meditation might lead to other benefits.

A 2007 NCCAM-funded review of the scientific literature found some evidence suggesting that meditation is associated with potentially beneficial health effects. However, the overall evidence was inconclusive. The reviewers concluded that future research needs to be more rigorous before firm conclusions can be drawn.

Side Effects and Risks

Meditation is considered to be safe for healthy people. There have been rare reports that meditation could cause or worsen symptoms in people who have certain psychiatric problems, but this question has not been fully researched.

People with physical limitations may not be able to participate in certain meditative practices involving physical movement. Individuals with existing mental or physical health conditions should speak with their health care providers prior to starting a meditative practice and make their meditation instructor aware of their condition.

If You Are Thinking about Using Meditation Practices

- Do not use meditation as a replacement for conventional care or as a reason to postpone seeing a doctor about a medical problem.

- Ask about the training and experience of the meditation instructor you are considering.

- Look for published research studies on meditation for the health condition in which you are interested.

- Tell your health care providers about any complementary and alternative practices you use. Give them a full picture of what you do to manage your health. This will help ensure coordinated and safe care.

NCCAM-Supported Research

Some recent NCCAM-supported studies have been investigating meditation for the following:

- Relieving stress in caregivers for elderly patients with dementia

- Reducing the frequency and intensity of hot flashes in menopausal women

- Relieving symptoms of chronic back pain

- Improving attention-related abilities (alerting, focusing, and prioritizing)

- Relieving asthma symptoms.

Chapter 48

Music Therapy

What is music therapy?

Music therapy is the clinical and evidence-based use of music interventions to accomplish individualized goals within a therapeutic relationship by a credentialed professional who has completed an approved music therapy program. (American Music Therapy Association definition, 2005)

What do music therapists do?

Music therapists assess emotional well-being, physical health, social functioning, communication abilities, and cognitive skills through musical responses; design music sessions for individuals and groups based on client needs using music improvisation, receptive music listening, song writing, lyric discussion, music and imagery, music performance, and learning through music; participate in interdisciplinary treatment planning, ongoing evaluation, and follow up.

Who can benefit from music therapy?

Children, adolescents, adults, and the elderly with mental health needs, developmental and learning disabilities, Alzheimer's disease and other aging related conditions, substance abuse problems, brain injuries, physical disabilities, and acute and chronic pain, including mothers in labor.

"Frequently Asked Questions About Music Therapy," © 2009 American Music Therapy Association (www.musictherapy.org). Reprinted with permission.

Where do music therapists work?

Music therapists work in psychiatric hospitals, rehabilitative facilities, medical hospitals, outpatient clinics, day care treatment centers, agencies serving developmentally disabled persons, community mental health centers, drug and alcohol programs, senior centers, nursing homes, hospice programs, correctional facilities, halfway houses, schools, and private practice.

What is the history of music therapy as a health care profession?

The idea of music as a healing influence which could affect health and behavior is at least as old as the writings of Aristotle and Plato. The 20th century discipline began after World War I and World War II when community musicians of all types, both amateur and professional, went to veterans' hospitals around the country to play for the thousands of veterans suffering both physical and emotional trauma from the wars. The patients' notable physical and emotional responses to music led the doctors and nurses to request the hiring of musicians by the hospitals. It was soon evident that the hospital musicians needed some prior training before entering the facility and so the demand grew for a college curriculum. The first music therapy degree program in the world, founded at Michigan State University in 1944, celebrated its 50th anniversary in 1994. The American Music Therapy Association was founded in 1998 as a union of the National Association for Music Therapy and the American Association for Music Therapy.

Who is qualified to practice music therapy?

Persons who complete one of the approved college music therapy curricula (including an internship) are then eligible to sit for the national examination offered by the Certification Board for Music Therapists. Music therapists who successfully complete the independently administered examination hold the music therapist-board certified credential (MT-BC).

The National Music Therapy Registry (NMTR) serves qualified music therapy professionals with the following designations: RMT [Registered Music Therapist], CMT [Certified Music Therapist], ACMT [Advanced Certified Music Therapist]. These individuals have met accepted educational and clinical training standards and are qualified to practice music therapy.

Is there research to support music therapy?

AMTA promotes a vast amount of research exploring the benefits of music as therapy through publication of the *Journal of Music Therapy*, *Music Therapy Perspectives*, and other sources. A substantial body of literature exists to support the effectiveness of music therapy.

What are some misconceptions about music therapy?

That the client or patient has to have some particular music ability to benefit from music therapy—they do not. That there is one particular style of music that is more therapeutic than all the rest—this is not the case. All styles of music can be useful in effecting change in a client or patient's life. The individual's preferences, circumstances and need for treatment, and the client or patient's goals help to determine the types of music a music therapist may use.

How can music therapy techniques be applied by healthy individuals?

Healthy individuals can use music for stress reduction via active music making, such as drumming, as well as passive listening for relaxation. Music is often a vital support for physical exercise. Music therapy assisted labor and delivery may also be included in this category since pregnancy is regarded as a normal part of women's life cycles.

How is music therapy utilized in hospitals?

Music is used in general hospitals to: alleviate pain in conjunction with anesthesia or pain medication; elevate patients' mood and counteract depression; promote movement for physical rehabilitation; calm or sedate, often to induce sleep; counteract apprehension or fear; and lessen muscle tension for the purpose of relaxation, including the autonomic nervous system.

How is music therapy utilized in nursing homes?

Music is used with elderly persons to increase or maintain their level of physical, mental, and social/emotional functioning. The sensory and intellectual stimulation of music can help maintain a person's quality of life.

How is music therapy utilized in schools?

Music therapists are often hired in schools to provide music therapy services listed on the Individualized Education Plan for mainstreamed special learners. Music learning is used to strengthen nonmusical areas such as communication skills and physical coordination skills which are important for daily life.

How is music therapy utilized in psychiatric facilities?

Music therapy allows persons with mental health needs to: explore personal feelings, make positive changes in mood and emotional states, have a sense of control over life through successful experiences, practice problem solving, and resolve conflicts leading to stronger family and peer relationships.

Is music therapy a reimbursable service?

Medicare: Since 1994, music therapy has been identified as a reimbursable service under benefits for Partial Hospitalization Programs (PHP). Falling under the heading of Activity Therapy, the interventions cannot be purely recreational or diversionary in nature and must be individualized and based on goals specified in the treatment plan. The current HCPCS [Healthcare Common Procedure Coding System] Code for PHP is G0176.

The music therapy must be considered an active treatment by meeting the following criteria:

- be prescribed by a physician;
- be reasonable and necessary for the treatment of the individual's illness or injury;
- be goal directed and based on a documented treatment plan;
- the goal of treatment cannot be to merely maintain current level of functioning—the individual must exhibit some level of improvement.

Medicaid: As Medicaid programs vary from state-to-state, so do the Medicaid coverage avenues for music therapy services. Some private practice music therapists have successfully applied for Medicaid provider numbers within their states. Some states offer waiver programs in which music therapy can be covered. In some situations, although music therapy is not specifically listed as a covered service, due to functional outcomes achieved, music therapy interventions can fall under an existing treatment category such as community support, rehabilitation, or habilitation.

Examples:

- **Arizona:** Medicaid coverage for music therapy provided to individuals with developmental disabilities; originally recognized as a habilitation service but also considered as a socialization service.

- **Minnesota:** Individual music therapist received provider number to service clients with mental illness and developmental disabilities. Waiver program for children with developmental disabilities provides coverage for music therapy.

- **Pennsylvania:** Department of Aging Waiver program allows Medicaid payment for music therapy provided in a community based setting. Music therapy is listed under health and mental health related counseling services.

- **North Carolina:** Medicaid reimbursement is available for music therapy services through the Community Alternatives Program (CAP) for clients with developmental disabilities.

- **Indiana:** Waiver program for children with developmental disabilities offers coverage for music therapy.

- **Michigan:** Music therapy is a covered service under the state's Medicaid Children's Waiver Program.

Private insurance: The number of success stories involving third party reimbursement for the provision of music therapy services continues to grow. Over the past 12 years a growing public demand for music therapy services has been accompanied by a demand for third party reimbursement. In response to the increasing demand the music therapy profession has worked to facilitate the reimbursement process for clients of music therapy services.

The American Music Therapy Association now estimates that at least 20% of music therapists receive third party reimbursement for the services they provide. This number is expected to increase exponentially as music therapy occupies a strong position in the health care industry.

Insurance companies are recognizing the advantages of including music therapy as a benefit as they respond to the increasing market demand for greater patient choice of health care services. Companies like Blue Cross/Blue Shield, Humana, Great West Life, Aetna, Metropolitan, and Provident have reimbursed for music therapy services on a case-by-case basis, based on medical necessity.

Music therapy is comparable to other health professions like occupational therapy and physical therapy in that individual assessments are provided for each client, service must be found reasonable and necessary for the individual's illness or injury, and interventions include a goal-directed documented treatment plan.

Like other therapies, music therapy is typically preapproved for coverage or reimbursement, and is found to be reimbursable when deemed medically necessary to reach the treatment goals of the individual patient. Therefore, reimbursement for services is determined on a case-by-case basis and is available in a large variety of health care settings, with patients with varying diagnoses.

Other sources: Additional sources for reimbursement and financing of music therapy services include: many state departments of mental health, state departments of mental retardation/developmental disabilities, state adoption subsidy programs, private auto insurance, employee worker's compensation, county boards of mental retardation/developmental disabilities, IDEA Part B related services funds, foundations, grants, and private pay.

What is the American Music Therapy Association?

The American Music Therapy Association is the largest professional association which represents over 5,000 music therapists, corporate members, and related associations worldwide. Founded in 1998, its mission is the progressive development of the therapeutic use of music in rehabilitation, special education, and community settings. AMTA sets the education and clinical training standards for music therapists. Predecessors to the American Music Therapy Association included the National Association for Music Therapy founded in 1950 and the American Association for Music Therapy founded in 1971.

What is a typical music therapy session like?

Since music therapists serve a wide variety of persons with many different types of needs there is no such thing as an overall typical session. Sessions are designed and music selected based on the individual client's treatment plan.

What is the future of music therapy?

The future of music therapy is promising because state of the art music therapy research in physical rehabilitation, Alzheimer's disease, and psychoneuroimmunology is documenting the effectiveness of music therapy in terms that are important in the context of a biological medical model.

Chapter 49

Prayer and Spirituality

General Information about Spirituality

Religious and spiritual values are important to patients coping with cancer.

The terms spirituality and religion are often used in place of each other, but for many people they have different meanings. Religion may be defined as a specific set of beliefs and practices, usually within an organized group. Spirituality may be defined as an individual's sense of peace, purpose, and connection to others, and beliefs about the meaning of life. Spirituality may be found and expressed through an organized religion or in other ways. Patients may think of themselves as spiritual or religious or both.

Spirituality and religion may have different meanings.

Studies have shown that religious and spiritual values are important to Americans. Most American adults say that they believe in God and that their religious beliefs affect how they live their lives. However, people have different ideas about life after death, belief in miracles, and other religious beliefs. Such beliefs may be based on gender, education, and ethnic background.

Many patients with cancer rely on spiritual or religious beliefs and practices to help them cope with their disease. This is called spiritual

PDQ® Cancer Information Summary. National Cancer Institute; Bethesda, MD. Spirituality in Cancer Care (PDQ®): Supportive Care—Patient. Updated 03/2009. Available at http://cancer.gov. Accessed December 9, 2009.

coping. Many caregivers also rely on spiritual coping. Each person may have different spiritual needs, depending on cultural and religious traditions. Some patients and their family caregivers may want doctors to talk about spiritual concerns, but may feel unsure about how to bring up the subject.

There is a growing understanding that doctors' support of spiritual well-being in very ill patients helps improve their quality of life. Health care providers who treat patients coping with cancer are looking at new ways to help them with religious and spiritual concerns. Doctors may ask patients which spiritual issues are important to them, not only for end-of-life issues but also during treatment.

Serious illness, such as cancer, may cause spiritual distress.

Serious illnesses like cancer may cause patients or family caregivers to have doubts about their beliefs or religious values and cause much spiritual distress. Some studies show that patients with cancer may feel that they are being punished by God or may have a loss of faith after being diagnosed. Other patients may have mild feelings of spiritual distress when coping with cancer.

Spirituality and Quality of Life

Spiritual and religious well-being may help improve quality of life.

It is not known for sure how spirituality and religion are related to health. Some studies show that spiritual or religious beliefs and practices create a positive mental attitude that may help a patient feel better and improve the well-being of family caregivers. Spiritual and religious well-being may help improve health and quality of life in the following ways:

- They may help decrease anxiety, depression, anger, and discomfort.
- They may help decrease the sense of isolation (feeling alone) and the risk of suicide.
- They may help decrease alcohol and drug abuse.
- They may lower blood pressure and the risk of heart disease.
- They may help the patient adjust to the effects of cancer and its treatment.
- They may increase the ability to enjoy life during cancer treatment.
- They may give a feeling of personal growth as a result of living with cancer.

- They may increase positive feelings, including the following:
  - Hope and optimism
  - Freedom from regret
  - Satisfaction with life
  - A sense of inner peace

Spiritual and religious well-being may also help a patient live longer.

Spiritual distress may also affect health. Spiritual distress may make it harder for patients to cope with cancer and cancer treatment. Health care providers may encourage patients to meet with experienced spiritual or religious leaders to help deal with their spiritual issues. This may improve their health, quality of life, and ability to cope.

Spiritual Assessment

A spiritual assessment may help the doctor understand how religious or spiritual beliefs will affect the way a patient copes with cancer.

A spiritual assessment is a method or tool used by doctors to understand the role that religious and spiritual beliefs have in the patient's life. This may help the doctor understand how these beliefs affect the way the patient responds to the cancer diagnosis and decisions about cancer treatment. Some doctors or caregivers may wait for the patient to bring up spiritual concerns. Others may use an interview or a questionnaire.

A spiritual assessment explores religious beliefs and spiritual practices.

A spiritual assessment may include questions about the following:

- Religious denomination, if any
- Beliefs or philosophy of life
- Important spiritual practices or rituals
- Using spirituality or religion as a source of strength
- Being part of a community of support
- Using prayer or meditation
- Loss of faith
- Conflicts between spiritual or religious beliefs and cancer treatments
- Ways that health care providers and caregivers may help with the patient's spiritual needs

- Concerns about death and afterlife
- Planning for the end of life

The health care team may not ask about every issue the patient feels is important. Patients should bring up other spiritual or religious issues that they think may affect their cancer care.

Meeting the Patient's Spiritual and Religious Needs

To help patients with spiritual needs during cancer care, medical staff will listen to the wishes of the patient.

Spirituality and religion are very personal issues. Patients should expect doctors and caregivers to respect their religious and spiritual beliefs and concerns. Patients with cancer who rely on spirituality to cope with the disease should be able to count on the health care team to give them support. This may include giving patients information about people or groups that can help with spiritual or religious needs. Most hospitals have chaplains, but not all outpatient settings do. Patients who do not want to discuss spirituality during cancer care should also be able to count on the health care team to respect their wishes.

Doctors and caregivers will try to respond to their patients' concerns, but may not take part in patients' religious practices or discuss specific religious beliefs.

The health care team will help with a patient's spiritual needs when setting goals and planning treatment.

The health care team may help with a patient's spiritual needs in the following ways:

- They may suggest goals and options for care that honor the patient's spiritual and/or religious views.

- They may support the patient's use of spiritual coping during the illness.

- They may encourage the patient to speak with his/her religious or spiritual leader.

- They may refer the patient to a hospital chaplain or support group that can help with spiritual issues during illness.

- They may refer the patient to other therapies that have been shown to increase spiritual well-being. These include mindfulness relaxation, such as yoga or meditation, or creative arts programs, such as writing, drawing, or music therapy.

Chapter 50

Relaxation Training

One of the most powerful tools a psychologist can use is actually nothing new, said Herbert Benson, MD, at APA's Annual Convention. In fact, it's an approach that's been around for millennia, yet its full potential remains untapped.

Benson was referring to the relaxation response, a physical state of deep rest that changes a person's physical and emotional responses to stress.

Benson, of Harvard Medical School and the Benson-Henry Institute for Mind Body Medicine at Massachusetts General Hospital, discovered the relaxation response's power to reduce stress in the 1960s. But his subsequent research found that the approach is really no different from what people have done for centuries through prayer, chanting, and repetitive motion.

Today, scientists have shown that such practices lower heart rates, blood pressure, and oxygen consumption, and they alleviate the symptoms associated with a vast array of conditions, including hypertension, arthritis, insomnia, depression, infertility, cancer, anxiety, even aging.

"You as psychologists can use the mind like you would use a drug," he said. "This should empower you in your practices."

His latest research, published in the online journal *Public Library of Science ONE* (July 2 [2008]), suggests that practicing the relaxation response can actually lead to genomic activity changes. In the study, his team of researchers looked at how the relaxation response affected each of the body's 40,000 genes and found that, compared with a control group, those who regularly used the relaxation response induced anti-oxidation and anti-inflammatory changes that counteracted the effects of stress on the body.

Everyday Meditation

Eliciting the relaxation response is simple, he explained: Once or twice a day for 10 to 20 minutes, sit in a relaxed position, eyes closed, and repeat a word or sound as you breathe. Some people use such words as "love" or "peace." Others say traditional prayers. If your thoughts stray—which is normal and expected—just refocus on the word repetition.

There are scores of other ways to summon the relaxation response, as well, said Benson. "Anything that breaks the train of everyday thought will evoke this physiological state."

That includes participating in repetitive sports such as running, letting go of tension through progressive muscular relaxation, practicing yoga, knitting, crocheting, even playing musical instruments.

"You know how when you play an instrument and you become 'one' with that instrument and the time flits away? That is the relaxation response," he said. "You know the high you get from running? That is the relaxation response coming about by the repetitive motion of your footfall."

Research into Practice

Benson recommended that psychology practitioners learn a variety of techniques so they can introduce their clients to the practice they'll be comfortable with. Catholics might want to try the "Hail Mary" prayer. Athletes can use repetitive sports.

Keep your mind open about the practice that will work for your clients, he said. "The damning thing about these techniques is that when you use them regularly, you come to believe that the one that was successful for you will be successful for everyone." Let your client find the technique that she or he believes in and encourage daily practice. "You can't simply save this for when they are under stress," he said.

With regular practice, clients develop quieter minds. So it's particularly beneficial when a client elicits the relaxation response before a therapy session.

"With less static, less noise, traditional cognitive restructuring enters," said Benson. "People listen better. It's a more fertile environment, so you can do what you are so well trained to do—the cognitive work, the positive ideation. It's a door opening to allow you to help change people's lives."

Given that 60 percent to 90 percent of health-care professional visits are stress-related, the potential of the relaxation response to help people is enormous, he said. "I believe this is going to change medicine."

Benson's invited address was sponsored by Div. 12 (Society of Clinical Psychology) and Div. 38 (Health).

Further Reading

For more information on Benson's work and the relaxation response, visit the Massachusetts General Hospital Benson-Henry Institute for Mind Body Medicine at www.massgeneral.org/bhi.

Benson's newest research, "Genomic Counter-Stress Changes Induced by the Relaxation Response," appears in the July 2 [2008] edition of PLoS Onc at www.plosone.org.

Chapter 51

Tai Chi

Tai chi, which originated in China as a martial art, is a mind-body practice in complementary and alternative medicine (CAM). Tai chi is sometimes referred to as "moving meditation"—practitioners move their bodies slowly, gently, and with awareness, while breathing deeply.

Overview

Tai chi developed in ancient China. It started as a martial art and a means of self-defense. Over time, people began to use it for health purposes as well.

Accounts of the history of tai chi vary. A popular legend credits its origins to Chang San-Feng, a Taoist monk, who developed a set of 13 exercises that imitate the movements of animals. He also emphasized meditation and the concept of internal force (in contrast to the external force emphasized in other martial arts, such as kung fu and tae kwon do).

The term "tai chi" (shortened from "tai chi chuan") has been translated in various ways, such as "internal martial art" and "supreme ultimate fist." It is sometimes called "taiji" or "taijiquan."

Tai chi incorporates the Chinese concepts of yin and yang (opposing forces within the body) and qi (a vital energy or life force). Practicing tai chi is said to support a healthy balance of yin and yang, thereby aiding the flow of qi.

Excerpted from "Tai Chi: An Introduction," by the National Center for Complementary and Alternative Medicine (NCCAM, nccam.nih.gov), part of the National Institutes of Health, April 2009.

349

People practice tai chi by themselves or in groups. In the Chinese community, people commonly practice tai chi in nearby parks—often in early morning before going to work. There are many different styles, but all involve slow, relaxed, graceful movements, each flowing into the next. The body is in constant motion, and posture is important. The names of some of the movements evoke nature (e.g., "Embrace Tiger, Return to Mountain"). Individuals practicing tai chi must also concentrate, putting aside distracting thoughts; and they must breathe in a deep and relaxed, but focused manner.

Use in the United States

A 2007 survey by the National Center for Health Statistics and the National Center for Complementary and Alternative Medicine (NCCAM) on Americans' use of CAM found that 1 percent of the more than 23,300 adults surveyed had used tai chi in the past 12 months. Adjusted to nationally representative numbers, this means more than 2.3 million adults.

People practice tai chi for various health-related purposes, such as the following:

- For benefits associated with low-impact, weight-bearing, aerobic exercise

- To improve physical condition, muscle strength, coordination, and flexibility

- To improve balance and decrease the risk of falls, especially in elderly people

- To ease pain and stiffness—for example, from osteoarthritis

- To improve sleep

- For overall wellness

The Status of Tai Chi Research

Scientific research on the health benefits of tai chi is ongoing. Several studies have focused on the elderly, including tai chi's potential for preventing falls and improving cardiovascular fitness and overall well-being. A 2007 NCCAM-funded study on the immune response to varicella-zoster virus (the virus that causes shingles) suggested that tai chi may enhance the immune system and improve overall well-being in older adults. Tai chi has also been studied for improving functional capacity in breast cancer patients and quality of life in people with HIV [human immunodeficiency virus] infection. Studies have also looked at tai chi's possible benefits for a variety of other conditions, including cardiovascular disease, hypertension, and osteoarthritis. In 2008, a review of published research, also funded by NCCAM, found that tai chi reduced participants' blood pressure in 22 (of 26) studies.

In general, studies of tai chi have been small, or they have had design limitations that may limit their conclusions. The cumulative evidence suggests that additional research is warranted and needed before tai chi can be widely recommended as an effective therapy.

Side Effects and Risks

Tai chi is a relatively safe practice. However, there are some cautions:

- As with any exercise regimen, if you overdo practice, you may have sore muscles or sprains.

- Tai chi instructors often recommend that you do not practice tai chi right after a meal, or when you are very tired, or if you have an active infection.

- If you are pregnant, or if you have a hernia, joint problems, back pain, fractures, or severe osteoporosis, your health care provider may advise you to modify or avoid certain postures in tai chi.

Training, Licensing, and Certification

Tai chi instructors do not have to be licensed, and the practice is not regulated by the federal government or individual states. In traditional tai chi instruction, a student learns from a master teacher. To become an instructor, an experienced student of tai chi must obtain a master teacher's approval. Currently, training programs vary. Some training programs award certificates; some offer weekend workshops. There is no standard training for instructors.

If You Are Thinking about Practicing Tai Chi

- Do not use tai chi as a replacement for conventional care or to postpone seeing a doctor about a medical problem.

- If you have a medical condition or have not exercised in a while, consult with your health care provider before starting tai chi.

- Keep in mind that learning tai chi from a video or book does not ensure that you are doing the movements correctly and safely.

351

- If you are considering a tai chi instructor, ask about the individual's training and experience.

- Look for published research studies on tai chi for the health condition you are interested in.

- Tell your health care providers about any complementary and alternative practices you use. Give them a full picture of what you do to manage your health. This will help ensure coordinated and safe care.

NCCAM-Funded Research

NCCAM has supported studies of tai chi's effects on the following:

- Bone loss in postmenopausal women

- Cancer survivors

- Depression in elderly patients

- Fibromyalgia symptoms, such as muscle pain, fatigue, and insomnia

- Osteoarthritis of the knee

- Patients with chronic heart failure

- Rheumatoid arthritis

Chapter 52

Yoga

Yoga is a mind-body practice in complementary and alternative medicine with origins in ancient Indian philosophy. The various styles of yoga that people use for health purposes typically combine physical postures, breathing techniques, and meditation or relaxation.

Overview

Yoga in its full form combines physical postures, breathing exercises, meditation, and a distinct philosophy. Yoga is intended to increase relaxation and balance the mind, body, and the spirit.

Early written descriptions of yoga are in Sanskrit, the classical language of India. The word "yoga" comes from the Sanskrit word yuj, which means "yoke or union." It is believed that this describes the union between the mind and the body. The first known text, *The Yoga Sutras,* was written more than 2,000 years ago, although yoga may have been practiced as early as 5,000 years ago. Yoga was originally developed as a method of discipline and attitudes to help people reach spiritual enlightenment. The *Sutras* outline eight limbs or foundations of yoga practice that serve as spiritual guidelines:

- Yama (moral behavior)

- Niyama (healthy habits)

Excerpted from "Yoga for Health: An Introduction," by the National Center for Complementary and Alternative Medicine (NCCAM, nccam.nih.gov), part of the National Institutes of Health, May 2008.

- Asana (physical postures)

- Pranayama (breathing exercises)

- Pratyahara (sense withdrawal)

- Dharana (concentration)

- Dhyana (contemplation)

- Samadhi (higher consciousness)

The numerous schools of yoga incorporate these eight limbs in varying proportions. Hatha yoga, the most commonly practiced in the United States and Europe, emphasizes two of the eight limbs: postures (asanas) and breathing exercises (pranayama). Some of the major styles of hatha yoga include Ananda, Anusara, Ashtanga, Bikram, Iyengar, Kripalu, Kundalini, and Viniyoga.

Use of Yoga for Health in the United States

According to the 2007 National Health Interview Survey (NHIS), which included a comprehensive survey of CAM use by Americans, yoga is one of the top 10 CAM modalities used. More than 13 million adults had used yoga in the previous year, and between the 2002 and 2007 NHIS, use of yoga among adults increased by 1 percent (or approximately 3 million people). The 2007 survey also found that more than 1.5 million children used yoga in the previous year.

People use yoga for a variety of health conditions including anxiety disorders or stress, asthma, high blood pressure, and depression. People also use yoga as part of a general health regimen—to achieve physical fitness and to relax.

The Status of Yoga Research

Research suggests that yoga might help with the following:

- Improve mood and sense of well-being

- Counteract stress

- Reduce heart rate and blood pressure

- Increase lung capacity

- Improve muscle relaxation and body composition

- Help with conditions such as anxiety, depression, and insomnia

- Improve overall physical fitness, strength, and flexibility

- Positively affect levels of certain brain or blood chemicals

More well-designed studies are needed before definitive conclusions can be drawn about yoga's use for specific health conditions.

Side Effects and Risks

- Yoga is generally considered to be safe in healthy people when practiced appropriately. Studies have found it to be well tolerated, with few side effects.

- People with certain medical conditions should not use some yoga practices. For example, people with disk disease of the spine, extremely high or low blood pressure, glaucoma, retinal detachment, fragile or atherosclerotic arteries, a risk of blood clots, ear problems, severe osteoporosis, or cervical spondylitis should avoid some inverted poses.

- Although yoga during pregnancy is safe if practiced under expert guidance, pregnant women should avoid certain poses that may be problematic.

Training, Licensing, and Certification

There are many training programs for yoga teachers throughout the country. These programs range from a few days to more than 2 years. Standards for teacher training and certification differ depending on the style of yoga.

There are organizations that register yoga teachers and training programs that have complied with minimum educational standards. For example, one nonprofit group requires at least 200 hours of training, with a specified number of hours in areas including techniques, teaching methodology, anatomy, physiology, and philosophy. However, there are currently no official or well-accepted licensing requirements for yoga teachers in the United States.

If You Are Thinking about Yoga

- Do not use yoga as a replacement for conventional care or to postpone seeing a doctor about a medical problem.

- If you have a medical condition, consult with your health care provider before starting yoga.

- Ask about the physical demands of the type of yoga in which you are interested, as well as the training and experience of the yoga teacher you are considering.

- Look for published research studies on yoga for the health condition you are interested in.

- Tell your health care providers about any complementary and alternative practices you use. Give them a full picture of what you do to manage your health. This will help ensure coordinated and safe care.

NCCAM-Funded Research

Recent studies supported by NCCAM have been investigating yoga's effects on the following:

- Blood pressure

- Chronic low-back pain

- Chronic obstructive pulmonary disease

- Depression

- Diabetes risk

- HIV [human immunodeficiency virus]

- Immune function

- Inflammatory arthritis and knee osteoarthritis

- Insomnia

- Multiple sclerosis

- Smoking cessation

Chapter 53

Other Mind-Body Medicine Therapies

Chapter Contents

Section 53.1—Color Therapy 358
Section 53.2—Dance Therapy 359

Section 53.1

Color Therapy

What other names is the therapy known by?

Chromotherapist, color medicine, color therapy, colorology

What is it?

Chromotherapy, or color therapy, is the use of color to treat medical conditions.

Is it effective?

Natural Medicines Comprehensive Database rates effectiveness based on scientific evidence according to the following scale: effective, likely effective, possibly effective, possibly ineffective, likely ineffective, and insufficient evidence to rate.

The effectiveness ratings for chromotherapy are as follows:

- Insufficient evidence to rate effectiveness for:

  - depression, anxiety, stress, fatigue, pain, cramps, headache, migraine headache, diabetes, hypertension, asthma, cough, and many other conditions.

How does it work?

Chromotherapy practitioners believe that color can be used to correct energy imbalances which are the cause of disease. A chromotherapist applies specific colors or lights to specific points on the body called "chakras." Different colors have different effects. For example, red is thought to increase pulse rate, blood pressure, and breathing rate. Therefore, it is often used for circulatory conditions. Blue is believed to cause relaxation and calm. Therefore, blue is used for headaches, pain, cramping, stress, and other conditions. There is no reliable scientific support for these beliefs.

Are there safety concerns?

There is not enough reliable information available to know if chromotherapy is safe or if there are any safety concerns.

Are there any interactions with medications?

It is not known if chromotherapy interacts with any medicines.

Before using chromotherapy, talk with your healthcare professional if you take any medications.

Section 53.2

Dance Therapy

"What Is Dance/Movement Therapy?" © 2009 American Dance Therapy Association (www.adta.org). Reprinted with permission.

Based on the understanding that the body and mind are interrelated, the American Dance Therapy Association [ADTA] defines dance/movement therapy as the psychotherapeutic use of movement to further the emotional, cognitive, physical, and social integration of the individual.

Dance/movement therapy is practiced in mental health, rehabilitation, medical, educational, and forensic settings, and in nursing home, day care center, disease prevention, private practice, and health promotion programs.

The dance/movement therapist focuses on movement behavior as it emerges in the therapeutic relationship. Expressive, communicative, and adaptive behaviors are all considered for both group and individual treatment. Body movement as the core component of dance simultaneously provides the means of assessment and the mode of intervention for dance/movement therapy.

Board Certified

The Dance/Movement Therapy Certification Board, Inc. follows standards of the National Organization for Competency Assurance, and awards the R-DMT (Registered-Dance/Movement Therapist) to individuals who have completed a master's degree in dance/movement therapy or a master's degree in a related field plus 45 credits of specific dance/movement therapy curriculum. All candidates must complete a 700-hour supervised clinical internship in dance/movement therapy. BC-DMT (Board Certified-Dance/Movement Therapist) is awarded only after the R-DMT has completed 3,640 hours of supervised, professional clinical work and passed a certification exam. BC-DMTs are qualified to teach, provide supervision, and engage in private practice. Many BC-DMTs hold state licenses, National Certified Counselor (NCC) status, and doctoral degrees.

Professional Training

Professional training of dance/movement therapists occurs on the graduate level. ADTA has established an approval procedure for granting recognition to those institutions that fulfill the guidelines for master's degree programs in dance/movement therapy. Prerequisite study includes Psychology, Anatomy and Kinesiology, and extensive dance experience.

Course content includes: Dance/Movement Therapy Theory; Development, Expressive, and Communicative Aspects of Verbal and Nonverbal Behavior; Methods for Observation, Analysis, and Assessment; Psychopathology and Diagnosis; Group Processes; Human Growth, Development, and Behavior; Research in Dance/Movement Therapy and Human Behavior; Clinical Applications of Dance/Movement Therapy and Related Psychological Theories; Clinical Fieldwork; Supervised Clinical Internship.

Part Six

Manipulative and
Body-Based Therapies

Chapter 54

Manipulative and Body-Based Therapies: An Overview

Under the umbrella of manipulative and body-based practices is a heterogeneous group of CAM interventions and therapies. These include chiropractic and osteopathic manipulation, massage therapy, Tui Na, reflexology, Rolfing, Bowen technique, Trager bodywork, Alexander technique, Feldenkrais method, and a host of others. Surveys of the U.S. population suggest that between 3 percent and 16 percent of adults receive chiropractic manipulation in a given year, while between 2 percent and 14 percent receive some form of massage therapy. In 1997, U.S. adults made an estimated 192 million visits to chiropractors and 114 million visits to massage therapists. Visits to chiropractors and massage therapists combined represented 50 percent of all visits to CAM practitioners. Data on the remaining manipulative and body-based practices are sparser, but it can be estimated that they are collectively used by less than 7 percent of the adult population.

Manipulative and body-based practices focus primarily on the structures and systems of the body, including the bones and joints, the soft tissues, and the circulatory and lymphatic systems. Some practices were derived from traditional systems of medicine, such as those from China, India, or Egypt, while others were developed within the last 150 years (e.g., chiropractic and osteopathic manipulation). Although many providers have formal training in the anatomy and physiology of humans, there is considerable variation in the training and the approaches of these

Excerpted from "Manipulative and Body-Based Practices: An Overview" by the National Center for Complementary and Alternative Medicine (NCCAM, nccam.nih.gov), part of the National Institutes of Health, March 2007.

providers both across and within modalities. For example, osteopathic and chiropractic practitioners, who use primarily manipulations that involve rapid movements, may have a very different treatment approach than massage therapists, whose techniques involve slower applications of force, or than craniosacral therapists. Despite this heterogeneity, manipulative and body-based practices share some common characteristics, such as the principles that the human body is self-regulating and has the ability to heal itself and that the parts of the human body are interdependent. Practitioners in all these therapies also tend to tailor their treatments to the specific needs of each patient.

Scope of the Research

Range of Studies

The majority of research on manipulative and body-based practices has been clinical in nature, encompassing case reports, mechanistic studies, biomechanical studies, and clinical trials. A cursory search in PubMed for research published in the last 10 years identified 537 clinical trials, of which 422 were randomized and controlled. Similarly, 526 trials were identified in the Cochrane database of clinical trials. PubMed also contains 314 case reports or series, 122 biomechanical studies, 26 health services studies, and 248 listings for all other types of clinical research published in the last 10 years. On the other hand, for this same time period, there have been only 33 published articles of research involving in vitro assays or employing animal models.

Primary Challenges

Different challenges face investigators studying mechanisms of action than those studying efficacy and safety. The primary challenges that have impeded research on the underlying biology of manual therapies include the following:

- Lack of appropriate animal models
- Lack of cross-disciplinary collaborations
- Lack of research tradition and infrastructure at schools that teach manual therapies
- Inadequate use of state-of-the-art scientific technologies

Clinical trials of CAM manual therapies face the same general challenges as trials of procedure-based interventions such as surgery, psychotherapy, or more conventional physical manipulative techniques (e.g., physical therapy). These include the following:

- Identifying an appropriate, reproducible intervention, including dose and frequency is a difficulty. This may be more difficult than in standard drug trials, given the variability in practice patterns and training of practitioners.

- Identifying an appropriate control group(s) is difficult. In this regard, the development of valid sham manipulation techniques has proven difficult.

- Randomizing subjects to treatment groups in an unbiased manner is difficult. Randomization may prove more difficult than in a drug trial, because manual therapies are already available to the public; thus, it is more likely that participants will have a preexisting preference for a given therapy.

- Maintaining investigator and subject compliance to the protocol is difficult. Group contamination (which occurs when patients in a clinical study seek additional treatments outside the study, usually without telling the investigators; this will affect the accuracy of the study results) may be more problematic than in standard drug trials, because subjects have easy access to manual therapy providers.

- Reducing bias by blinding subjects and investigators to group assignment can be problematic. Blinding of subjects and investigators may prove difficult or impossible for certain types of manual therapies. However, the person collecting the outcome data should always be blinded.

- Identifying and employing appropriate validated, standardized outcome measures can be a problem.

- Employing appropriate analyses, including the intent-to-treat paradigm, can be difficult.

Summary of the Major Threads of Evidence

Preclinical Studies

The most abundant data regarding the possible mechanisms underlying chiropractic manipulation have been derived from studies in animals, especially studies on the ways in which manipulation may affect the nervous system. For example, it has been shown, by means of standard neurophysiological techniques, that spinal manipulation evokes changes in the activity of proprioceptive primary afferent neurons in paraspinal tissues. Sensory input from these tissues has the capacity to reflexively alter the neural outflow to the autonomic nervous system. Studies are under way to determine whether input from the paraspinal tissue also modulates pain processing in the spinal cord.

Animal models have also been used to study the mechanisms of massage-like stimulation. It has been found that antinociceptive and cardiovascular effects of massage may be mediated by endogenous opioids and oxytocin at the level of the midbrain. However, it is not clear that the massage-like stimulation is equivalent to massage therapy.

Although animal models of chiropractic manipulation and massage have been established, no such models exist for other body-based practices. Such models could be critical if researchers are to evaluate the underlying anatomical and physiological changes accompanying these therapies.

Clinical Studies: Mechanisms

Biomechanical studies have characterized the force applied by a practitioner during chiropractic manipulation, as well as the force transferred to the vertebral column, both in cadavers and in normal volunteers. In most cases, however, a single practitioner provided the manipulation, limiting generalizability. Additional work is required to examine interpractitioner variability, patient characteristics, and their relation to clinical outcomes.

Studies using magnetic resonance imaging (MRI) have suggested that spinal manipulation has a direct effect on the structure of spinal joints; it remains to be seen if this structural change relates to clinical efficacy.

Clinical studies of selected physiological parameters suggest that massage therapy can alter various neurochemical, hormonal, and immune markers, such as substance P in patients who have chronic pain, serotonin levels in women who have breast cancer, cortisol levels in patients who have rheumatoid arthritis, and natural killer (NK) cell numbers and CD4+ T-cell counts in patients who are HIV [human immunodeficiency virus]-positive. However, most of these studies have come from one research group, so replication at independent sites is necessary. It is also important to determine the mechanisms by which these changes are elicited.

Despite these many interesting experimental observations, the underlying mechanisms of manipulative and body-based practices are poorly understood. Little is known from a quantitative perspective. Important gaps in the field, as revealed by a review of the relevant scientific literature, include the following:

- Lack of biomechanical characterization from both practitioner and participant perspectives

- Little use of state-of-the-art imaging techniques

- Few data on the physiological, anatomical, and biomechanical changes that occur with treatment

- Inadequate data on the effects of these therapies at the biochemical and cellular levels

- Only preliminary data on the physiological mediators involved with the clinical outcomes

Clinical Studies: Trials

Forty-three clinical trials have been conducted on the use of spinal manipulation for low-back pain, and there are numerous systematic reviews and meta-analyses of the efficacy of spinal manipulation for both acute and chronic low-back pain. These trials employed a variety of manipulative techniques. Overall, manipulation studies of varying quality show minimal to moderate evidence of short-term relief of back pain. Information on cost-effectiveness, dosing, and long-term benefit is scant. Although clinical trials have found no evidence that spinal manipulation is an effective treatment for asthma, hypertension, or dysmenorrhea, spinal manipulation may be as effective as some medications for both migraine and tension headaches and may offer short-term benefits to those suffering from neck pain. Studies have not compared the relative effectiveness of different manipulative techniques.

Although there have been numerous published reports of clinical trials evaluating the effects of various types of massage for a variety of medical conditions (most with positive results), these trials were almost all small, poorly designed, inadequately controlled, or lacking adequate statistical analyses. For example, many trials included co-interventions that made it impossible to evaluate the specific effects of massage, while others evaluated massage delivered by individuals who were not fully trained massage therapists or followed treatment protocols that did not reflect common (or adequate) massage practice.

There have been very few well-designed controlled clinical trials evaluating the effectiveness of massage for any condition, and only three randomized controlled trials have specifically evaluated massage for the condition most frequently treated with massage—back pain. All three trials found massage to be effective, but two of these trials were very small. More evidence is needed.

Risks

There are some risks associated with manipulation of the spine, but most reported side effects have been mild and of short duration. Although rare, incidents of stroke and vertebral artery dissection have been reported following manipulation of the cervical spine. Despite the fact that some forms of massage involve substantial force, massage is generally considered to have few adverse effects. Contraindications for massage include deep vein thrombosis, burns, skin infections, eczema, open wounds, bone fractures, and advanced osteoporosis.

Utilization/Integration

In the United States, manipulative therapy is practiced primarily by doctors of chiropractic, some osteopathic physicians, physical therapists, and physiatrists. Doctors of chiropractic perform more than 90 percent of the spinal manipulations in the United States, and the vast majority of the studies that have examined the cost and utilization of spinal manipulation have focused on chiropractic.

Individual provider experience, traditional use, or arbitrary payer capitation decisions—rather than the results of controlled clinical trials—determine many patient care decisions involving spinal manipulation. More than 75 percent of private payers and 50 percent of managed care organizations provide at least some reimbursement for chiropractic care. Congress has mandated that the Department of Defense (DOD) and the Department of Veterans Affairs provide chiropractic services to their beneficiaries, and there are DOD medical clinics offering manipulative services by osteopathic physicians and physical therapists. The State of Washington has mandated coverage of CAM services for medical conditions normally covered by insurance. The integration of manipulative services into health care has reached this level despite a dearth of evidence about long-term effects, appropriate dosing, and cost-effectiveness.

Although the numbers of Americans using chiropractic and massage are similar, massage therapists are licensed in fewer than 40 states, and massage is much less likely than chiropractic to be covered by health insurance. Like spinal manipulation, massage is most commonly used for musculoskeletal problems. However, a significant fraction of patients seek massage care for relaxation and stress relief.

Cost

A number of observational studies have looked at the costs associated with chiropractic spinal manipulation in comparison with the costs of conventional medical care, with conflicting results. Smith and Stano found that overall health care expenditures were lower for patients who received chiropractic treatment than for those who received medical care in a fee-for-service environment. Carey and colleagues found chiropractic spinal manipulation to be more expensive than primary medical care, but less expensive than specialty medical care. Two randomized trials comparing the costs of chiropractic care with the costs of physical therapy failed to find evidence of cost savings through chiropractic treatment. The only study of massage that measured costs found that the costs for subsequent back care following massage were 40 percent lower than those following acupuncture or self-care, but these differences were not statistically significant.

Patient Satisfaction

Although there are no studies of patient satisfaction with manipulation in general, numerous investigators have looked at patient satisfaction with chiropractic care. Patients report very high levels of satisfaction with chiropractic care. Satisfaction with massage treatment has also been found to be very high.

Chapter 55

Alexander Technique

Why do I need the Alexander Technique?

You may be mystified by your back pain, excess tension, or lack of co-ordination. You might have a chronic physical problem you'd like to solve. Perhaps you see your problem as hereditary, structural, unchangeable. You may be unaware that how you move could be creating or compounding your problem. You may not realize that how you go through your daily activities needlessly strains your joints and muscles.

How can the Alexander Technique help me?

The Technique offers you a way to streamline what you do, making your activities less stressful and more pleasurable. You come to understand how your body can move most efficiently. As you learn to move more easily, you make surprising improvements in how you look and feel. As you learn to apply Alexander's principles, you practice an effective, lasting method of self-care.

What is the Alexander Technique?

The Alexander Technique is an intelligent way to solve the common movement problems that cause chronic pain and stress. It is a way to notice your movement habits, release compression, and move with ease

"Frequently Asked Questions," by Joan Arnold and Hope Gillerman, Certified Teachers of the Alexander Technique, © 2009. For additional information, visit the website of the American Society for the Alexander Technique, www.alexandertech.org.

and expansion. A proven self-care method, it is a set of skills that you learn to relieve pain, prevent injury, and enhance performance.

How is the Alexander Technique different from other approaches?

It is not a treatment, such as chiropractic or massage. Any treatment has its own unique benefits. The Alexander Technique's unique contribution is a mode of self-management that gives you independence in maintaining your health. Rather than being solely a recipient, you learn to soothe your own nervous system, release your own muscles, and balance your own structure. Alexander skills also make you a more informed, receptive patient when you do need any kind of treatment.

It is not a set of exercises such as those you might learn in yoga, physical therapy, Feldenkrais, Pilates, or the gym. Because the Alexander Technique is a way to heighten awareness of how you move and to better coordinate your body during activity, it helps you do specific postures, procedures, or exercises with less strain and more comfort. Since it is a tool to improve your overall coordination, you become a more intelligent exerciser who can focus effort during a strenuous challenge. You learn more about the body, and bring that refined understanding to a class or set of stretches.

What are the Alexander Technique's benefits?

People who learn the Alexander Technique can better handle daily stress and develop a long-term solution to chronic pain and muscular tension. They acquire an enduring way to perceive tensions as they arise and to restore their own balance.

- **Self-care**—As the premiere form of self-care, the Alexander Technique helps people prevent injury and recover from chronic back, hip and neck disorders, traumatic or repetitive strain injuries, balance and coordination disorders, arthritis, and muscle spasms. It can also be helpful for people with asthma and stress-related disorders, such as migraine headaches, sleep disorders, and panic attacks.

- **Skill enhancement**—Athletes use the Technique to help them improve strength, endurance, flexibility, and responsiveness. Performing artists use it to lessen performance anxiety while improving concentration and stage presence. Public speakers use it to improve vocal projection and voice quality. Those in business find it enhances presentation skills and increases confidence.

- **Mental health**—As your posture and movement style improve, you look and feel better. As your breathing capacity expands, you have a greater resource of energy. Physicians recommend the Alexander Technique to lessen the depression and anxiety associated with chronic conditions. Psychotherapists also refer their patients to Alexander Technique teachers. While you unravel muscular tensions, you may perceive an emotional link to your physical symptom. Study of the Alexander Technique can help release emotion, can provoke deeper understanding of the self, and can complement psychotherapy.

Who studies the Alexander Technique?

People of all types are Alexander students. They might come to recuperate from an injury or surgery or for relief from chronic pain. They may hear of the Technique from friends, physicians, or other health professionals. Here are some examples of the many who have used the Alexander Technique to improve their comfort level, professional achievement, and their lives:

- Performing artists
- Parents
- Executives
- Computer users
- The wheelchair bound

What problems and conditions can the Alexander Technique help me resolve?

- **Stress in daily life**—Because the Alexander Technique helps you change your response to stress, it can help you relieve or eliminate stress-related conditions. The body's reaction to threat—a fear reflex marked by a tight neck and contracted body—is a natural, adaptive response. But if the body does not unwind from this contraction and stays in a constant state of emergency, we pay a physical price. You can learn to restabilize and recuperate from stress with the Alexander Technique: A set of body/mind skills that helps you release contracted muscles, calm the nervous system, and handle stressors more easily.

- **Chronic pain**—Chronic pain can be the result of injury, disease, structural abnormality, or muscular tension. Though the Technique is not a miracle cure for medical conditions, by reducing the stress response it can often provide a surprising degree of relief. For conditions that cannot be changed—such as rheumatoid arthritis—it can still help the individual release the muscular tension and fear response that accompany injury or disease.

- **Back problems**—One of the most effective approaches to chronic back problems, the Technique can address the underlying cause and often relieve the condition completely. When there are unchangeable factors of disease or structure, the Alexander teacher's soothing hands and helpful guidance enables you—whatever your limitation—to reach your full potential for function. A 2008 *British Medical Journal* study reported a randomized trial that showed Alexander Technique to be the most effective tool in reducing or eliminating back pain (http://www.bmj.com/cgi/content/full/337/aug19_2/a884).

- **Arthritis**—Studying the Alexander Technique will help you relieve pain, retain mobility, and increase range of motion. The Alexander Technique teacher helps you see what in your movement style causes joint compression and might exacerbate your condition. As you re-educate your overall coordination, the torso muscles support rather than compress the spine. Reduced compression allows your body to expand during daily activities and can help reduce pain.

- **Postural problems**—Many people develop unhealthy posture and movement habits that become deep-seated patterns of strain. These habits are typically expressed by tight back and neck muscles and collapsed stature. With the hands-on guidance of a trained Alexander Technique teacher, you learn to elicit the primary control—an easy, dynamic relationship between the head and spine. You gain access to the body's elegant power steering. You learn that finding poise can help to ease discomfort and streamline movement. With greater fluidity and stability, you gain confidence and a more positive self-image.

- **Asthma and other breathing disorders**—Asthma is the body's respiratory reflex gone awry. Neck muscles tighten, shoulders yank up to the ears, and the abdominal muscles contract. Sufferers say the greatest problem is rising panic at an attack's onset—the fear that they won't win the fight for the next breath. These responses are elements of the startle pattern. With the Alexander Technique, asthmatics can halt the startle pattern and calm the nervous system, inviting an easier balance in body and mind. They can control or conquer their symptoms. Expanded space in the torso and information about how to breathe can help anyone who wants to improve breathing capacity and, with it, overall vitality.

- **Repetitive strain injury and carpal tunnel syndrome—** The Alexander Technique addresses the cause of these widespread injuries: Lack of postural support and excess joint compression while working. With the Alexander Technique, you learn to eliminate strain and perform repetitive movements with ease and comfort. Much of our current epidemic of repetitive strain injury and carpal tunnel syndrome could be alleviated if more people learned how to:
  - sit upright easily;
  - do repeated motions with less muscular tension in the shoulders, arms, and wrists;
  - tap the keyboard and mouse lightly;
  - attune to their bodies' signals.

How do I learn the Alexander Technique?

You learn the Technique from a highly trained professional in a series of one-on-one sessions. Some teachers offer group classes, but the Technique is most commonly offered privately. The teacher gives you expert coaching tailored to your specific needs.

What happens in an Alexander Technique session?

In an Alexander Technique session, your teacher instructs you—with words and touch—to approach movement differently. Using a mirror, s/he helps you recognize your ingrained patterns and highlights how your movement style relates to your symptoms. Your teacher uses a specialized hands-on method to help you release areas of tension and elicit your body's capacity for dynamic expansion. With this expert guidance, you learn the skills to replicate that ease and expansion on your own. Over a course of sessions, you strip away the movement habits at the root of your discomfort. You acquire a way to guide yourself through daily activities that stays with you for the rest of your life.

What do I wear?

You come to your Alexander lesson wearing loose, comfortable clothing.

What is an Alexander studio like?

The Alexander teacher's studio is a low-tech environment with a chair, bodywork table, and a mirror.

How long are sessions?

Usually 45–60 minutes, the Alexander lesson is instruction tailored to your needs.

What's the point of a lesson?

An Alexander Technique session is an opportunity for you to unwind and observe how your mind and body work. Your teacher gives you focused, supportive coaching on how to use your increased awareness to calm your system and raise your level of functioning.

What will we do?

Your Alexander teacher observes you doing simple actions, such as sitting, standing, or walking. Using a mirror, s/he helps you see and sense how your movement style relates to your problem. There are two aspects to an Alexander lesson:

- **Table work**—While you lie clothed on a bodywork table and settle into restful state, the teacher gently moves your head and limbs, encouraging expansion. S/he guides you with a unique, informative touch that does not intrude or manipulate, but suggests soothing release and an enlivened kinesthetic sense.

- **Guidance during activity**—While you perform ordinary movements, the teacher gives you verbal, visual, and conceptual cues to help you sit, stand, walk, or reach more comfortably. You consider activities you would like to enhance, such as public speaking, lifting and carrying, computer work, practicing yoga or a martial art, playing your favorite sport, or even sleeping comfortably. Performers can choose to work on a monologue, an aria, or a dance movement. If you would like to refine a specialized activity— such as how you swing a tennis racket, lift a child, or play an instrument—the teacher can help you reduce compression and increase overall physical support as you do it.

How can an Alexander Technique teacher help me?

Your Alexander Technique teacher offers personally tailored instruction with a unique hands-on approach, helping you see what in your individual movement style contributes to your recurring problem. As he or she helps you to release muscular tension and restore your body's original poise, you learn to sit, stand, and move with safety, balance, and ease. Your teacher can point out the source of your problem. With anatomical pictures s/he helps you to better understand the body's functioning. S/he considers your entire body—not just segments—and looks at you as the dynamic creature you are.

Who can benefit from learning the Alexander Technique?

- **Computer users**—In the current epidemic of repetitive strain injury, carpal tunnel syndrome, chronic back pain, headaches, and stress-related disorders, many computer users suffer. While ergonomic design can improve the work station—chair design, monitor, and keyboard placement—the Alexander Technique enables you to use your own body's design, even when the work station is not ideal. By understanding the Technique's basic alphabet of movement, you can avoid injury and often relieve the agonizing symptoms associated with computer use.

  Your Alexander Technique teacher guides you to:

  - sit upright without strain;
  - prevent spinal compression and muscular tension in the neck, shoulders, and upper back;
  - encourage freer range of motion in the joints and muscles;
  - tap the keyboard and mouse lightly to reduce stress on the wrist and carpal tunnel;
  - attune to your body's signals, heed early warning stress signs, and ward off pain before it escalates;
  - breathe properly to prevent fatigue and soothe the nervous system;
  - restore balance in your back—during and after work—each day.

- **Singers, dancers, actors, and musicians**—Performing artists study the Technique to reduce performance anxiety, lessen the likelihood of injury, and enhance stage presence. The Alexander Technique gives them sharp focus, a highly refined sensory awareness, efficient use of their energy, excellent balance and coordination and an inner sense of calm. Some of the renowned actors and musicians who have been using the Alexander Technique since the beginning of this century are: Julie Andrews,

William Hurt, Jeremy Irons, James Earl Jones, Paul McCartney, Kelley McGillis, Patti Lupone, Paul Newman, Sting, Maggie Smith, Mary Steenbergen, Robin Williams, Joanne Woodward, and members of the New York Philharmonic.

- **Athletes and fitness enthusiasts**—Though the Technique is a wonderful stress reducer, you can also use it during vigorous activities. If you work out, proper form and degree of muscular tension are just as important as how strenuously or how often you exercise. By demonstrating principles of efficient movement, the Alexander teacher offers the fitness enthusiast a way to prevent injury and gain better results. Studying the Technique gives you the skills to prevent pain while you improve breathing, balance, and posture. Together, you and your Alexander teacher can explore how to solve movement problems and optimize your performance, adding to your achievement and enjoyment. You can apply the Technique to any activity—tennis, golf, skiing, baseball, horseback riding, basketball, etc.

- **Pregnant women**—The Alexander Technique has much to offer women before, during, and after childbirth.

  - Before pregnancy, you can use the Technique to unlearn harmful postural habits while improving balance and coordination. This enables you to manage your body during the changes pregnancy brings.

  - During pregnancy, the Alexander teacher can help eliminate lower back pain caused by increased weight in front of the body. The baby's growth limits the mother's internal space and her organs become compressed. This can result in digestive problems and shortness of breath. Use of the Alexander Technique will allow more internal space for both mother and baby. With more breath and mobility, the mother can stay active. To help the mother prepare for labor and delivery, Alexander Technique lessons coordinate breathing and strengthen pelvic muscles.

  - During childbirth, the Alexander Technique can help the mother manage the physical challenges.

  - After childbirth, a mother can continue to use the Technique to help focus on her own self care while nourishing and caring for her child. Both parents can learn how to manage the constant lifting and carrying that come with parenthood.

How did the Alexander Technique begin?

The Alexander Technique was developed by F.M. Alexander (1869–1955). As a young Australian actor, he suffered from a vocal problem that interrupted his burgeoning career as a Shakespearean actor. Frustrated by this limitation, he studied his own movement for the cause of his problem. Through a long process of self-observation and experiment, he evolved a way to restore full use of his voice. In exploring how to help himself and others, he discovered the crucial importance of the relationship between the head, neck, and spine. He named this relationship the primary control because he perceived it as primary in controlling posture, breath, and movement. He developed a way to teach people how to elicit the primary control in their daily lives.

What are the Alexander Technique's basic ideas?

Though your body is much more elaborate and subtle than any machine, you can understand the Alexander Technique's basic ideas by comparing it to driving a car. You use the mirrors (awareness), the brake (inhibition), and the gas (direction). As you develop each of these skills and learn to use them all together, you gain access to your body's power steering—the primary control. Just as you don't have to focus on every detail of a car's operation, you learn about your body's capacity to respond and coordinate each of its systems to work together, as an integrated whole.

- **Primary control**—The primary control is the relationship between the head, neck, and spine. The quality of that relationship—compressed or free—determines the quality of our overall movement and functioning. When the neck is not overworking, the head balances lightly atop the spine, the torso expands and breath comes more easily. We restore the efficacy of the postural reflex—a natural, dynamic force that counters gravity and easily guides the torso upward. You elicit your body's primary control by developing three interlocking skills:

  - Awareness—Many people don't realize the source of their limitation, aches, or chronic pain. You acquire a powerful tool when you refine awareness of your habitual tendencies, observe how you operate moment to moment, and understand how your body works best.

  - Inhibition—Though we often tend to think we're not doing enough, Alexander found that our habits of tension and compression interfere with our body's ingenious design. By

379

catching ourselves as we move with compression and reducing excess muscular effort, we can inhibit (or stop) compressive habits and stress responses. We can actually accomplish more by doing less.

- Direction—Each of us has the capacity to visualize movement and mentally guide the flow of force through the body. Rather than gunning the motor and muscling our way through an activity, we can use the mind to direct—or envision—dynamic expansion while moving. By doing so, the body's reflexive coordination seems to handle the action by itself, gracefully and effortlessly.

How long will it be before I see results?

Each lesson will bring new insights that you can apply immediately, and you will probably feel the effects of your Alexander Technique work within the first 6–10 lessons. As you continue and your understanding grows, you will be able to apply what you've learned to a wider range of activities. Instead of a quick fix with a fleeting effect, you will experience a gradual change and long-term results.

How long should I take lessons to get the full benefit?

Like any skill, it takes practice. A series of 30 lessons, once or twice a week for 3 to 6 months, is the best way for you to learn the Technique.

Does everyone need the same number of lessons?

The number of lessons you need depends upon your goals, interests, and physical condition. Some students study for 3–5 months, others continue taking lessons after reaching their initial goals and continue for years. Duration of study is up to you.

Do the Alexander Technique's benefits wear off when I stop taking lessons?

Not if you continue to use what you have learned! While taking lessons, you reclaim your body's natural sense of ease and increase your understanding of how you function. This practice enables you to take the mind/body process wherever you go and apply it to anything you do, such as riding a bike, sitting through a long meeting, playing an instrument, swinging a racket, or carrying luggage. You can continue to build your skills on your own after you stop taking lessons.

Since F.M. Alexander was not a physician, why should the medical field take the Alexander Technique seriously?

Because it works! The Alexander Technique is a proven, safe, self-care method to stop pain, muscle tension, and stress cause by everyday misuse of the body.

- **Endorsed by physicians and health care professionals**—The Alexander Technique is offered in wellness centers and health education programs. Medical professionals of every kind recommend the Alexander Technique for chronic back pain, migraines, repetitive stress injuries, balance and coordination problems, and for the depression and anxiety that often accompanies chronic pain and stress.

- **Endorsed by scientists**—Alexander's findings are supported by behavioral scientists and physiologists including Nobel laureate Sir Charles Sherrington, Dr. Rudolph Magnus, G.E. Coghill, Frank Pierce Jones, and Nikolaus Tinbergen, who noted Alexander's discoveries in his Nobel Prize acceptance speech.

- **An established record of success**—Clinical studies have shown that the Technique modifies stress responses while improving breathing capacity and posture. In a 1988 study of chronic pain sufferers, the Alexander Technique was chosen as patients' preferred method of reducing pain.

Is the Alexander Technique just another health fad?

Now over 100 years old, the Alexander Technique has a long track record of helping people with back problems, chronic pain and tension, posture and movement disorders, asthma, migraines, and whiplash. As its wide applications are understood and its successes continue to multiply, the reputation of the Technique is growing. Today there are about 2,500 teachers worldwide, with about 700 in the United States.

What are Alexander Technique teachers like?

Many have come from the performing arts, such as dance, theater, or music. Some are physical therapists, massage therapists, or teachers in another field.

What training is required to be an Alexander Technique teacher?

AmSAT-certified Alexander Technique teachers must complete 1,600 hours of training over a minimum of 3 years in an AmSAT-approved training program. To assure quality instruction, each Alexander Teaching Training Program maintains a five-to-one student/teacher ratio.

Alexander teachers must practice what they teach: the ability to integrate and streamline their own movement while guiding their clients toward improved functioning. They acquire this ability from expert mentors through long hours of intense, focused hands-on training.

Alexander practitioners are trained in careful visual observation to spot the source of movement problems. They are schooled in teaching skills that encourage learning in a non-judgmental, supportive atmosphere. And they are trained in the unique Alexander touch, a complex combination of kinesthetic receptivity and the subtle suggestion of expansion and lightness in movement. Additional studies include anatomy, study of F.M. Alexander's theoretical writings, literature, and research by Alexander scholars and those in related fields.

What is AmSAT?

The American Society of the Alexander Technique is the largest professional association of certified Alexander Technique teachers in the United States. Its mission is to maintain the integrity of the Alexander Technique as developed by F.M. Alexander (1869–1955). AmSAT maintains the nation's highest standards for teacher training, certification, and membership and maintains affiliations with similar credentialing bodies worldwide. Since its formation in 1987, over 1,200 teachers have completed a rigorous training process to earn AmSAT certification.

Chapter 56

Aquatic Therapy (Hydrotherapy)

The Standards and Steering Committees of the Aquatic Therapy and Rehabilitation Industry Certification define aquatic therapy and rehabilitation as: "The use of water and specifically designed activity by qualified personnel to aid in the restoration, extension, maintenance and quality of function for persons with acute, transient, or chronic disabilities, syndromes or diseases."

Definition of Hydrotherapy

Hydrotherapy is the use of water by external applications, either for its pressure effect or as a means of applying physical energy to a tissue. The term often refers to the use of water in wound management, such as whirlpool baths, but can be used interchangeably with the term, "aquatic therapy."

Definition of Adapted Aquatics

Adapted aquatics are techniques that emphasize swimming skills modified or adapted to accommodate individual abilities. Usually used with people with disabilities, adapted aquatics focuses on skills including pool entry and exit and swimming skill development, and should also encompass community referral.

Indications for Aquatic Therapy

- Sensory disorders
- Limited range of motion
- Weakness
- Poor motor coordination
- Pain
- Spasticity
- Perceptual/spatial problems
- Balance deficits
- Respiratory problems
- Circulatory problems
- Depression/poor self-esteem
- Cardiac diseases
- Joint replacement
- Motor learning
- Orthopedic injuries/trauma
- Obesity
- Prenatal
- Neurological (MS [multiple sclerosis])
- Osteoporosis
- Rheumatology (arthritis/fibromyalgia)

Aquatic Therapy Techniques

Ai Chi

Created by Jun Konno of Japan, ai chi is a combination of deep breathing and slow broad movements of the arms, legs, and torso, using concepts of T'ai Chi, Shiatsu, and Qigong. Ai Chi is performed standing in shoulder-depth water with an ideal pool temperature of 88 degrees Fahrenheit to 96 degrees Fahrenheit.

Ai Chi Ne

Ai Chi Ne (pronounced Eye Chee Knee) is a partner stretching program. "Ne" is the Japanese word for "two." Ai Chi Ne involves breathing techniques to increase relaxation and therefore enhance the stretch abilities. Using the breathing techniques decreases stress, joint tension, muscular tension, and the stretch reflex response.

BackHab

This is an integrated program that the individual can do on his or her own. It was developed for people with back problems but is now being used by group programs for people with disabilities. Rather than focusing on healing one part of the body, all the body parts coordinate to work on healing and fixing the affected area. BackHab is an aquatic walking program using various strides to accomplish a variety of benefits. It is excellent for gait re-training.

Bad Ragaz

This technique originated in Germany in 1957 and was introduced by a German therapist to the therapeutic thermal pools of Bad Ragaz in Switzerland. The technique has since become more clearly defined as the Bad Ragaz Ring Method. Bad Ragaz is a method of muscle re-education utilizing specific patterns of resistance, endurance, elongation, relaxation, range of motion, and tonal reduction.

The Burdenko Method

The Burdenko Method is used for athletic training and as a therapeutic method for people with disabilities. The basic concepts include integrating land and water therapy, using a vertical position, focusing on the whole body, and homework.

Feldenkrais

Developed by Dr. Moshe Feldenkrais, this method uses gentle movement and directed attention to improve movement and enhance human functioning. This method aims to increase ease and range of motion, improve flexibility and coordination, and encourage the individual to rediscover innate capacity for graceful, efficient movement. These improvements will often generalize to enhance functioning in other aspects of life.

Halliwick

The Halliwick concept is an approach to teaching people with physical and/or learning difficulties to participate in water activities, to move independently in water, and to swim. The practice utilizes the Ten Point Program, which includes essential components of motor learning, and eventually leads to independence in the water. The Ten Point Program includes the concepts of mental adjustment, balance control, and movement.

Lyu Ki Dou

Lyu Ki Dou developed from studies of various hands-on healing modalities, along with Ai Chi, Tai Chi, and Qi Gong. The name was derived from the Japanese translation of "Floating Life Energy Pathways." Lyu Ki Dou emphasizes the facilitator's self-care, which in turn will benefit the clients/patients that are receiving any type of therapy or exercise programming from an individual who has literally "turned on" this vital life-giving energy source that is inside each of us.

Massage

Massage therapists have moved their practice to the water to expand the benefits and applications of massage. Water massage, the use of soft tissue manipulation and body mobilization techniques in water warmer than skin temperature (92 degrees Fahrenheit–93 degrees Fahrenheit), is evolving as a therapeutic method. Practitioners find that the use of massage in water is creative, innovative, and individualized, and no two practitioners have the same approach.

Proprioceptive Neuromuscular Facilitation (PNF)

PNF is an approach to therapeutic exercise which aims to improve motor skill through positive motor transfer, using the principles of facilitation/inhibition, irradiation/reinforcement, and reciprocal innervation. Exercises consist of spiral and diagonal patterns and must incorporate three components of motion: flexion or extension, adduction or abduction, and rotation.

Water Pilates

Pilates exercises have been adapted for the pool. Created by Joseph Pilates, this body conditioning program is designed to improve strength, flexibility, and range of motion, and also encourages musculoskeletal alignment. The main tenets are resisting your own weight, controlled breathing, spine alignment, and abdominal strengthening.

Unpredictable Command Technique (UCT)

Created by David Ogden, a PT [physical therapist] from Phoenix, AZ, UCT has a goal of progressing the client(s) so that two or more motor movements are done simultaneously. Improved somatic awareness and motor control can be achieved through the challenge to do a variety of constantly-changing familiar and unfamiliar activities. Using the UCT, the author and others have observed client(s) demonstrating improved voluntary control, awareness of movement and body in space, and enhanced mental concentration.

Wassertanzen

Wassertanzen is a dynamic movement therapy that includes work below the water surface with the aid of nose clips. Wassertanzen means "water dance" and was created in 1987 by Swiss-Germans Arjana Brunschwiler and Aman Schroter. "Wassertanzen is very different from watsu because of the challenge it presents for a person to surrender control of his breath to go underwater," says Harold Dull, creator of Watsu.

Water Yoga

Hatha yoga poses performed in warm, waist- to chest-depth water develop strength and static balance simultaneously. In addition, range of motion increases in coordination with diaphragmatic breathing and long exhalations.

Watsu

Developed by Harold Dull, watsu (water + shiatsu) is a cradling, one-on-one program that is experienced in a very warm (approx. 94 degrees Fahrenheit) pool. The client is held in the water by the practitioner and moved using the water to massage the body. Shiatsu (acupressure) points are stimulated along the meridians of the body during the massage. Watsu is used for pain reduction, increased range of motion, increased circulation, psychological problems, relaxation, and reduction of stress. It has been used in rehabilitation programs for people with orthopedic problems or physical disabilities, for pregnant mothers, and the elderly.

Yogalates

Fluid Yogalates, developed by Dr. Mary Wykle, combines Iyengar Yoga, Pilates, and Ai Chi. Static poses and core stabilization exercises are transitioned with circular movements and emphasis on deep breathing to create a continual fluid program. The objectives are increased body awareness, strength, range of motion, relaxation, and an inward focus.

Adaptations and Modifications

- Equipment
- Begin slowly.
- Use progressive overload (pushing a muscle past its normal capacity. This is a basic principle of exercise and is necessary to increase strength, flexibility, and conditioning.)
- Begin with conservative ROM [range of motion].
- Consider wearing aqua-shoes for protection and slip resistance.
- Use good technique as tolerated (stop with poor technique).

Exercise Session Format

- Start with 10 to 15 minutes and increase in 5-minute intervals.
- Use deep breathing to increase vital capacity.
- Use gradual progressive overload.
- Work on balance.
- Work on strength.
- Work on flexibility.
- Longer cool down

Program Modifications

- Use fewer reps of the same muscle group when beginning.
- Center the body between transitions.
- Reach across the midline and overhead across.
- Use hands behind head and body.
- Move backward as well as forward.
- Exercise to improve posture.
- Use slow, controlled movement.
- Begin weight-bearing issues in deeper water and progress to shallower.
- Enter water slowly so all systems have an opportunity to gradually accommodate the environment.
- Keep medications at pool edge.

Sample Aquatic Therapy Exercise Program I

Begin at pool edge with spinal alignment and postural awareness with Water Pilates.

Exercise: The Hundred

1. In waist-deep water at the side of the pool, sit in an imaginary chair. Thighs are parallel to the bottom of the pool and knees align over the ankles. The back is against the pool wall and remains immobile throughout the exercise. Arms are at the sides with palms facing backward and shoulders are relaxed. The head faces straight ahead.
2. Begin pumping the arms forward and back about 6 inches.
3. Inhale for five counts and exhale for five counts.
4. Keep the back against the pool wall.

Challenges: Learning to "scoop" the stomach in to set the back to the wall is the main concern. Encourage full breaths.

Progression: Gradually increase the pumping action with the arms coordinated with the breath until you count to 100.

Exercise: Single Leg Circles

1. In waist-deep water at the side of the pool, sit in an imaginary chair. Thighs are parallel to the bottom of the pool and knees align over the ankles. The back is against the pool wall and remains immobile throughout the exercise. Arms are at the sides with palms facing backward and against the wall. Shoulders should be relaxed. The head looks straight ahead.
2. Lift the right leg about 12 inches and straighten. Turn the leg out slightly from the hip socket.
3. Begin the leg circle by moving the leg across the body, then circling it down, around, and back to the starting position. The back does not move from the wall. Complete five circles. Inhale as you begin the motion and exhale to return to the starting position.
4. Reverse the direction of the circle starting outward, continuing down, then across the body, and return to the starting position.
5. Repeat the leg circles with the left leg.

Challenges: Emphasize that only the leg moves with the back, hips, and arms staying stable against the pool wall.

Progression: Gradually increase the size of the circles while maintaining control throughout the movement.

Sample Aquatic Therapy Exercise Program II

Use BackHab exercises for integrating cardio, mobility, coordination, balance, ROM, and motor skills.

Exercise: On Toes

- Goal: Balance, coordination, experience of axial elongation
- Considerations: Eliminate leaning forward; keep flowing (not jerky)
- Progression: Lengthen stride

Exercise: On Heels

- Goal: Balance, stretch of calf muscles (gastrocnemius), endurance of tibialis anterior
- Considerations: Keep torso upright, keep flowing (not jerky)
- Progression: No arms

Exercise: High Knee

- Goal: Gluteal and hamstring endurance, flexibility
- Considerations: Lift both knees equally, press foot back when moving backward
- Progression: Heavy, add pause or stop

Exercise: Side Lifts (Hip Abduction)

- Goal: Strengthen abductors and adductors, balance, structural stability for knee
- Considerations: Eliminate external hip rotation, equal lift and stride length
- Progression: Pause or stop

Exercise: Dips (Lunge)

- Goal: Bending skills, increase muscle tone and flexibility
- Considerations: Maintain upright stance on lunge, lunge without "slamming"
- Progression: Use explosive power on abduction

Sample Aquatic Therapy Exercise Program III

Use Fluid Yogalates and Ai Chi for re-patterning and to further develop coordination, balance, ROM, and pain-free movement. These can also be used for relaxation unless a trained practitioner is available to offer Watsu.

Fluid Yogalates

Pose—Warrior II:

1. In waist- to chest-deep water, separate legs approximately 4 feet.

2. Turn the right foot to the side and come into a lunge position. The right ankle and knee align. The right thigh should be almost parallel to the bottom of the pool. The back leg (left) continues to bear weight, pushing the energy flow up to the torso.

3. The torso remains upright and facing forward. It does not rotate.

4. The arms extend out from the shoulders. Extension continues through the fingertips. The shoulders remain relaxed and down.

5. The head turns to look through the fingers of the leading arm. Maintain this position for five or more slow breaths.

6. Repeat to the left side.

Challenges: It is difficult to adequately separate the legs and maintain balance. The leading knee has a tendency to rotate inward. The body leans forward or backward if the weight is not distributed between the legs.

Progression: Hold for longer periods. Add variations such as Side Angle Pose.

Pose—Warrior I:

1. In waist- to chest-deep water, separate legs approximately 4 feet.

2. Turn the right foot and leg to the side. Rotate the entire body to the same side. The left leg and foot also turn in the same direction. Insure the pelvis is squared to the side.

3. Bend the right knee, aligning the knee over the ankle. The left leg remains straight.

4. Extend the arms above the head with palm facing each other and hold for approximately five breaths.

5. Repeat to the left side.

Challenges: Maintaining balance in the water with the arms extended out of the water. Caution to limit extension of the back and discourage hyperextension.

Progression: Extend the left (back) heel to the bottom of the pool. Progress to other poses such as Warrior III.

Pose—Tree:

1. Stand erect in waist- to chest-deep water. Look straight ahead.

2. Balancing on one leg, flex the knee of the opposite leg and lift that foot to the inside of the supporting leg.

3. Arms bend into prayer position at chest level.

4. Gradually extend the arms overhead, keeping the palms together. Body stays straight and appears to lengthen.

5. Begin by trying to hold the position for five breaths. Repeat on the other side.

Challenges: Do not place the foot of the bent leg against the supporting knee. Extend the arms overhead only when balance is secure. Watch the body position because of a tendency to shift one hip to the side to assist with balance.

Progression: Hold for longer periods. Lengthen body and arms upward.

Ai Chi

Accepting:

1. Exhale easily through your mouth, turn your palms down, bring the right arm over to the left so the thumbs of both hands touch each other, while pivoting both feet 90 degrees left so you're facing the left side. Your weight is evenly balanced between both legs.

2. While still facing left, inhale through your nose, turn your palms up, and pull both arms back so that your rib cage feels fully opened. At the same time, shift your weight back on the right leg so that you're leaning back slightly. The trunk must be stable.

3. While still facing left, exhale through your mouth, turn your palms down, and bring both arms together so the thumbs of both hands touch each other. At the same time, shift your weight forward onto the left leg so you're leaning forward slightly.

4. Repeat steps two and three, flowing smoothly 5 to 10 times.

5. Inhale through your nose, turn your palms up, bring the right arm back to the right side, while pivoting both feet 90 degrees right so you're facing front.

6. Exhale easily through your mouth, turn your palms down, bring the left arm over to the right so the thumbs of both hands touch each other, while pivoting both feet 90 degrees right so you're facing the right side. Your weight is evenly balanced between both legs.

7. While still facing right, inhale through your nose, turn your palms up, and pull both arms back so that your rib cage feels fully opened. At the same time, shift your weight back on the left leg so that you're leaning back slightly.

8. While still facing right, exhale through your mouth, turn your palms down, and bring both arms together so the thumbs of both hands touch each other. At the same time, shift your weight forward onto the right leg so you're leaning forward slightly.

9. Repeat steps seven and eight, flowing smoothly 5 to 10 times.

10. Inhale through your nose, turn your palms up, bring the left arm back to the left side, while pivoting both feet 90 degrees left so you're facing front.

Rounding:

1. Exhale easily through your mouth, turn your palms down, bring the right arm over to the left so the thumbs of both hands touch each other, while pivoting both feet 90 degrees left so you're facing the left side. Your weight is evenly balanced between both legs.

2. While still facing left, inhale through your nose, turn your palms up, pull arms back so that your rib cage feels fully opened. At the same time, step your right leg back and shift your weight back so you're leaning back slightly.

3. While still facing left, exhale through your mouth, turn your palms down, and bring both arms together so the thumbs of both hands touch each other. At the same time, lift your right leg straight in front of you and lean forward slightly. Bring toes to fingertips.

4. Repeat steps two and three, flowing smoothly 5 to 10 times.

5. Inhale through your nose, turn your palms up, bring the right arm back to the right side, while pivoting both feet 90 degrees right so you're facing front.

6. Exhale easily through your mouth, turn your palms down, bring the left arm over to the right so the thumbs of both hands touch each other, while pivoting both feet 90 degrees right so you're facing the right side. Your weight is evenly balanced between both legs.

7. While still facing right, inhale through your nose, turn your palms up, pull arms back so that your rib cage feels fully opened. At the same time step your left leg back and shift your weight back so you're leaning back slightly.

8. While still facing right, exhale through your mouth, turn your palms down, and bring both arms together so the thumbs of both hands touch each other. At the same time, lift your left leg straight in front of you and lean forward slightly. Bring toes and fingertips together.

9. Repeat steps seven and eight, flowing smoothly 5 to 10 times.

10. Inhale through your nose, turn your palms up, bring the left arm back to the left side, while pivoting both feet 90 degrees left so you're facing front.

Balancing:

1. Exhale easily through your mouth, turn your palms down, bring the right arm over to the left so the thumbs of both hands touch each other, while pivoting both feet 90 degrees left so you're facing the left side. Your weight is evenly balanced between both legs.

2. While still facing left, inhale through your nose, turn your palms up, and press both arms down and back (bilateral shoulder extension) with hands supinated. At the same time, lift your right (back) leg forward and lean forward slightly.

3. While still facing left, exhale through your mouth, turn your palms down, and lift both arms forward and up (bilateral shoulder flexion with hands pronated). At the same time, stretch the right leg back but do not step it down. Lean forward. Repeat steps two and three, flowing smoothly 5 to 10 times without stepping the right leg down. Inhale through your nose, turn your palms up, bring the right arm back to the right side,

while stepping the right foot down and pivoting both feet 90 degrees right so you're facing front.

4. Exhale easily through your mouth, turn your palms down, bring the left arm over to the right so the thumbs of both hands touch each other, while pivoting both feet 90 degrees right so you're facing the right side. Your weight is evenly balanced between both legs.

5. While still facing right, inhale through your nose, turn your palms up, and press both arms down and back (bilateral shoulder extension with hands supinated). At the same time, lift your left (back) leg forward and lean forward slightly.

6. While still facing right, exhale through your mouth, turn your palms down, and lift both arms forward and up (bilateral shoulder flexion with hands pronated). At the same time, stretch the left leg back but do not step it down. Lean forward.

7. Repeat steps seven and eight, flowing smoothly 5 to 10 times without stepping the left leg down.

8. Inhale through your nose, turn your palms up, bring the left arm back to the left side, while pivoting both feet 90 degrees left so you're facing front.

About the Author

An internationally recognized leader in the health and fitness industry, Ruth Sova is dedicated to the growth and betterment of the industry through her tireless research and development efforts. She has founded eight successful businesses and holds numerous honors and awards in the industry. She educates and energizes audiences with her presentations on personal growth, entrepreneurship, health, fitness, wellness, running a business, and aquatic rehab and fitness.

In 1994, she founded the Aquatic Therapy and Rehab Institute, Inc. (ATRI), a non-profit educational organization dedicated to the professional development of health care professionals involved with aquatic therapy. ATRI, with headquarters in Chassell, MI, offers continuing education courses at conferences and workshops that advance the knowledge and skills of the aquatic therapist. She is also the founder and past president of the Aquatic Exercise Association (AEA), a non-profit international association serving as a clearinghouse for all aspects of the aquatics industry.

Organizations

1. American Alliance for Health, Physical Education, Recreation, and Dance [http://www.ncpad.org/organizations/index.php?id=1056&state=Virginia&city=Reston], Reston, Virginia

2. American Red Cross [http://www.ncpad.org/organizations/index.php?id=974&state=District of Columbia&city=Washington], Washington, District of Columbia

3. Aquatic Exercise Association (AEA) [http://www.ncpad.org/organizations/index.php?id=876&state=Florida&city=North Venice], North Venice, Florida

4. Aquatic Resources Network [http://www.ncpad.org/organizations/index.php?id=1517&state=Wisconsin&city=Amery], Amery, Wisconsin

5. Aquatic Therapy and Rehab Institute (ATRI) [http://www.ncpad.org/organizations/index.php?id=877&state=Florida&city=West Palm Beach], West Palm Beach, Florida

6. International Council for Aquatic Therapy and Rehabilitation [http://www.ncpad.org/organizations/index.php?id=1518&state=Washington&city=Spokane], Spokane, Washington

7. Jeff Ellis & Associates [http://www.ncpad.org/organizations/index.php?id=1058&state=Texas&city=Kingwood], Kingwood, Texas

8. National Therapeutic Recreation Society [http://www.ncpad.org/organizations/index.php?id=920&state=Virginia&city=Ashburn], Ashburn, Virginia

9. Worldwide Aquatic Bodywork Association [http://www.ncpad.org/organizations/index.php?id=1520&state=California&city=Middletown], Middletown, California

10. Aquatic Consulting & Education Resource Services [http://www.ncpad.org/organizations/index.php?id=1521&state=Wisconsin&city=Milwaukee], Milwaukee, Wisconsin

11. Aquatic Consulting Services [http://www.ncpad.org/organizations/index.php?id=1522&state=California&city=San Diego], San Diego, California

12. Aquatic Healing Services [http://www.ncpad.org/organizations/index.php?id=1523&state=Virginia&city=Charlottesville], Charlottesville, Virginia

13. Burdenko Water and Sports Therapy Institute [http://www.ncpad .org/organizations/index.php?id=1525&state=Massachusetts&cit y=Wayland], Wayland, Massachusetts

14. Essert Associates—Aquatic Therapy [http://www.ncpad.org/ organizations/index.php?id=1527&state=Arkansas&city=Conwa y], Conway, Arkansas

15. MW Aquatics [http://www.ncpad.org/organizations/index.php?id= 1530&state=Virginia&city=Burke], Burke, Virginia

16. Therapeutic Aquatics, Inc. [http://www.ncpad.org/organizations/ index.php?id=1534&state=Wyoming&city=Jackson], Jackson, Wyoming

Suppliers

1. Adolf Kiefer and Associates [http://www.ncpad.org/suppliers/ index.php?id=651&state=Illinois&city=Zion], Zion, Illinois

2. Aqua Gear, Inc. [http://www.ncpad.org/suppliers/index.php?id= 752&state=Florida&city=West Palm Beach], West Palm Beach, Florida

3. Blue Moon Aqua Products, TRMN Enterprises, Inc. [http:// www.ncpad.org/suppliers/index.php?id=753&state=Ohio&city= Columbus], Columbus, Ohio

4. Danmar Products, Inc. [http://www.ncpad.org/suppliers/index .php?id=351&state=Michigan&city=Ann Arbor], Ann Arbor, Michigan

5. Ferno-Washington, Inc. [http://www.ncpad.org/suppliers/index .php?id=754&state=Ohio&city=Wilmington], Wilmington, Ohio

6. Fitness Mart Country Technology, Inc. [http://www.ncpad.org/ suppliers/index.php?id=755&state=Wisconsin&city=Gays Mills], Gays Mills, Wisconsin

7. Hydro-Fit, Inc. [http://www.ncpad.org/suppliers/index.php?id=6 54&state=Oregon&city=Eugene], Eugene, Oregon

8. Orthopedic Physical Therapy Products (OPTP) [http://www .ncpad.org/suppliers/index.php?id=756&state=Minnesota&city =Minneapolis], Minneapolis, Minnesota

9. Recreonics, Inc. [http://www.ncpad.org/suppliers/index.php?id= 757&state=Kentucky&city=Louisville], Louisville, Kentucky

10. Water Gear [http://www.ncpad.org/suppliers/index.php?id=758& state=California&city=Pismo Beach], Pismo Beach, California

11. WaterWear, Inc. [http://www.ncpad.org/suppliers/index. php?id=759&state=New Hampshire&city=Wilton], Wilton, New Hampshire

12. Water Warm-Ups [http://www.ncpad.org/suppliers/index.php?id =760&state=California&city=Corona del Mar], Corona del Mar, California

13. The Wet Wrap DK Douglas Company, Inc. [http://www.ncpad.org/ suppliers/index.php?id=761&state=Massachusetts&city=Longme adow], Longmeadow, Massachusetts

Books

1. Sova, R. *Ai Chi: Balance, Harmony and Healing.*

2. Sova, R. & Harpt, S. (1996). *BACKHAB: The Water Way to Mobility and Pain Free Living.* Washington, Wisconsin: DSL, Ltd.

3. Wykle, M. *Transitioning Yoga and Pilates to the Water.*

4. Grosse, Susan J. *The Halliwick Method: Water Freedom for Individuals with Disabilities.*

5. Grosse, Susan. *Sponges, Splashes, and Sprinkles.*

Chapter 57

Chiropractic Care and Osteopathic Manipulation

Chiropractic is a health care approach that focuses on the relationship between the body's structure—mainly the spine—and its functioning. Although practitioners may use a variety of treatment approaches, they primarily perform adjustments to the spine or other parts of the body with the goal of correcting alignment problems and supporting the body's natural ability to heal itself.

Overview and History

The term "chiropractic" combines the Greek words cheir (hand) and praxis (action) to describe a treatment done by hand. Hands-on therapy—especially adjustment of the spine—is central to chiropractic care. Chiropractic, which in the United States is considered part of complementary and alternative medicine (CAM), is based on these key concepts:

- The body has a powerful self-healing ability.

- The body's structure (primarily that of the spine) and its function are closely related, and this relationship affects health.

- Therapy aims to normalize this relationship between structure and function and assist the body as it heals.

Excerpted from "Chiropractic: An Introduction," by the National Center for Complementary and Alternative Medicine (NCCAM, nccam.nih.gov), part of the National Institutes of Health, November 2007.

While some procedures associated with chiropractic care can be traced back to ancient times, the modern profession of chiropractic was founded by Daniel David Palmer in 1895 in Davenport, Iowa. Palmer, a self-taught healer, believed that the body has a natural healing ability. Misalignments of the spine can interfere with the flow of energy needed to support health, Palmer theorized, and the key to health is to normalize the function of the nervous system, especially the spinal cord.

Patterns of Use

According to the 2007 National Health Interview Survey, which included a comprehensive survey of CAM use by Americans, about 8 percent of American adults and nearly 3 percent of children had received chiropractic or osteopathic manipulation in the past 12 months. Adjusted to nationally representative numbers, these percentages mean that more than 18 million adults and 2 million children received chiropractic or osteopathic manipulation in the previous year.

Many people who seek chiropractic care have chronic, pain-related health conditions. Low-back pain, neck pain, and headache are common conditions for which people seek chiropractic treatment.

What to Expect from Chiropractic Visits

During the initial visit, chiropractors typically take a health history and perform a physical examination, with a special emphasis on the spine. Other examinations or tests such as x-rays may also be performed. If chiropractic treatment is considered appropriate, a treatment plan will be developed.

During followup visits, practitioners may perform one or more of the many different types of adjustments used in chiropractic care. Given mainly to the spine, a chiropractic adjustment (sometimes referred to as a manipulation) involves using the hands or a device to apply a controlled, sudden force to a joint, moving it beyond its passive range of motion. The goal is to increase the range and quality of motion in the area being treated and to aid in restoring health. Other hands-on therapies such as mobilization (movement of a joint within its usual range of motion) also may be used.

Chiropractors may combine the use of spinal adjustments with several other treatments and approaches such as the following:

- Heat and ice
- Electrical stimulation
- Rest

- Rehabilitative exercise
- Counseling about diet, weight loss, and other lifestyle factors
- Dietary supplements

Side Effects and Risks

Side effects and risks depend on the specific type of chiropractic treatment used. For example, side effects from chiropractic adjustments can include temporary headaches, tiredness, or discomfort in parts of the body that were treated. The likelihood of serious complications, such as stroke, appears to be extremely low and related to the type of adjustment performed and the part of the body treated.

If dietary supplements are a part of the chiropractic treatment plan, they may interact with medicines and cause side effects. It is important that people inform their chiropractors of all medicines (whether prescription or over-the-counter) and supplements they are taking.

Qualifications to Practice

To practice chiropractic care in the United States, a practitioner must earn a Doctor of Chiropractic (D.C.) degree from a college accredited by the Council on Chiropractic Education (CCE). CCE is the agency certified by the U.S. Department of Education to accredit chiropractic colleges in the United States. Admission to a chiropractic college requires a minimum of 90 semester hour credits (approximately 3 years) of undergraduate study, mostly in the sciences.

Chiropractic training is a 4-year academic program that includes both classroom work and direct experience caring for patients. Coursework typically includes instruction in the biomedical sciences, as well as in public health and research methods. Some chiropractors pursue a 2- to 3-year residency for training in specialized fields.

Regulation

Chiropractic is regulated individually by each state and the District of Columbia. Board examinations are required for licensing and include a mock patient encounter. Most states require chiropractors to earn annual continuing education credits to maintain their licenses. Chiropractors' scope of practice varies by state in areas such as laboratory tests or diagnostic procedures, the dispensing or selling of dietary supplements, and the use of other CAM therapies such as acupuncture or homeopathy.

Insurance Coverage

Compared with other CAM therapies, insurance coverage for chiropractic services is extensive. Many HMOs (health maintenance organizations) and private health care plans cover chiropractic treatment, as do all state workers' compensation systems. Chiropractors can bill Medicare, and many states cover chiropractic treatment under Medicaid. If you have health insurance, check whether chiropractic services are covered before you seek treatment.

Other Points to Consider

Research to expand the scientific understanding of chiropractic treatment is ongoing. If you decide to seek chiropractic care, talk to your chiropractor about the following:

- His education, training, and licensing

- Whether he has experience treating the health conditions for which you are seeking care

- Any special medical concerns you have and any medicines or dietary supplements you are taking

Tell all of your health care providers about any complementary and alternative practices you use. Give them a full picture of what you do to manage your health. This will help ensure coordinated and safe care.

NCCAM-Funded Research

Recent research projects on chiropractic care supported by the National Center for Complementary and Alternative Medicine (NCCAM) have focused on the following:

- Effectiveness of chiropractic treatments for back pain, neck pain, and headache, as well as for other health conditions such as temporomandibular disorders

- Development of a curriculum to increase the number of chiropractors involved in research

- Influence of people's satisfaction with chiropractic care on their response to treatment

Chapter 58

Craniosacral Therapy

Discovering the best form of therapy for your condition can be an enlightening moment. That "aha" moment for many of our patients comes when we introduce craniosacral therapy.

Craniosacral therapy is an effective treatment for:

- headaches and migraines;

- chronic neck and back pain;

- anxiety and nervousness;

- insomnia;

- depression;

- TMJ [temporomandibular joint disorder];

- dizziness and tinnitus.

Craniosacral therapy is a powerful alternative in cases where other therapies have not provided relief. In addition, craniosacral therapy promotes relaxation and immune system function, thereby enhancing healing throughout your body.

How It Works

The craniosacral system consists of the brain, spinal cord, membranes, and the fluid within it. This fluid has a pulse or rhythm not unlike the pulse of the circulatory or respiratory systems.

After the body experiences a trauma such as a fall or accident or has been in a cycle of repeated stress, the rhythm within the craniosacral system can be disrupted and a restriction can occur in the natural flow of this fluid. Because the system that is affected is the central nervous system, a variety of different symptoms can occur from headaches to chronic pain and many other neurological complaints.

Through light touch and gentle manipulation of areas on the head and throughout the body including the spine, a trained practitioner can detect where the natural flow is restricted and facilitate a release where flow is then restored. The natural healing ability of the body is the key to the effectiveness of this therapy.

This complementary therapy is gaining popularity due to its gentle and non-invasive treatment of a variety of symptoms. In addition, craniosacral therapy works well in conjunction with other therapeutic techniques to promote balance and recovery for a variety of symptoms.

Case Study #1

A woman in her 50s came for an appointment with allergies that developed into ear infections several months ago. The ear infections cleared up but one ear remained plugged and filled with fluid and the patient stated that she couldn't hear out of it.

The patient's ear, nose, and throat specialist recommended surgery but the patient wanted to try an alternative approach instead. Our therapist saw her a total of three times for craniosacral therapy. On the third visit the patient stated that she could hear out of her ear and it was no longer plugged. She also stated that she had her energy back as well.

Case Study #2

A female patient in her 50s came for an appointment complaining of chronic low back pain that kept her from being able to sit for long periods of time. This was difficult for her as she had a desk job. The pain had been with her for many years. She had a history of several falls on her tailbone as well as fractures to the tailbone.

After two sessions of craniosacral therapy, the client reported that the pain was gone and she could sit at her desk for the length of her shift. A monthly follow-up was recommended and the client continues to be pain free.

What a Session Is Like

In a typical session the patient lies on a padded table on their back, fully clothed and usually covered with a blanket. Light touch no heavier than the weight of a nickel is used to detect the rhythm of the craniosacral system and gentle techniques are used on the head, spine, and throughout the body to release a restriction.

A client can expect to feel relaxed, sleepy, or even energized. Some clients report that they become more aware of their body and the restrictions within it. A typical craniosacral therapy session lasts approximately 1 hour.

Health Reference Series *Medical Advisor's Notes and Updates*

The effectiveness of craniosacral therapy for the disorders listed remains controversial. Few good-quality scientific trials have been performed, and there have been conflicting results. Additional research is needed to determine whether the effects of craniosacral therapy are unique or can be attributed to other factors.

In the How It Works section, the explanations for the effects of craniosacral therapy are those stated by its practitioners. Scientific study of the underlying assumptions has produced mixed results.

Chapter 59

Feldenkrais Method

What is the Feldenkrais Method?

The Feldenkrais Method is named after its originator, Dr. Moshe Feldenkrais, D.Sc. (1904–1984) [about], a Russian born physicist, judo expert, mechanical engineer, and educator.

The Feldenkrais Method is a form of somatic education that uses gentle movement and directed attention to improve movement and enhance human functioning. Through this method, you can increase your ease and range of motion, improve your flexibility and coordination, and rediscover your innate capacity for graceful, efficient movement. These improvements will often generalize to enhance functioning in other aspects of your life.

The Feldenkrais Method is based on principles of physics, biomechanics, and an empirical understanding of learning and human development. By expanding the self-image through movement sequences that bring attention to the parts of the self that are out of awareness, the method enables you to include more of yourself in your functioning movements. Students become more aware of their habitual neuromuscular patterns and rigidities and expand options for new ways of moving. By increasing sensitivity the Feldenkrais Method assists you to live your life more fully, efficiently, and comfortably.

"Frequently Asked Questions," © 2009 Feldenkrais Educational Foundation of North America (www.feldenkrais.com). Reprinted with permission.

The improvement of physical functioning is not necessarily an end in itself. Such improvement is based on developing a broader functional awareness which is often a gateway to more generalized enhancement of physical functioning in the context of your environment and life.

Who benefits from the Feldenkrais Method?

Anyone—young or old, physically challenged or physically fit—can benefit from the method. Feldenkrais is beneficial for those experiencing chronic or acute pain of the back, neck, shoulder, hip, legs, or knee, as well as for healthy individuals who wish to enhance their self-image. The method has been very helpful in dealing with central nervous system conditions such as multiple sclerosis, cerebral palsy, and stroke. Musicians, actors, and artists can extend their abilities and enhance creativity. Many seniors enjoy using it to retain or regain their ability to move without strain or discomfort.

Through lessons in this method you can enjoy greater ease of movement, an increased sense of vitality, and feelings of peaceful relaxation. After a session you often feel taller and lighter, breathe more freely, and find that your discomforts have eased. You experience relaxation, and feel more centered and balanced.

Successful Students: Here are examples of recent successes students have accomplished after work with the Feldenkrais Method:

- A 42-year-old computer programmer with incipient wrist problems is able to increase his speed on the keyboard after learning how to use his arms and hands more efficiently.

- A 28-year-old woman goes through her third pregnancy, but the first one without back pain.

- A 55-year-old woman is able to lift her affectionate 2-year-old granddaughter without straining her back.

- A 40-year-old cellist becomes so creative in developing new, less strained positions to play in that she is able to extend her musical repertoire.

- A 9-year-old with learning disabilities can read a full page competently and gains self-confidence in his intelligence.

- A 19-year-old diver is able to visualize and perform the complex series of movements needed to accomplish an intricate endeavor more proficiently.

- A 78-year-old man walks a mile daily, free of chronic knee pain he's had for 30 years.

- A 32-year-old man learns to reuse his hands after a crippling auto accident.

Professional athletes who have enjoyed the benefits of Feldenkrais include basketball star Julius Erving and PGA golfers Rick Acton and Duffy Waldorf. Celebrities who have used Feldenkrais include Norman Cousins, Margaret Mead, former Israeli Prime Minister David Ben-Gurion, Helen Hayes, and Whoopi Goldberg. Famous musicians include violinist Yehudi Menuhin and cellist Yo Yo Ma.

What happens in a Feldenkrais Method session?

Feldenkrais work is done in two formats.

In group classes, called Awareness Through Movement, the Feldenkrais teacher verbally leads you through a sequence of movements in basic positions: sitting or lying on the floor, standing or sitting in a chair.

Private Feldenkrais lessons, called Functional Integration, are tailored to each student's individual learning needs; the teacher guides your movements through touch.

People learning the Feldenkrais Method are usually referred to as "students" rather than clients or patients. This reinforces our view of the work as primarily being an educational process.

What happens in an Awareness Through Movement® lesson?

Awareness Through Movement (ATM) consists of verbally directed movement sequences presented primarily to groups. A lesson generally lasts from 30 to 60 minutes. The lessons consist of comfortable, easy movements that gradually evolve into movements of greater range and complexity. These precisely structured movement explorations involve thinking, sensing, moving, and imagining. Many are based on developmental movements and ordinary functional activities (reaching, standing, lying to sitting, looking behind yourself, etc.); some are based on more abstract explorations of joint, muscle, and postural relationships. There are hundreds of ATM lessons, varying in difficulty and complexity, for all levels of movement ability.

The emphasis is on learning which movements work better and noticing the quality of these changes in your body. Through increased awareness, you will learn to abandon habitual patterns of movement and develop new alternatives, resulting in improved flexibility and coordination.

How do you learn in an Awareness Through Movement lesson?

- Using slow, gentle movement and directing students to move within the limits of safety by avoiding pain and strain

- Orienting to the process of learning and doing rather than working toward a goal

- Directing awareness toward sensing differences and perceiving whole interconnected patterns in movement

- Allowing the student to find his/her own way with a lesson

What happens in a Functional Integration® lesson?

As Feldenkrais practitioners guide you through movement sequences verbally in Awareness Through Movement lessons, they also guide you through movement in Functional Integration lessons with gentle non-invasive touching.

Functional Integration is performed with the student fully clothed, usually lying on a table or with the student in sitting or standing positions. At times, various props (pillows, rollers, blankets) are used in an effort to support the person's body configuration or to facilitate certain movements. The learning process is carried out without the use of any invasive or forceful procedure.

Functional Integration is a hands-on form of tactile, kinesthetic communication. The practitioner communicates how you organize your body and, through gentle touching and movement, conveys the experience of comfort, pleasure, and ease of movement while you learn how to reorganize your body and behavior in new and more expanded functional motor patterns.

In Functional Integration the practitioner/teacher develops a lesson for you, custom-tailored to your unique configuration at that particular moment, relating to a desire, intention, or need you have. Through rapport and respect for your abilities, qualities, and integrity, the practitioner/teacher creates an environment in which you can learn comfortably.

How does the Feldenkrais Method differ from massage and chiropractic?

The similarity is that both practices touch people, but beyond that our method is very different. In massage, the practitioner is working directly with the muscles, in chiropractic, with the bones. These are structural approaches that seek to affect change through changes in structure (muscles and spine). The Feldenkrais Method works with your ability to regulate and coordinate your movement; which means working with the nervous system. We refer to this as a functional approach wherein you can improve your use of self inclusive of whatever structural considerations are present.

How can I find a certified Feldenkrais® practitioner?

The Feldenkrais Guild® of North America can refer you to a practitioner in your area, or see the online directory [http://www.feldenkrais.com/practitioners/find]. Visit the International Feldenkrais Federation [http://feldenkrais-method.org/en/node/580] for international associations.

How are Feldenkrais practitioners trained?

All Feldenkrais practitioners must complete 740–800 hours of training over a 3- to 4-year period. Trainees participate in Awareness Through Movement and Functional Integration lessons, lectures, discussions, group process, and videos of Dr. Feldenkrais teaching. Eventually students teach Awareness Through Movement and Functional Integration under supervision. Trainees gradually acquire knowledge of how movement and function are formed and organized. This extensive subjective experience forms the basis from which she/he will learn to work with others.

The main purpose of the training is for the trainees to acquire for themselves a deep understanding of movement and its formation, to become aware of their own movement, to become astute observers of movement in others, and to be able to teach other people to enlarge their awareness and movement skills.

The training process is based upon the vast body of knowledge Dr. Feldenkrais introduced. Since he integrated into his body of learning theory aspects from a variety of scientific fields such as Newtonian mechanics, physics, neurophysiology, movement development, biology, and learning theories, we present some of these aspects in the training program for the trainee to comprehend the theoretical background of the method.

Who was Moshe Feldenkrais?

Feldenkrais was born in Russia. At the age of 13 he left his home and travelled alone for a year until he reached Palestine, where he worked as a laborer, cartographer, and tutor in mathematics. He also became active in sports (gymnastics, soccer) and the martial arts (jiujitsu). During his mid twenties he left for France and eventually became a graduate of l'Ecole des Travaux Publiques de Paris, in Mechanical and Electrical Engineering. Later he earned his Doctor of Science in Physics from the Sorbonne in Paris, where he assisted Nobel Prize winner Joliot-Curie in early nuclear research.

In Paris, Feldenkrais also met Jigaro Kano, the creator of modern Judo, and Feldenkrais became one of the first Europeans to earn a

Black Belt in Judo (1936) and to introduce Judo in the West through his teaching and books on the subject. In the early 1940s, while working in anti-submarine warfare for the British Admiralty, he patented a number of sonar devices.

After suffering crippling knee injuries, Feldenkrais used his own body as his laboratory and merged his acquired knowledge with his deep curiosity about biology, perinatal development, cybernetics, linguistics, and systems theory. He taught himself to walk again and in the process developed an extraordinary system for accessing the power of the central nervous system to improve human functioning.

Feldenkrais studied intensively in psychology, neurophysiology, and other health-related disciplines, and in 1949 he returned to Israel where he continued to integrate and refine his ideas into the system known as the Feldenkrais Method.

Chapter 60

Massage Therapy

Chapter Contents

Section 60.1—Massage Therapy Overview 414

Section 60.2—Lymphatic Drainage Massage 419

Section 60.3—Tui Na: Chinese Massage 421

Section 60.1

Massage Therapy Overview

Excerpted from "Massage Therapy: An Introduction," by the National Center for Complementary and Alternative Medicine (NCCAM, nccam.nih.gov), June 2009.

Massage therapy has a long history in cultures around the world. Today, people use many different types of massage therapy for a variety of health-related purposes. In the United States, massage therapy is often considered part of complementary and alternative medicine (CAM), although it does have some conventional uses.

History of Massage

Massage therapy dates back thousands of years. References to massage appear in writings from ancient China, Japan, India, Arabic nations, Egypt, Greece (Hippocrates defined medicine as "the art of rubbing"), and Rome.

Massage became widely used in Europe during the Renaissance. In the 1850s, two American physicians who had studied in Sweden introduced massage therapy in the United States, where it became popular and was promoted for a variety of health purposes. With scientific and technological advances in medical treatment during the 1930s and 1940s, massage fell out of favor in the United States. Interest in massage revived in the 1970s, especially among athletes.

Use of Massage Therapy in the United States

According to the 2007 National Health Interview Survey, which included a comprehensive survey of CAM use by Americans, an estimated 18 million U.S. adults and 700,000 children had received massage therapy in the previous year.

People use massage for a variety of health-related purposes, including to relieve pain, rehabilitate sports injuries, reduce stress, increase relaxation, address anxiety and depression, and aid general wellness.

Defining Massage Therapy

The term "massage therapy" encompasses many different techniques. In general, therapists press, rub, and otherwise manipulate the muscles and other soft tissues of the body. They most often use their hands and fingers, but may use their forearms, elbows, or feet.

In Swedish massage, the therapist uses long strokes, kneading, deep circular movements, vibration, and tapping. Sports massage is similar to Swedish massage, adapted specifically to the needs of athletes. Among the many other examples are deep tissue massage; trigger point massage, which focuses on myofascial trigger points—muscle "knots" that are painful when pressed and can cause symptoms elsewhere in the body; and reflexology, which applies pressure to the feet (or sometimes the hands or ears), to promote relaxation or healing in other parts of the body.

The Practice of Massage Therapy

Massage therapists work in a variety of settings, including private offices, hospitals, nursing homes, studios, and sport and fitness facilities. Some also travel to patients' homes or workplaces. They usually try to provide a calm, soothing environment.

Therapists usually ask new patients about symptoms, medical history, and desired results. They may also perform an evaluation through touch, to locate painful or tense areas and determine how much pressure to apply.

Typically, the patient lies on a table, either in loose-fitting clothing or undressed (covered with a sheet, except for the area being massaged). The therapist may use oil or lotion to reduce friction on the skin. Sometimes, people receive massage therapy while sitting in a chair. A massage session may be fairly brief, but may also last an hour or even longer.

Research Status

Although scientific research on massage therapy—whether it works and, if so, how—is limited, there is evidence that massage may benefit some patients. Conclusions generally cannot yet be drawn about its effectiveness for specific health conditions.

According to one analysis, however, research supports the general conclusion that massage therapy is effective. The studies included in the analysis suggest that a single session of massage therapy can reduce "state anxiety" (a reaction to a particular situation), blood pressure, and heart rate, and multiple sessions can reduce "trait anxiety" (general anxiety-proneness), depression, and pain. In addition, recent studies suggest that massage may benefit certain conditions, for example:

- A 2008 review of 13 clinical trials found evidence that massage might be useful for chronic low-back pain. Clinical practice guidelines issued in 2007 by the American Pain Society and the American College of Physicians recommend that physicians consider using certain CAM therapies, including massage (as well as acupuncture, chiropractic, progressive relaxation, and yoga), when patients with chronic low-back pain do not respond to conventional treatment.

- A multisite study of more than 300 hospice patients with advanced cancer concluded that massage may help to relieve pain and improve mood for these patients.

- A study of 64 patients with chronic neck pain found that therapeutic massage was more beneficial than a self-care book, in terms of improving function and relieving symptoms.

There are numerous theories about how massage therapy may affect the body. For example, the "gate control theory" suggests that massage may provide stimulation that helps to block pain signals sent to the brain. Other examples include theories suggesting that massage might stimulate the release of certain chemicals in the body, such as serotonin or endorphins, or cause beneficial mechanical changes in the body. However, additional studies are needed to test the various theories.

Safety

Massage therapy appears to have few serious risks—if it is performed by a properly trained therapist and if appropriate cautions are followed. The number of serious injuries reported is very small. Side effects of massage therapy may include temporary pain or discomfort, bruising, swelling, and a sensitivity or allergy to massage oils.

Cautions about massage therapy include the following:

- Vigorous massage should be avoided by people with bleeding disorders or low blood platelet counts, and by people taking blood-thinning medications such as warfarin.

- Massage should not be done in any area of the body with blood clots, fractures, open or healing wounds, skin infections, or weakened bones (such as from osteoporosis or cancer), or where there has been a recent surgery.

- Although massage therapy appears to be generally safe for cancer patients, they should consult their oncologist before having a massage that involves deep or intense pressure. Any direct pressure over a tumor usually is discouraged. Cancer patients should discuss any concerns about massage therapy with their oncologist.

- Pregnant women should consult their health care provider before using massage therapy.

Training, Licensing, and Certification

There are approximately 1,500 massage therapy schools and training programs in the United States. In addition to hands-on practice of massage techniques, students generally learn about the body and how it works, business practices, and ethics. Massage training programs generally are approved by a state board. Some may also be accredited by an independent agency, such as the Commission on Massage Therapy Accreditation (COMTA).

As of 2007, 38 states and the District of Columbia had laws regulating massage therapy. In some states, regulation is by town ordinance.

The National Certification Board for Therapeutic Massage and Bodywork (NCBTMB) certifies practitioners who pass a national examination. Increasingly, states that license massage therapists require them to have a minimum of 500 hours of training at an accredited institution, pass the NCBTMB exam, meet specific continuing education requirements, and carry malpractice insurance.

In addition to massage therapists, health care providers such as chiropractors and physical therapists may have training in massage.

Some common licenses or certifications for massage therapists include the following:

- LMT: Licensed Massage Therapist

- LMP: Licensed Massage Practitioner

- CMT: Certified Massage Therapist

- NCTMB: Has met the credentialing requirements (including passing an exam) of the National Certification Board for Therapeutic Massage and Bodywork, for practicing therapeutic massage and bodywork

- NCTM: Has met the credentialing requirements (including passing an exam) of the National Certification Board for Therapeutic Massage and Bodywork, for practicing therapeutic massage

If You Are Thinking about Using Massage Therapy

- Do not use massage therapy to replace your regular medical care or as a reason to postpone seeing a health care provider about a medical problem.

- If you have a medical condition and are unsure whether massage therapy would be appropriate for you, discuss your concerns with your health care provider. Your health care provider may also be able to help you select a massage therapist. You might also look for published research articles on massage therapy for your condition.

- Before deciding to begin massage therapy, ask about the therapist's training, experience, and credentials. Also ask about the number of treatments that might be needed, the cost, and insurance coverage.

- If a massage therapist suggests using other CAM practices (for example, herbs or other supplements, or a special diet), discuss it first with your regular health care provider.

- Tell your health care providers about any complementary and alternative practices you use. Give them a full picture of what you do to manage your health. This will ensure coordinated and safe care.

Section 60.2

Lymphatic Drainage Massage

What Is Lymphatic Drainage Massage?

Lymphatic drainage massage is a specialized massage technique for the purpose of reducing swelling in the body and increasing the flow of lymph. Lymph is the fluid that seeps out of the cells and must be returned to the bloodstream. It flows through vessels very similar to blood vessels. In the process, the lymph nodes filter and purify the lymph. The lymphatic system is an integral part of the immune system, so in stimulating the flow of lymph, you are also stimulating the immune system, leading to better overall health.

Swelling in the body often occurs because there is an imbalance, injury, or disease that reduces, overloads, or blocks the flow of lymph. Lymphatic drainage massage very gently opens and stretches the initial lymphatic vessels just under the skin, facilitating the flow of the lymph and reducing the swelling. It also very lightly flushes the lymph nodes, encouraging a smoother, more effective flow of the lymph through them. It can also speed the healing of injuries and reduce the size of scar tissue.

Benefits of Lymphatic Drainage Massage

- Reduces swelling and edema
- Enhances immune function
- Speeds healing of injuries and surgeries
- Reduces scarring
- Reduces stress and tension
- Relieves headaches

- Relieves sinus problems
- Improves the condition of the skin
- Rejuvenates the skin on the face and neck
- Improves the client's overall energy level

The Technique

Lymphatic drainage massage uses very light pressure of the fingers and hands, just slightly moving the skin, a technique quite different from the long deeper flowing strokes of regular massages. The pattern of strokes in lymphatic drainage massage is very small and precise, moving very slowly and rhythmically, and repeating over and over. Because of this, lymphatic drainage massage is very relaxing and therefore excellent for reducing the effects of stress and tension.

What Is a Session of Lymphatic Drainage Massage Like?

A session of lymphatic drainage massage is very restful. The client lies comfortably on a massage table under a sheet while the therapist very lightly massages the skin, working one area thoroughly before moving to another area.

Sessions can involve massaging all the major areas of the body, which take an hour and a half or more. They can also be shorter sessions, between 30 to 60 minutes, focusing on one particular area of the body. For example, if someone has an injured arm, the therapist could massage just the arm and torso.

Facial Lymphatic Drainage

Facial lymphatic drainage sessions are very popular. Facial lymphatic drainage reduces swelling in the face and neck as well as improving and rejuvenating the skin. This helps the skin look younger. Facial lymphatic drainage works very well in conjunction with facial rejuvenation acupuncture, improving skin tone and reducing the signs of aging. This combination of therapies has proven successful results. Facial lymphatic drainage is also very beneficial in relieving headaches and sinus problems.

Section 60.3

Tui Na: Chinese Massage

"The mind, the spirit, and the hands are the most fundamental tools of healing we possess. Tui Na makes use of all three to promote health and well being through the individual's muscular, skeletal, and energetic systems."—Christopher Reilly, L.Ac., MSA.

Tui Na is perhaps the oldest branch of traditional Chinese medicine (TCM). The first written record of Tui Na dates to 2700 BCE [Before the Common Era], and the official Tui Na department was established in the State Office of Imperial Physicians in China's Sui and Tang Dynasties (581–907 CE [Common Era]). Literally translated as "pushing and grasping," Tui Na encompasses an extremely broad set of hands-on techniques whose applications are guided by the same theory and physiological concepts that govern acupuncture and herbal therapy. Throughout the past 5,000 years, Tui Na experts have developed methods of bone-setting, joint manipulation, trauma therapy, massage therapy, pediatric therapy, preventive therapy, and topical herbal applications.

The Tui Na form of bodywork differs from most Swedish and western styles in the speed and vigor with which certain techniques are applied, the TCM theory and philosophy embedded within the Tui Na, and an emphasis on the stimulation of acupuncture points and meridians. There are a variety of techniques, such as dragon and phoenix rolling, zhen's single finger pushing, and trembling that are unique to Tui Na. In modern terms, Tui Na as it is practiced in America can be understood as a hands-on form of bodywork which uses acupressure and traditional Chinese medical theory to achieve a variety of wellness goals, including pain relief and muscular health.

Tui Na is often the treatment of choice for TCM practitioners, and is used in place of acupuncture in children. The first treatise on pediatric Tui Na in China dates to 1601 CE. Areas of the body that are of particular relevance to pediatric sessions have been documented over hundreds of years with names such as sky river, wood gate, the three fences, and the six fu. During very brief sessions (about 5 to 10 minutes), gentle techniques are applied to the extremities and trunk to relieve poor appetite, loose stools, low-grade fevers, etc. Very simple techniques are taught to the child's caregivers, who can perform them at home to enhance and boost the effectiveness of the Tui Na. In the case of children and adults, Tui Na provides a non-invasive and well-tolerated means to apply traditional Chinese medical theory to contemporary health challenges.

Chapter 61

Pilates

Pilates (pronounced: puh-lah-teez) improves your mental and physical well-being, increases flexibility, and strengthens muscles. Pilates uses controlled movements in the form of mat exercises or equipment to tone and strengthen the body. For decades, it's been the exercise of choice for dancers and gymnasts (and now Hollywood actors), but it was originally used to rehabilitate bedridden or immobile patients during World War I.

What Is Pilates?

Pilates is a body conditioning routine that seeks to build flexibility, strength, endurance, and coordination without adding muscle bulk. In addition, Pilates increases circulation and helps to sculpt the body and strengthen the body's "core" or "powerhouse" (torso). People who do Pilates regularly feel they have better posture, are less prone to injury, and experience better overall health.

Joseph H. Pilates, the founder of the Pilates exercise method, was born in Germany. As a child he was frail, living with asthma in addition to other childhood conditions. To build his body and grow stronger, he took up several different sports, eventually becoming an accomplished athlete. As a nurse in Great Britain during World War I, he designed exercise methods and equipment for immobilized patients and soldiers.

In addition to his equipment, Pilates developed a series of mat exercises that focus on the torso. He based these on various exercise methods from around the world, among them the mind-body formats of yoga and Chinese martial arts.

Joseph Pilates believed that our physical and mental health are intertwined. He designed his exercise program around principles that support this philosophy, including concentration, precision, control, breathing, and flowing movements.

There are two ways to exercise in Pilates. Today, most people focus on the mat exercises, which require only a floor mat and training. These exercises are designed so that your body uses its own weight as resistance. The other method of Pilates uses a variety of machines to tone and strengthen the body, again using the principle of resistance.

Getting Started

The great thing about Pilates is that just about everyone—from couch potatoes to fitness buffs—can do it. Because Pilates has gained lots of attention recently, there are lots of classes available. You'll probably find that many fitness centers and YMCAs offer Pilates classes, mostly in mat work. Some Pilates instructors also offer private classes that can be purchased class by class or in blocks of classes; these may combine mat work with machine work. If your health club makes Pilates machines available to members, make sure there's a qualified Pilates instructor on duty to teach and supervise you during the exercises.

The fact that Pilates is hot and classes are springing up everywhere does have a downside, though: inadequate instruction. As with any form of exercise, it is possible to injure yourself if you have a health condition or don't know exactly how to do the moves. Some gyms send their personal trainers to weekend-long courses and then claim they're qualified to teach Pilates (they're not!), and this can lead to injury.

So look for an instructor who is certified by a group that has a rigorous training program. These instructors have completed several hundred hours of training just in Pilates and know the different ways to modify the exercises so new students don't get hurt.

The Pilates mat program follows a set sequence, with exercises following on from one another in a natural progression, just as Joseph Pilates designed them. Beginners start with basic exercises and build up to include additional exercises and more advanced positioning.

Keep these tips in mind so that you can get the most out of your Pilates workout.

- **Stay focused.** Pilates is designed to combine your breathing rhythm with your body movements. Qualified instructors teach ways to keep your breathing working in conjunction with the exercises. You will also be taught to concentrate on your muscles and what you are doing. The goal of Pilates is to unite your mind and body, which relieves stress and anxiety.

- **Be comfortable.** Wear comfortable clothes (as you would for yoga—shorts or tights and a T-shirt or tank top are good choices), and keep in mind that Pilates is usually done without shoes. If you start feeling uncomfortable, strained, or experience pain, you should stop.

- **Let it flow.** When you perform your exercises, avoid quick, jerky movements. Every movement should be slow, but still strong and flexible. Joseph Pilates worked with dancers and designed his movements to flow like a dance.

- **Don't leave out the heart.** The nice thing about Pilates is you don't have to break a sweat if you don't want to—but you can also work the exercises quickly (bearing in mind fluidity, of course!) to get your heart rate going. Or, because Pilates is primarily about strength and flexibility, pair your Pilates workout with a form of aerobic exercise like swimming or brisk walking.

Most fans of Pilates say they stick with the program because it's diverse and interesting. Joseph Pilates designed his program for variety—people do fewer repetitions of a number of exercises rather than lots of repetitions of only a few. He also intended his exercises to be something people could do on their own once they've had proper instruction, cutting down the need to remain dependent on a trainer.

Before you begin any type of exercise program, it's a good idea to talk to your doctor, especially if you have a health problem.

Chapter 62

Qigong

Qigong is an ancient Chinese health care system that integrates physical postures, breathing techniques, and focused intention.

The word Qigong (Chi Kung) is made up of two Chinese words. Qi is pronounced chee and is usually translated to mean the life force or vital energy that flows through all things in the universe.

The second word, Gong, pronounced gung, means accomplishment, or skill that is cultivated through steady practice. Together, Qigong (Chi Kung) means cultivating energy; it is a system practiced for health maintenance, healing, and increasing vitality.

Qigong is an integration of physical postures, breathing techniques, and focused intentions.

Qigong practices can be classified as martial, medical, or spiritual. All styles have three things in common: They all involve a posture (whether moving or stationary), breathing techniques, and mental focus. Some practices increase the Qi; others circulate it, use it to cleanse and heal the body, store it, or emit Qi to help heal others. Practices vary from the soft internal styles such as Tai Chi; to the external, vigorous styles such as Kung Fu. However, the slow gentle movements of most Qigong forms can be easily adapted, even for the physically challenged and can be practiced by all age groups.

"What is Qigong?" © 2009 National Qigong Association (www.nqa.org). Reprinted with permission.

Like any other system of health care, Qigong is not a panacea, but it is certainly a highly effective health care practice. Many health care professionals recommend Qigong as an important form of alternative complementary medicine.

Qigong creates an awareness of and influences dimensions of our being that are not part of traditional exercise programs. Most exercises do not involve the meridian system used in acupuncture nor do they emphasize the importance of adding mind intent and breathing techniques to physical movements. When these dimensions are added, the benefits of exercise increase exponentially.

The gentle, rhythmic movements of Qigong reduce stress, build stamina, increase vitality, and enhance the immune system. It has also been found to improve cardiovascular, respiratory, circulatory, lymphatic, and digestive functions.

Those who maintain a consistent practice of Qigong find that it helps one regain a youthful vitality, maintain health even into old age, and helps speed recovery from illness. Western scientific research confirms that Qigong reduces hypertension and the incidence of falling in the aged population. One of the more important long-term effects is that Qigong reestablishes the body/mind/soul connection.

People do Qigong to maintain health, heal their bodies, calm their minds, and reconnect with their spirit.

When these three aspects of our being are integrated, it encourages a positive outlook on life and helps eliminate harmful attitudes and behaviors. It also creates a balanced life style, which brings greater harmony, stability, and enjoyment.

There are a wide variety of Qigong practices. They vary from the simple, internal forms to the more complex and challenging external styles. They can interest and benefit everyone, from the most physically challenged to the super athlete. There are Qigong classes for children, senior citizens, and every age group in between. Since Qigong can be practiced anywhere or at any time, there is no need to buy special clothing or to join a health club.

Qigong's great appeal is that everyone can benefit, regardless of ability, age, belief system, or life circumstances.

Anyone can enrich their lives by adding Qigong to their daily routine: Children learning to channel their energy and develop increased concentration; office workers learning Qigong to reduce stress; seniors participating in gentle movements to enhance balance and their quality of life; caregivers embracing a practice to develop their ability to help others; prisons instituting Qigong programs to restore balance in inmates lives; midwives using Qigong techniques to ease childbirth.

When an individual or group assumes responsibility and takes action for their health and healing, we all benefit. It is best to get referrals from people whose judgment you have confidence in. Check the Yellow Pages for Tai Chi schools, acupuncturists, or martial art academies. The National Qigong Association (NQA) directory is also an excellent source for finding instructors.

Keep in mind the following criteria for choosing a qualified instructor: What is their background and experience; are they of good character; do they treat everyone fairly and with respect; do they live what they teach; do they refrain from making wild, unsubstantiated claims; do they encourage and bring out a student's highest potential? While keeping these points in mind, remember to trust your intuition in finding an instructor who is right for you.

How can I learn if there aren't any teachers near me?

If there are no instructors in your area, many teachers regularly travel to give workshops in all regions of the country. Many excellent instructional books and videos are also available.

Begin by familiarizing yourself with the many resources available for learning Qigong. The internet is one of the best tools today for learning about Qigong.

Seek referrals in your area and visit local classes. Attending the annual NQA conference also provides an introduction to many styles of Qigong and practitioners from around the world.

After you have looked into some of these resources, find a style you feel comfortable with, and develop a consistent daily practice. It is recommended by experienced teachers to stay with a form for at least 100 days. A consistent practice is the most important asset you can develop.

When beginners ask, "What is the most important aspect of practicing Qigong?" The answer is always "just do it."

Chapter 63

Reflexology

A Brief History of Foot Reflexology

Modern Reflexology is based on the work of two American physicians, Dr. William Fitzgerald and Dr. Joe Shelby Riley of the 1920s, and on that of physiotherapist Eunice D. Ingham who developed Fitzgerald and Riley's knowledge into a usable therapy, calling it Foot Reflexology and took it to the public in the late 1930s through the early 70s.

The scientific basis to Reflexology begins in the last century. In the 1890s knighted research scientist and medical doctor, Sir Henry Head, demonstrated the neurological relationship that exists between the skin and the internal organs. Nobel prizewinner, Sir Charles Sherrington, proved that the whole nervous system and body adjusts to a stimulus when it is applied to any part of the body. Around the same time in Germany, Dr. Alfons Cornelius observed that pressure to certain spots triggered muscle contractions, changes in blood pressure, variation in warmth and moisture in the body as well as directly affecting the psychic processes, or mental state of the patient. The Russians, beginning with Drs. Ivan Pavlov and Vladimir Bekhterev, have also been exploring reflex responses in the body for nearly a century.

In the last 30 years, because of Eunice Ingham's traveling around the country teaching groups of people her method of Reflexology, a grassroots following of Reflexology emerged in the United States. In that time practicing Reflexologists have emerged, more than 40 Reflexology books have been published, and the number of magazine articles published has risen by 500 percent since 1982. Television appearances by Reflexologists have increased by 500 percent since 1988.

Today recent research studies have been conducted around the world, including in the United States, which are validating the effectiveness of Reflexology on a wide variety of conditions. Chronic conditions seem to respond especially well to Reflexology. In China, where Reflexology is accepted by the central government as a means of preventing and curing diseases and preserving health, over 300 research studies have shown Reflexology provided some improvement to 95 percent of the over 18,000 cases covering 64 illnesses studied. In Japan and Denmark, Reflexology has been incorporated into the employee health programs of several large corporations saving each company thousands of dollars annually in paid sick leave benefits.

Many of our health problems can be linked to stress. It is an acknowledged fact by the medical community that a body trying to function while under the influence of prolonged stress is less capable of organizing its defenses against illnesses and repair damage caused by injury. Stress can be mentally, emotionally, physically, or environmentally induced. Reflexology is primarily a relaxation technique. Reflexology can negate the effects of stress while it helps the body relax and balance. Through the relaxation process the body is more capable of dealing with the stresses placed on it by daily living and those associated with illness. Reflexology gently nudges the body toward better functioning by improving lymphatic drainage and venous circulation, stimulation to the nerve pathways, and muscle relaxation, helping the body to balance itself.

While historically Reflexology has anecdotally been found to have a positive effect on the body suffering from a wide variety of chronic problems, it is not a panacea for all ills. Reflexology is not a substitute for medical treatment, but can be used as a complement to any type of medical approach or therapy. Reflexology can also be incorporated into an overall healthy lifestyle, which includes attention to diet, moderate exercise, and different forms of stress reduction and relaxation.

The Differences between Reflexology and Massage

Some people confuse Reflexology with massage, but they are two different modalities—each with its own strengths. Both, like many other therapies, such as chiropractics, osteopathy, and other somatic practices, involve the use of the hands to apply their techniques. The aim with both Reflexology and massage is to enhance the well-being of the client. [See Table 63.1 for a comparison of reflexology and massage.]

Table 63.1. Comparison of Reflexology and Massage

Reflexology	Massage
Application	
Applied to specific areas (usually feet, hands and ears); to promote a response from an area far removed from the tissue stimulated via the nervous systems and acupuncture meridians.	Applied to the whole body; muscles and connective tissue locally for local benefit, or when applied to muscles located all over the body, benefits the entire body.
Only the footwear comes off, as only the feet, hands, and ears are touched.	All the clothing comes off, as most of the body is touched.
Techniques	
Uses small muscle movements; primarily thumbs and fingers are used.	Uses large muscle movement; hands (either opened or closed), and sometimes feet, arms, and elbows.
Purpose	
To improve the function of organs and glands and all systems of the body. Works with the function of the body.	Primarily to change the soft tissue directly stimulated. Works with the structure of the body.
Benefit	
Total body relaxation leading to the balancing of all internal and external body systems; improving circulation via stimulation to the nervous and subtly, energy systems.	Local muscle relaxation or if the entire body is massaged then to muscular system improving circulation and reducing muscular tension.

It is not necessary for Reflexology practitioners to study working on a naked body when all they work on are the feet, hands, and ears of a fully clothed person.

Chapter 64

Structural Integration Techniques

Chapter Contents

Section 64.1—Hellerwork Structural Integration..................... 436

Section 64.2—Rolfing 438

Section 64.1

Hellerwork Structural Integration

"What Hellerwork Structural Integration Is," © 2009
Hellerwork International (www.hellerwork.com).
Reprinted with permission.

Hellerwork Structural Integration (SI) is a powerful system of somatic education and structural bodywork, based on the inseparability of body, mind, and spirit. Following Ida Rolf's lineage of Structural Integration bodywork, Joseph Heller incorporated movement education/awareness and body-centered human development processes creating Hellerwork.

Deep tissue bodywork combined with movement education and dialogue of the mind/body connection guides you to new options, both physically and emotionally. Hellerwork SI encourages you to make the connection between movement and body alignment. Hellerwork restores your body's natural balance from the inside out.

During the 11 section series, the structural balance of your body is realized through the systematic release and reorganization of muscle and connective tissue using a variety of deep-tissue bodywork techniques. When your body comes into alignment within the field of gravity chronic pain and tension dissipate. A comfortable sense of support replaces the stress and strain of carrying your body through life. Movement education is incorporated to enhance fluidity and ease of motion and helps you develop a deeper awareness of your body and its expression in the world.

Self-awareness facilitated through dialogue is an important component of the Hellerwork SI series. As your body releases patterns of tension and stress, new options of support and fluidity become available. Emotionally, new options also become available. Guided dialogue enhances a deeper awareness of your emotional and cultural patterns allowing for choice and change.

Hellerwork Structural Integration is based on the assumption that every person is innately healthy. Your results are maximized by creating a deeper experience of the integrity in your body, your movement, and in your relationship with yourself and the world around you.

What to Expect in a Hellerwork SI Session

A session starts with a check-in to discuss how your body has been assimilating the work, what changes you have noticed, and what is getting your attention in the moment. This followed by an assessment of your structure and movement patterns. The practitioner utilizes this information to individualize the session to address your particular needs.

The bodywork is received primarily while lying on a massage table, although seated and standing work may be included. Hellerwork generally feels like slow deep pressure followed by a pleasant sense of ease and release. As a client you may be asked to make slow movements while the practitioner guides the tissue, releasing patterns of strain and tension. Sensations may range from pleasure to temporary discomfort depending on the condition of the tissue. Hellerwork practitioners are skilled in working sensitively with you to determine an appropriate level of pressure, depth, and speed.

An important part of the session involves movement education and body/mind awareness. The Dialogue component of a Hellerwork session helps to enhance your awareness of the inseparable connection of mind, body, emotion, and spirit. Movement exercises are designed and taught to meet your individual needs. Proper mechanics involved in walking, sitting, and standing are emphasized.

In general, clients report feeling a sense of lightness, length, and well-being upon completion of a session. The release and rebalancing of your structure will continue between sessions. Your body continues to integrate your newfound awareness, new relationship with gravity, new way of being, and new sense of "excellence with ease."

Section 64.2

Rolfing

Who should consider Rolfing?

According to Dr. Rolf, all bodies have some degree of disorder and
compensation in their structure; therefore she believed that everyone
should receive Rolfing structural integration. In fact, in her global vision, she imagined a more evolved and structurally efficient human
species as a result of Rolfing. However, we realize that most potential
clients need more compelling reasons to undergo this powerful transformative sequence of session. It is possible to divide those who come
to Rolfing into two groups.

The first and largest group who should consider Rolfing are those
who have a history of injury or trauma and notice that the effects of
their often minor injuries are beginning to interfere with their everyday lives. In many cases these individuals have tried traditional
medical treatments or exercise to reduce or counteract the long-term
effects of old injuries with varying degrees of success. This group might
include former and current athletes, musicians, performers, or those
engaged in physically demanding jobs who choose not to accept the
notion that the quality of their lives must suffer simply because they
are aging. In fact, all adults of any age who suffer from any limiting
physical discomfort can absolutely benefit from Rolfing as long as
the pains themselves are in the neuromuscular system and not signs
of a nervous disorder or a deeper pathology. For most of us, Rolfing
combined with appropriate movement therapy and exercise offers a
long-lasting solution for connective tissue problems.

The second group are those who are on a spiritual path and who
find that their physical limitations prevent them from attaining a
higher level of spiritual or emotional peace. Frequently, many on this
path assume that the body is something to be transcended rather
than something to be honored and loved. For these individuals, Rolfing can serve as an educational resource which allows them a more

intimate and comfortable relationship with their physical body, which in turn allows a greater ability to experience greater serenity. Interestingly enough, as the body transforms physically it transforms on other planes as well, so that, while Rolfing's primary focus is the muscular and connective tissue system, it frequently has an even more dramatic effect in seemingly unrelated areas such as the spiritual. Exactly how this happens is still a matter of much debate and speculation. However, the results of the work were of much greater importance than the how or why for Dr. Rolf. The genius of Rolfing is that it can affect so many people in so many ways and continue to reveal new possibilities for such a rich diversity of individuals.

Does Rolfing hurt?

When most people think of Rolfing, one of the first words that come to their mind is pain. Often, this perception is based on anecdotal accounts of sessions performed during Rolfing's infancy, when it tended to be often a less subtle and more intense discipline, frequently linked to popular emotionally intense types of therapies in the late 1960s and early 70s. Part of this reputation can be attributed to an often-quoted complaint of Dr. Rolf during her training classes that her students failed to work deep enough. Apparently, many assumed that what she meant was that they needed to work harder and deeper. However, we now realize that deep work is not necessarily synonymous with physical intensity.

Several factors determine the level of comfort or discomfort during a Rolfing session. One is the degree of trauma in the system; the other is how long fascial distortions have been in the client's body. Long-term distortions create more tenacious and widespread compensatory patterns, which may require more sustained pressure to release.

Another factor is the degree of emotional charge associated with an area of injury or strain. Dr. Rolf made the point that during the therapeutic process, emotional pain is often experienced when deeply held emotional traumas and memories are brought to surface and processed. Similarly, she reasoned, deep touch can result in transitory experience of pain that is healing and transformative. However, there is actually a fair amount of variation in the level of intensity. Various practitioners feel it is appropriate to affect the necessary level of change. It is recommended that the potential Rolfing client speak to all Rolfers about this issue and try the various work of practitioners, judging both the level of intensity and the quality of the results you experience.

A general guideline for the vast majority of Rolfing clients is that the intensity experienced is transitory, moving quickly from brief intensity to a decrease in sensation and finally to an easing of long-standing holdings which can prove both profound and transformative. To paraphrase Peter Schwind, a Certified Advanced Rolfer from Munich, Germany, "The art of Rolfing is to master a wide range of styles of touch and know when a lighter and more intense touch is required." Continuous communication with the client and pacing the level of intensity are essential, profoundly affecting the client's reaction to the transitory discomfort when seriously restricted tissue is softened, discriminated, and reintegrated.

What is the difference between massage and Rolfing?

One of the most common misconceptions about Rolfing is that it is a nothing more than a type of very deep massage. There are many varieties of massage, which are particularly effective for loosening tight tissue, reducing stress, detoxing the body, and an increased feeling of relaxation and well-being. Since these benefits are also a byproduct of Rolfing, the general public experience confusion as to the precise difference between our work and the proliferation of effective touch modalities currently available. Ray McCall, an Advanced Rolfer in Boulder and former student of Dr. Rolf, once said that what Rolfers do can be summed up in three words: palpation, discrimination, and integration. We palpate, or touch the tissue, feeling for imbalances in tissue texture, quality, and temperature to determine where we need to work. We discriminate, or separate fascial layers that adhere and muscles that have been pulled out of position by strain or injury. Finally, we integrate the body, relating its segments in an improved relationship, bringing physical balance in the gravitational field. Other soft-tissue manipulation methods, including massage, are quite good at the first two, but do not balance the body in gravity. As Dr. Rolf used to say: "Anyone can take a body apart, very few know how to put it back together." The true genius of her method is the art and science of reshaping and reorganizing human structure according to clearly defined principles in a systematic and consistent manner.

In addition to our skill as structural integrators, we are also educators, a point Dr. Rolf stressed frequently in her training classes. The role of teacher is something every Rolfer takes seriously. In each session, Rolfers seek to impart insights to clients to increase their awareness and understanding, to help the client make the work we do their own. Our job is to make ourselves obsolete, by empowering our clients to take charge of their own physical and emotional health. Influencing the structural evolution of man on a global level was Dr. Rolf's fondest dream.

How does Rolfing work?

Rolfing strives to align and balance the body's components until the entire system is a smoothly functioning coordinated whole. For example, the legs are aligned to the hips, shoulders to rib cage, the body is positioned over the feet, and then all of these joints and related tissue are integrated to one another. A few of the many benefits people experience are reduced pain, increased flexibility, an enhanced sense of body awareness, and improved posture.

These wonderful transformations are possible because Rolfing addresses the body's internal system of flexible support, otherwise known as fascia. These connective tissues surround every muscle fiber, encase all joints, and even have a role in the nervous system. Think of the fascial system as an intricate internal guide wire network for the body. And if one set of support wires becomes tight or out of place, the excess tension may appear as nagging joint pain, muscle soreness, or a postural shift.

To correct internal misalignments, a Rolfing practitioner uses mild, direct pressure to melt or release facial holdings and allow the body to find health through the reestablishment of balance. It is currently believed that the slow, deep strokes of Rolfing stimulate intra-fascial mechanoreceptors (sensory neurons of the muscle nerve), which in turn triggers the nervous system to reduce the tension of the related muscles and fascia.

Put another way, Rolfing allows the brain and nervous system to "re-boot" areas of the body that are receiving too much electrical stimulation (chronically tight or sore muscles). And once a healthy level of muscle contraction is established, someone's entire structure is free to express a pain-free form.

What is the Rolfing Ten Series?

The hallmark of Rolfing Structural Integration is a standardized "recipe" known as the Ten Series, the goal of which is to systematically balance and optimize both the structure (shape) and function (movement) of the entire body over the course of 10 Rolfing sessions.

Each session focuses on freeing restrictions or holdings trapped in a particular region of the body. A practitioner also maintains a holistic view of the client's entire system during each session, thus ensuring the transformational process evolves in a comfortable and harmonious way.

The Ten Series can be divided into three distinct units.

Sessions 1–3: Called the "sleeve" sessions, numbers one through three strive to loosen and balance surface layers of connective tissue.

Specifically, the first session is devoted to enhancing the quality of breath with work on the arms, ribcage, and diaphragm. Opening is also started along the upper leg, hamstrings, neck, and spine. The second session helps give the body a stable foundation by balancing the foot and muscles of the lower leg. Number three typically involves a "side view" for an understanding of how the head, shoulder girdle, and hips are positionally related to one another when standing under the influence of gravity. Then, the body is addressed within the context of this new vision.

Sessions 4–7: Four through seven are referred to as "core" sessions and examine terrain found between the bottom of the pelvis and top of the head. The idea of core also includes the deep tissue of the legs for its role in support.

Session four begins this journey; its territory extends from the inside arch of the foot and up the leg, to the bottom of the pelvis. The fifth session is concerned with balancing surface and deep abdominal muscles to the curve of the back. Number six seeks to enlist more support and momentum from the legs, pelvis, and lower back, while the seventh session turns its sole attention to the neck and head.

Session 8–10: "Integration" is emphasized throughout the remaining three sessions, as eight, nine, and ten provide an opportunity for the practitioner to blend previously established advancements, and ones yet to be made, into the body in a way that encourages smooth movement and natural coordination.

During sessions eight and nine, the practitioner is free to decide how best to achieve this integration, as the protocol is unique for each individual. The tenth and final session is also one of integration, but more importantly, serves to inspire a sense of order and balance. Once completed, the wisdom of the Rolfing Ten Series will drive and support the body with health for years to come.

Does Rolfing relieve stress?

When people come to Rolfers, they frequently complain about their high level of stress and how it affects their everyday life. They are seeking some means of reducing their stress. Often, they have explored allopathic means such as muscle relaxants, painkillers, liniments, balms, and other topical treatments. When these treatments fail to achieve a satisfactory level of improvement, those still suffering seek other forms of relief such as exercise, meditation, yoga, visualization, and chanting.

They may also seek a myofascial (neuromuscular) solution and start receiving regular massages or some other similar soft tissue therapy. In many cases, these therapies are good at providing transitory relief of the physical causes of chronic stress. Those seeking a more permanent solution to the problem are more likely to have success with Rolfing.

What most potential clients fail to understand is that Rolfing is not a method which focuses on stress reduction. What the Rolfing method does is create a higher level of integration in the body, balancing and educating the body and the psyche. As the body approaches balance, it is more comfortable in the gravitational field. As the body becomes more comfortable, physical and emotional stress diminish. This chain of events is a more typical sequence of events as a body changes during the Rolfing process. Ultimately, however, the results as experienced by the client are more important than the process. All clients experience benefits from Rolfing, an important one for most is that they are less stressed and more at ease in their bodies.

What about the emotional and psychological effects of Rolfing?

It is impossible to touch the physical body without touching the emotional body. All individuals develop compensatory patterns, ways of holding and defending against a variety of physical and emotional insults to form.

During the Rolfing process, we offer options and new modes of physical expression. Resultant emotional changes are quite common. There is a well-documented "cellular memory," a memory of experience stored in the tissue at a cellular level. Touching the body will frequently help the client access these physical memories encoded in the fascial (or connective tissue) matrix. Anecdotal reports of major cathartic releases during Rolfing sessions are very common and often act as an impediment to some individuals entering into the Rolfing process.

For most Rolfers, this catharsis is not something consciously desired nor intended. Rather, the person is approached with reverence and compassion. When emotionally charged areas of the body have been identified by the client, or intuited by the practitioner, they are normally accessed slowly and with constant communication between the Rolfer and the client.

Sometimes, however, repressed memories or experiences will arise for which the client and the Rolfer may not have any advanced warning. In this situation, the goal of the Rolfer is to provide a safe container for the release and take the requisite time to integrate the experience into the physical and emotional body in a way that promotes maximum resolution and minimal trauma to the system.

Rolfers are trained to ease a client through such an experience but not always trained as therapists. The nature and quality of accessing and resolution of emotionally charged material may be the most profound portion of a client's Rolfing experience. However, the client should not enter the Rolfing process anticipating such a major release but should remember that a Rolfer's actual expertise is integrating and balancing connective tissue. The emotional component, as attractive or dreaded as it may be, remains an ancillary aspect of the Rolfing process and not its primary intention.

Where can I find a Rolfer in my area?

Call 800-530-8875 to receive a list in the mail, or go to Find a Rolfer at http://www.rolf.org/find/locate.asp.

What are some books I can read to learn about Rolfing?

Selected annotated bibliography on Rolfing:

Anson, Briah. Rolfing: *Stories of Personal Empowerment* (Berkeley, CA: North Atlantic Press, 1998). Inspiring and insightful accounts of the Rolfing experience as reported by numerous former Rolfing clients.

Bond, Mary. *Balancing Your Body: A Self-Help Approach to Rolfing to Balancing the Body* (Rochester, VT: Healing Arts Press, 1993).

Cottingham, John T. *Healing Through Touch* (Boulder, CO, The Rolf Institute, 1985). Exploration of methods of healing going back 5,000 years.

Fahey, Brian W., PhD. *The Power of Balance: A Rolfing View of Health* (Portland, OR: Metamorphous Press, 1995). A very accessible summary of the basic Rolfing theory and movement.

Feitus, Rosemary, ed. *Remembering Ida Rolf* (Berkeley, CA, North Atlantic Books, 1996). Collection of stories from people who knew Dr. Rolf.

Maitland, Jeffrey, PhD. *Spacious Body: Explorations in Somatic Ontology* (Berkeley, CA: North Atlantic Books, 1995). Philosophical consideration of embodiment, Buddhism, and the Rolfing experience.

Ida Rolf Talks about Rolfing and Physical Reality. Rosemary Feitis, ed. Reprinted ed. (Boulder, CO, The Rolf Institute, 1978). A collection of quotes on bodywork and a variety of topics of interest to Dr. Rolf.

Rolf, Ida. *Rolfing: Reestablishing the Natural Alignment and Structural Integration of the Human Body for Vitality and Well-being.* Reprinted Ed. (Rochester, VT: Healing Arts Press, 1989). The bible of Rolfing completed late in Dr. Rolf's long career.

Schultz, R. Louis, PhD. *Out in the Open: The Complete Male Pelvis* (Berkeley, CA: North Atlantic Books, 1999). A unique look at the structural and psychological issues involved in the male pelvis from a Rolfing perspective.

What is Rolf Movement®?

Toward the end of her life, Dr. Rolf felt that a movement training component would be a valuable adjunct to her structural Ten Series. In her lifetime, Dr. Rolf collaborated with first Dorothy Nolte and then Judith Aston to develop this aspect of Rolfing. Since Dr. Rolf's death in 1979, others, including Jane Harrington, Heather Starsong, Gael Ohlgren, and Vivian Jaye have elevated this less familiar style of Rolfing to a level of high art with tremendous transformative value. Currently, approximately 25% of all Rolfers have been certified in Rolf Movement and employ their training as a way of enriching their work. The purpose of Rolfing Movement is to work with the client to help her identify movement patterns that promote strain and asymmetry in her system. Once the patterns are identified, the Rolf Movement practitioner does not seek to change those patterns, which have served the client well, but rather to offer more economical solutions which promote greater balance and efficiency in the gravitational field.

Like the structural Ten Series, Rolfing Movement is taught as a sequence of sessions devoted to specific structural and movement themes. In a classic movement series, the first session is devoted to exploring breathing patterns and using the breath to promote ease and release holdings in the ribs, lungs, and respiratory diaphragm. Subsequent sessions address movement patterns in the foot, ankle, and knee joints, the hip joint, the arms, and head and neck. These sessions are normally repeated to access deeper holding patterns and achieve higher levels of order just as structural Rolfers return to the extremities and upper and lower girdles (the shoulder and pelvis) in the latter sessions to more fully integrate structure and function. Rolfing movement can be explored by clients who have completed a structural series and can serve equally well as an autonomous tool for achieving higher levels of self-awareness and coherence.

Is Rolfing helpful to musicians?

Musicians often face a number of unique physical challenges brought on by years of diligent practice and performing. Sometimes, even the best musicians develop habits which lead to chronic pain, mostly in their hands and wrists, forearms, neck and shoulders and lower back. Rolfing and Rolfing movement can help in a number of ways. Physical adaptations to a musician's chosen instrument, including the voice, which often lead to discomfort and imbalance, are normalized in a traditional Rolfing Ten Series. The Rolfing Ten Series can be specifically adapted to address such patterns as carpal tunnel, chronic muscle imbalances, and long-term effects of odd stances and body position caused by the exigencies of playing a given instrument. Musicians who have experienced the basic series have consistently noticed profound changes in their level of physical comfort, energy level, and internal awareness. This increased freedom of movement noticeably impacts the performer's pleasure in performing and often leads to greater creative abilities. Another tool many Rolfers employ is movement work. Those trained in this modality observe you in the act of playing and call your attention to subtle ways you hold or translate force through your body which reinforce strain patterns that interfere with your performance. The movement teacher's intention is not to change how you play or to inhibit your unique approach to the instrument. Rather, they help you find creative alternatives to stressful patterns in your current mode of performance.

Is Rolfing suitable for children?

A common misunderstanding about Rolfing is that its main value is in correcting long-standing structural patterns. Rolfing can also serve as a prophylactic measure to reverse potentially problematic patterns in the young. One of the things children learn from watching us is how we carry ourselves and they will naturally imitate their parent's language, movement, and other modes of expression. These patterns can be seen in family photos and are as much a part of a child's makeup as his hair color, height, and predisposition to certain hereditary illnesses. Rolfing can begin to correct patterns, such as hip imbalances which may limit the child's development and mobility.

Also, when children are injured from falls or minor accidents, they may seem to be fine on the outside since the cut or bruise healed. However, as Dr. Rolf pointed out, they are not really the same. Minor changes have taken place in the connective tissue, in their joints, and in the muscles that were injured. Small tears or pulls cause the tissue to thicken. Soon, muscles begin to adhere to each other and are less able to function as discrete entities. These changes may express themselves as a slight limp, lower energy, a decrease in range of motion or strength. Early intervention by a Rolfer aware of the unique needs of children can make a profound difference in a child's awareness, comfort level, and self-esteem. The importance of receiving loving supportive touch in and of itself is of immeasurable value to a developing child. Rolfing, however, can accomplish so much more, creating palpable change in the child's connective tissue matrix. We have also found that Rolfing adolescents during and after puberty, a time of great insecurity and emotional turmoil for most of us, besides the obvious structural benefits, frequently has a profound effect on the developing child's awareness and comfort in his or her rapidly changing body and mind.

Chapter 65

Other Manipulative and Body-Based Therapies

Chapter Contents

Section 65.1—Applied Kinesiology.. 448

Section 65.2—Bowcn Technique... 449

Section 65.3—Trager Approach.. 450

447

Section 65.1

Applied Kinesiology

From "Applied Kinesiology," © 2009 Natural Medicines Comprehensive Database (www.naturaldatabase.com). Reprinted with permission.

What other names is the therapy known by?

AK, applied kinesiology, educational kinesiology, health kinesiology, kinesiology muscle test

What is it?

Kinesiology is an alternative medicine system used to diagnose and treat medical conditions.

Is it effective?

Natural Medicines Comprehensive Database rates effectiveness based on scientific evidence according to the following scale: effective, likely effective, possibly effective, possibly ineffective, likely ineffective, and insufficient evidence to rate.

The effectiveness ratings for kinesiology are as follows:

- Likely ineffective for:

  - disease diagnosis.

- Insufficient evidence to rate effectiveness for:

  - learning disabilities;

  - mastalgia (breast pain).

How does it work?

Kinesiology is an alternative medicine system used to diagnose and treat conditions based on the belief that build up of toxins around muscles results in weakness in that area. By identifying muscle weakness, the practitioner is able to identify areas of disease. However, there is no reliable scientific evidence that kinesiology is an accurate indicator of medical conditions or disease.

Are there safety concerns?

There are no known safety concerns; however, this technique should not be relied upon to identify or diagnose medical conditions in place of modern diagnostic techniques.

Are there any interactions with medications?

It is not known if kinesiology interacts with any medicines. Before using kinesiology, talk with your healthcare professional if you take any medications.

Section 65.2

Bowen Technique

What other names is the therapy known by?

Bowen manipulative therapy, Bowen therapist, Bowen therapy, BT

What is it?

The Bowen technique is a manipulative technique.

Is it effective?

Natural Medicines Comprehensive Database rates effectiveness based on scientific evidence according to the following scale: effective, likely effective, possibly effective, possibly ineffective, likely ineffective, and insufficient evidence to rate.

The effectiveness ratings for the Bowen technique are as follows:

- Insufficient evidence to rate effectiveness for:

    - pain, fatigue, relaxation, frozen shoulder, and other conditions.

How does it work?

The Bowen technique is a manipulative therapy that uses light pressure applied to specific locations throughout the body. Practitioners of the Bowen technique believe that applying pressure in these areas can stimulate the body's own healing ability. However, there is no reliable scientific support for this belief.

Are there safety concerns?

There is not enough reliable information available to know if the Bowen technique is safe or if there are any safety concerns.

Are there any interactions with medications?

It is not known if the Bowen technique interacts with any medicines.

Before using the Bowen technique, talk with your healthcare professional if you take any medications.

Section 65.3

Trager Approach

"What Is the Trager Approach?" © 2005 Trager International (www.trager.com). Reprinted with permission. Reviewed by David A. Cooke, MD, FACP, December 25, 2009.

The Trager Approach is the innovative approach to movement education, created and developed over a period of 65 years by Milton Trager, MD.

There are two aspects of the Trager Approach; one in which you, the client, are passive and the other in which you are active. The passive aspect is usually referred to as the table work, and the active aspect is called Mentastics.

Utilizing gentle, non-intrusive, natural movements, the Trager Approach helps release deep-seated physical and mental patterns and facilitates deep relaxation, increased physical mobility, and mental clarity. These patterns may have developed in response to accidents, illnesses, or any kind of physical or emotional trauma, including the stress of everyday life.

A session usually lasts from 60 to 90 minutes. No oils or lotions are used and the client is dressed for their comfort, with a minimum of swimwear or briefs, and are additionally draped appropriately.

During the table work session the client is passive and lying on a comfortably padded table. The practitioner moves the client in ways they naturally move, and with a quality of touch and movement such that the recipient experiences the feeling of moving that effortlessly and freely on his/her own.

The movements are never forced so that there is no induced pain or discomfort to the client.

This quality of effortless movement is maintained and reinforced by Mentastics. These are simple, active, self-induced movements which you, the client, can do on your own, during your daily activities. They have the same intent as the table work in terms of releasing deep-seated patterns.

For many people, Mentastics becomes a part of their life in taking care of themselves, and relieving themselves of stress and tension.

Because many of the effects of the Trager Approach are cumulative, clients most often appreciate and will benefit most from a series of sessions.

One of the most potent aspects of the Trager Approach is the ability to recall the feeling of deep relaxation, and how it feels to move freely and easily.

Who does it?

Certified Practitioners of the Trager Approach have successfully completed the certification program provided by Trager International, and have maintained continuing education, and other requirements of Trager International. Trager International maintains a database of Certified Practitioners worldwide. If you have any question about someone's credentials, you are advised to contact Trager International for verification.

Part Seven

Energy-Based Therapies

Chapter 66

Energy Medicine: An Overview

Energy medicine is a domain in CAM that deals with energy fields of two types:

- Veritable, which can be measured
- Putative, which have yet to be measured

The veritable energies employ mechanical vibrations (such as sound) and electromagnetic forces, including visible light, magnetism, monochromatic radiation (such as laser beams), and rays from other parts of the electromagnetic spectrum. They involve the use of specific, measurable wavelengths and frequencies to treat patients.

In contrast, putative energy fields (also called biofields) have defied measurement to date by reproducible methods. Therapies involving putative energy fields are based on the concept that human beings are infused with a subtle form of energy. This vital energy or life force is known under different names in different cultures, such as qi in traditional Chinese medicine (TCM), ki in the Japanese Kampo system, doshas in Ayurvedic medicine, and elsewhere as prana, etheric energy, fohat, orgone, odic force, mana, and homeopathic resonance. Vital energy is believed to flow throughout the material human body, but it has not been unequivocally measured by means of conventional instrumentation. Nonetheless, therapists claim that they can work

Excerpted from text by the National Center for Complementary and Alternative Medicine (NCCAM, nccam.nih.gov), part of the National Institutes of Health, March 2007.

with this subtle energy, see it with their own eyes, and use it to effect changes in the physical body and influence health.

Practitioners of energy medicine believe that illness results from disturbances of these subtle energies (the biofield). For example, more than 2,000 years ago, Asian practitioners postulated that the flow and balance of life energies are necessary for maintaining health and described tools to restore them. Herbal medicine, acupuncture, acupressure, moxibustion, and cupping, for example, are all believed to act by correcting imbalances in the internal biofield, such as by restoring the flow of qi through meridians to reinstate health. Some therapists are believed to emit or transmit the vital energy (external qi) to a recipient to restore health.

Examples of practices involving putative energy fields include the following:

- Reiki and Johrei, both of Japanese origin

- Qi gong, a Chinese practice

- Healing touch, in which the therapist is purported to identify imbalances and correct a client's energy by passing his or her hands over the patient

- Intercessory prayer, in which a person intercedes through prayer on behalf of another

In the aggregate, these approaches are among the most controversial of CAM practices because neither the external energy fields nor their therapeutic effects have been demonstrated convincingly by any biophysical means. Yet, energy medicine is gaining popularity in the American marketplace and has become a subject of investigations at some academic medical centers. A recent National Center for Health Statistics survey indicated that approximately 1 percent of the participants had used Reiki, 0.5 percent had used qi gong, and 4.6 percent had used some kind of healing ritual.

Scope of the Research

Veritable Energy Medicine

There are many well-established uses for the application of measurable energy fields to diagnose or treat diseases: electromagnetic fields in magnetic resonance imaging, cardiac pacemakers, radiation therapy, ultraviolet light for psoriasis, laser keratoplasty, and more. There are many other claimed uses as well. The ability to deliver quantifiable amounts of energies across the electromagnetic spectrum is an advantage to studies of their mechanisms and clinical effects. For example, both static and pulsating electromagnetic therapies have been employed.

Magnetic therapy: Static magnets have been used for centuries in efforts to relieve pain or to obtain other alleged benefits (e.g., increased energy). Numerous anecdotal reports have indicated that individuals have experienced significant, and at times dramatic, relief of pain after the application of static magnets over a painful area. Although the literature on the biological effects of magnetic fields is growing, there is a paucity of data from well-structured, clinically sound studies. However, there is growing evidence that magnetic fields can influence physiological processes. It has recently been shown that static magnetic fields affect the microvasculature of skeletal muscle. Microvessels that are initially dilated respond to a magnetic field by constricting, and microvessels that are initially constricted respond by dilating. These results suggest that static magnetic fields may have a beneficial role in treating edema or ischemic conditions, but there is no proof that they do.

Pulsating electromagnetic therapy has been in use for the past 40 years. A well-recognized and standard use is to enhance the healing of nonunion fractures. It also has been claimed that this therapy is effective in treating osteoarthritis, migraine headaches, multiple sclerosis, and sleep disorders. Some animal and cell culture studies have been conducted to elucidate the basic mechanism of the pulsating electromagnetic therapy effect, such as cell proliferation and cell-surface binding for growth factors. However, detailed data on the mechanisms of action are still lacking.

Millimeter wave therapy: Low-power millimeter wave (MW) irradiation elicits biological effects, and clinicians in Russia and other parts of Eastern Europe have used it in past decades to treat a variety of conditions, ranging from skin diseases and wound healing to various types of cancer, gastrointestinal and cardiovascular diseases, and psychiatric illnesses. In spite of an increasing number of in vivo and in vitro studies, the nature of MW action is not well understood. It has been shown, for example, that MW irradiation can augment T-cell mediated immunity in vitro. However, the mechanisms by which MW irradiation enhances T-cell functions are not known. Some studies indicate that pretreating mice with naloxone may block the hypoalgesic and antipruritic effects of MW irradiation, suggesting that endogenous opioids are involved in MW therapy-induced hypoalgesia. Theoretical and experimental data show that nearly all the MW energy is absorbed in the superficial layers of skin, but it is not clear how the energy absorbed by keratinocytes, the main constituents of epidermis, is transmitted to elicit the therapeutic effect. It is also unclear whether MW yields clinical effects beyond a placebo response.

Sound energy therapy: Sound energy therapy, sometimes referred to as vibrational or frequency therapy, includes music therapy as well as wind chime and tuning fork therapy. The presumptive basis of its effect is that specific sound frequencies resonate with specific organs of the body to heal and support the body. Music therapy has been the most studied among these interventions, with studies dating back to the 1920s, when it was reported that music affected blood pressure. Other studies have suggested that music can help reduce pain and anxiety. Music and imagery, alone and in combination, have been used to entrain mood states, reduce acute or chronic pain, and alter certain biochemicals, such as plasma beta-endorphin levels. These uses of energy fields truly overlap with the domain of mind-body medicine.

Light therapy: Light therapy is the use of natural or artificial light to treat various ailments, but unproven uses of light extend to lasers, colors, and monochromatic lights. High-intensity light therapy has been documented to be useful for seasonal affective disorder, with less evidence for its usefulness in the treatment of more general forms of depression and sleep disorders. Hormonal changes have been detected after treatment. Although low-level laser therapy is claimed to be useful for relieving pain, reducing inflammation, and helping to heal wounds, strong scientific proof of these effects is still needed.

Energy Medicine Involving Putative Energy Fields

The concept that sickness and disease arise from imbalances in the vital energy field of the body has led to many forms of therapy. In TCM, a series of approaches are taken to rectify the flow of qi, such as herbal medicine, acupuncture (and its various versions), qi gong, diet, and behavior changes.

Acupuncture: Of these approaches, acupuncture is the most prominent therapy to promote qi flow along the meridians. Acupuncture has been extensively studied and has been shown to be effective in treating some conditions, particularly certain forms of pain. However, its mechanism of action remains to be elucidated. The main threads of research on acupuncture have shown regional effects on neurotransmitter expression, but have not validated the existence of an "energy" per se.

Qi gong: Qi gong, another energy modality that purportedly can restore health, is practiced widely in the clinics and hospitals of China.

Most of the reports were published as abstracts in Chinese, which makes accessing the information difficult. But Sancier has collected more than 2,000 records in his qi gong database which indicates that qi gong has extensive health benefits on conditions ranging from blood pressure to asthma. The reported studies, however, are largely anecdotal case series and not randomized controlled trials. Few studies have been conducted outside China and reported in peer-reviewed journals in English. There have been no large clinical trials.

Whole medical systems and energy medicine: Although modalities such as acupuncture and qi gong have been studied separately, TCM uses combinations of treatments (e.g., herbs, acupuncture, and qi gong) in practice. Similarly, Ayurvedic medicine uses combinations of herbal medicine, yoga, meditation, and other approaches to restore vital energy, particularly at the chakra energy centers.

Homeopathy: One Western approach with implications for energy medicine is homeopathy. Homeopaths believe that their remedies mobilize the body's vital force to orchestrate coordinated healing responses throughout the organism. The body translates the information on the vital force into local physical changes that lead to recovery from acute and chronic diseases. Homeopaths use their assessment of the deficits in vital force to guide dose (potency) selection and treatment pace, and to judge the likely clinical course and prognosis. Homeopathic medicine is based on the principle of similars, and remedies are often prescribed in high dilutions. In most cases, the dilution may not contain any molecules of the original agents at all. As a consequence, homeopathic remedies, at least when applied in high dilutions, cannot act by pharmacological means. Theories for a potential mechanism of action invoke the homeopathic solution, therefore, postulating that information is stored in the dilution process by physical means. Other than a study reported by the Benveniste laboratory and other smaller studies, this hypothesis has not been supported by scientific research. There have been numerous clinical studies of homeopathic approaches, but systematic reviews point out the overall poor quality and inconsistency of these studies.

Therapeutic touch and related practices: Numerous other practices have evolved over the years to promote or maintain the balance of vital energy fields in the body. Examples of these modalities include Therapeutic Touch, healing touch, Reiki, Johrei, vortex healing, and polarity therapy. All these modalities involve movement of the practitioner's hands over the patient's body to become attuned to the condition of the patient, with the idea that by so doing, the practitioner is able to strengthen and reorient the patient's energies.

459

Many small studies of Therapeutic Touch have suggested its effectiveness in a wide variety of conditions, including wound healing, osteoarthritis, migraine headaches, and anxiety in burn patients. In a recent meta-analysis of 11 controlled Therapeutic Touch studies, 7 controlled studies had positive outcomes, and 3 showed no effect; in one study, the control group healed faster than the Therapeutic Touch group. Similarly, Reiki and Johrei practitioners claim that the therapies boost the body's immune system, enhance the body's ability to heal itself, and are beneficial for a wide range of problems, such as stress-related conditions, allergies, heart conditions, high blood pressure, and chronic pain. However, there has been little rigorous scientific research. Overall, these therapies have impressive anecdotal evidence, but none has been proven scientifically to be effective.

Distant healing: Proponents of energy field therapies also claim that some of these therapies can act across long distances. For example, the long-distance effects of external qi gong have been studied in China and summarized in the book *Scientific Qigong Exploration,* which has been translated into English. The studies reported various healing cases and described the nature of qi as bidirectional, multifunctional, adaptable to targets, and capable of effects over long distances. But none of these claims has been independently verified. Another form of distant healing is intercessory prayer, in which a person prays for the healing of another person who is a great distance away, with or without that person's knowledge. Review of eight nonrandomized and nine randomized clinical trials published between 2000 and 2002 showed that the majority of the more rigorous trials do not support the hypothesis that distant intercessory prayer has specific therapeutic effects.

Physical properties of putative energy fields: There has always been an interest in detecting and describing the physical properties of putative energy fields. Kirlian photography, aura imaging, and gas discharge visualization are approaches for which dramatic and unique differences before and after therapeutic energy attunements or treatments have been claimed. However, it is not clear what is being detected or photographed. Early results demonstrated that gamma radiation levels markedly decreased during therapy sessions in 100 percent of subjects and at every body site tested, regardless of which therapist performed the treatment. Recently replicated studies identified statistically significant decreases in gamma rays emitted from patients during alternative healing sessions with trained practitioners.

It has been hypothesized that the body's primary gamma emitter, potassium-40 (K40), represents a "self-regulation" of energy within the body and the surrounding electromagnetic field. The body's energy adjustment may result, in part, from the increased electromagnetic fields surrounding the hands of the healers. Furthermore, an extremely sensitive magnetometer called a superconducting quantum interference device (SQUID) has been claimed to measure large frequency-pulsing biomagnetic fields emanating from the hands of Therapeutic Touch practitioners during therapy. In one study, a simple magnetometer measured and quantified similar frequency-pulsing biomagnetic fields from the hands of meditators and practitioners of yoga and qi gong. These fields were 1,000 times greater than the strongest human biomagnetic field and were in the same frequency range as those being tested in medical research laboratories for use in speeding the healing process of certain biological tissues. This range is low energy and extremely low frequency, spanning from 2 Hz to 50 Hz. However, there are considerable technical problems in such research. For example, SQUID measurement must be conducted under a special shielded environment, and the connection between electromagnetic field increases and observed healing benefits reported in the current literature is missing.

Other studies of putative energies suggested that energy fields from one person can overlap and interact with energy fields of other people. For example, when individuals touch, one person's electrocardiographic signal is registered in the other person's electroencephalogram (EEG) and elsewhere on the other person's body. In addition, one individual's cardiac signal can be registered in another's EEG recording when two people sit quietly opposite one another.

Additional theories: Thus far, electromagnetic energy has been demonstrated and postulated to be the energy between bioenergy healers and patients. However, the exact nature of this energy is not clear. Among the range of ideas emerging in this field is the theory of a Russian researcher who recently hypothesized that "torsion fields" exist and that they can be propagated through space at no less than 109 times the speed of light in vacuum; that they convey information without transmitting energy; and that they are not required to obey the superposition principle.

There are other extraordinary claims and observations recorded in the literature. For example, one report claimed that accomplished meditators were able to imprint their intentions on electrical devices (IIED), which when placed in a room for 3 months, would elicit these intentions, such as changes in pH and temperature, in the room even when the IIED was removed from the room. Another claim is that water will crystallize into different forms and appearances under the influence of written intentions or types of music.

For research, questions remain about which of the above theories and approaches can be and should be addressed using existing technologies, and how.

Chapter 67

Magnet Therapy

Magnets have been used for health purposes for centuries. Static, or permanent, magnets are widely marketed for pain control and are considered part of complementary and alternative medicine (CAM).

About Magnets

A magnet produces a measurable force called a magnetic field. Static magnets have magnetic fields that do not change (unlike another type called electromagnets, which generate magnetic fields only when electrical current flows through them). Magnets are usually made from metals (such as iron) or alloys (mixtures of metals, or of a metal and a nonmetal).

Magnets come in different strengths, often measured in units called gauss (G) or, alternatively, units called tesla (1 tesla = 10,000 G). Magnets marketed for pain usually claim strengths of 300 to 5,000 G—many times stronger than the Earth's magnetic field (about 0.5 G) and much weaker than the magnets used for MRI [magnetic resonance imaging] machines (approximately 15,000 G or higher).

Various products with magnets in them are marketed for health purposes, including shoe insoles, bracelets and other jewelry, mattress pads, bandages, headbands, and belts. These products are often placed in contact with painful areas of the body with the goal of providing relief.

From "Magnets for Pain," by the National Center for Complementary and Alternative Medicine (NCCAM, nccam.nih.gov), part of the National Institutes of Health, March 2009.

History of Magnets for Health Uses

Magnets have been used for many centuries for a variety of health purposes. By various accounts, magnets were discovered when people first noticed the presence of naturally magnetized stones, also called lodestones. By the third century AD [Anno Domini], Greek physicians were using magnetic rings to treat arthritis and magnetized pills made of amber to stop bleeding. In the Middle Ages, doctors used magnets to treat gout, arthritis, poisoning, and baldness; to clean wounds; and to retrieve arrowheads and other iron-containing objects from the body.

In the United States, magnetic devices (such as hairbrushes and insoles), magnetic ointments, and clothes with magnets attached came into wide use after the Civil War, especially in some rural areas where few doctors were available. Healers claimed that magnetic fields existed in the blood, and that people became ill when their magnetic fields were depleted. Thus, healers marketed magnets as a means of replenishing these magnetic fields. Magnets were promoted as cures for a wide range of health conditions, including paralysis, headache, backache, sleeplessness, upset stomach, and liver and kidney problems.

The use of magnets to treat medical problems remained popular well into the 20th century. Today, magnets are used for many different types of pain, including foot pain and back pain from conditions such as arthritis and fibromyalgia.

What the Science Says

What Studies Have Shown

Overall, the scientific evidence does not support the use of magnets for pain relief. Preliminary studies looking at different types of pain— such as knee, hip, wrist, foot, back, and pelvic pain—have had mixed results. Some of these studies, including a recent NIH [National Institutes of Health]-sponsored clinical trial that looked at back pain in a small group of people, have suggested a benefit from using magnets. The majority of rigorous trials, however, have found no effect on pain.

Some research results suggest that effects may depend on the type of pain treated. For example, results from a few studies suggest that magnets might provide some relief specifically from osteoarthritis pain. Effects may also depend on the type and strength of the magnets used, the frequency of use, and the length of time the magnet was applied during the study.

Many studies were not high-quality because they included a small number of participants, were too short, and/or were poorly designed.

More rigorous research is needed before reaching any firm conclusions about the effectiveness of magnets for pain.

Challenges Facing Researchers

Researchers face challenges when studying magnets in clinical trials:

- Something other than the magnet may relieve a study participant's pain. For example, relief could come from a placebo effect or from a warm bandage or cushioned insole that holds the magnet in place.

- It can be difficult to design a sham magnet that participants cannot distinguish from an active magnet. If participants know whether they are using an active magnet, study findings may be less reliable.

- It is possible that the magnetic properties of low-strength magnets, which are sometimes used as shams, can actually have a therapeutic effect.

- Opinions differ about how to administer magnet therapy, including what strength magnet to use, where to place the magnets on the body, and how long to use them. These factors have not been fully studied in humans. Clinical trials that look at these factors are needed.

How Magnets Might Work

No scientific theory or manufacturer claim about how magnets might work has been conclusively proven. Although some preliminary research has been conducted in animals and in small clinical trials, the mechanisms by which magnets might affect the human body are not yet known.

Scientific researchers and magnet manufacturers have proposed that magnets might work by the following methods:

- Changing how nerve cells function and blocking pain signals to the brain

- Restoring the balance between cell death and growth

- Increasing the flow of blood and the delivery of oxygen and nutrients to tissues

- Increasing the temperature of the area of the body being treated

Findings from preliminary studies in healthy people—including one study funded by NIH—suggest that magnets may not affect blood flow or nerve function.

Side Effects and Risks

Magnets may not be safe for some people to use, including those who meet the following conditions:

- Use a medical device such as a pacemaker, defibrillator, or insulin pump, because magnets may interfere with the functioning of the medical device

- Have a wound that has not healed

Otherwise, magnets are generally considered safe when applied to the skin. Reports of side effects or complications have been rare.

It is important not to use magnets in place of proven treatments for serious medical conditions. Tell your health care providers about any complementary and alternative practices you use. Give them a full picture of what you do to manage your health. This will help ensure coordinated and safe care.

Chapter 68

Polarity Therapy

What Is Polarity Therapy?

Energy fields and currents exist everywhere in nature. Polarity Therapy asserts that the flow and balance of energy in the human body is the foundation of good health.

In the Polarity model, health is experienced when:

1. energy systems function in their natural state; and

2. energy flows smoothly without significant blockage or fixation.

When energy is unbalanced, blocked or fixed due to stress or other factors, pain and disease arise.

Blockages generally manifest in sequence from the subtle to the dense levels of the field. Polarity Therapy seeks to find the blockages and release energy to normal flow patterns, and to maintain the Energy Field in an open, flexible condition.

A blend of modern science and complementary medicine, Polarity Therapy is a comprehensive health system involving energy-based bodywork, diet, exercise, and self-awareness. Scientifically, it works with the Human Energy Field, electromagnetic patterns expressed in mental, emotional, and physical experience. In Polarity Therapy, health is viewed as a reflection of the condition of the energy field, and therapeutic methods are designed to balance the field for health benefit. There are three types of energy fields in the human body: long line currents that run north to south on the body; transverse currents that run east-west in the body; and spiral currents that start at the navel and expand outward.

In the healing arts, Polarity Therapy is special in its comprehensive exploration of the different dimensions of the human condition (physical, mental, and emotional). Polarity Therapy seeks to bridge the full spectrum of body, mind, and spirit: The body is designed by nature to heal itself. Polarity Therapy assists in this natural occurrence. Applying the Polarity Therapy system can take diverse forms, always based on the underlying intention to support the client's inherent self-healing intelligence as expressed in its energetic patterns.

Polarity Therapy was developed by Dr. Randolph Stone, DO, DC, ND (1890–1981), who conducted a thorough investigation of energy in the healing arts over the course of his 60-year medical career. Drawing on information from a wide range of sources, he found that the Human Energy Field is affected by touch, diet, movement, sound, attitudes, relationships, life experience, trauma, and environmental factors. Since Polarity Therapy lends an energy-based perspective to all these subjects, the scope of Polarity practice is often very broad, with implications for health professionals in many therapeutic disciplines.

As a result, Polarity supports strong connections to many other healing and holistic health systems. For example, basic characteristics of the Human Energy Field are described in many sources, both ancient and modern. From the Ayurvedic tradition, Polarity integrates the "Three Principles and Five Chakras" and has been called the modern manifestation of ancient Hermetic Philosophy. Polarity is experienced as the universal pulsation of expansion/contraction or repulsion/attraction known as Yang and Yin in Oriental therapies. Energy moves out from a central source—which is repulsion, then back to the source—which is attraction. Polarity practitioners use this natural phenomenon as a way of tracking energy flow.

What Can I Expect in a Typical Polarity Therapy Session?

In a typical session, the practitioner assesses energetic attributes using palpation, observation, and interview methods. Sessions usually take 60–90 minutes, do not require disrobing, and involve soft touch, some rocking, as well as point specific touch.

Energetic Touch is the work Polarity practitioners perform with clients—verbal interaction is energetic communication which has to do with reading the energy in people's words and staying neutral vs. engaging in the emotions of the patient and verbal interaction. Contact may be light, medium, or firm. In the session, the practitioner supports the client in increasing self-awareness of subtle energetic sensations, which are often experienced as tingling, warmth, expansion, or wavelike movement. The results of Polarity Therapy sessions vary, and may include profound relaxation, an understanding of energetic patterns and their implications, and relief from numerous specific problematic situations such as hypertension, anxiety attacks, and breathing disorders.

Chapter 69

Reiki

Reiki is a healing practice that originated in Japan. Reiki practitioners place their hands lightly on or just above the person receiving treatment, with the goal of facilitating the person's own healing response. In the United States, Reiki is part of complementary and alternative medicine (CAM).

History

The word "Reiki" is derived from two Japanese words: rei, or universal, and ki, or life energy. Current Reiki practice can be traced to the spiritual teachings of Mikao Usui in Japan during the early 20th century. Usui's teachings included meditative techniques and healing practices. One of Usui's students, Chujiro Hayashi, further developed the healing practices, placing less emphasis on the meditative techniques. An American named Hawayo Takata learned Reiki from Hayashi in Japan and introduced it to Western cultures in the late 1930s.

The type of Reiki practiced and taught by Hayashi and Takata may be considered traditional Reiki. Numerous variations (or schools) of Reiki have since been developed and are currently practiced.

From "Reiki: An Introduction," by the National Center for Complementary and Alternative Medicine (NCCAM, nccam.nih.gov), part of the National Institutes of Health, July 2009.

Practice

Reiki is based on the idea that there is a universal (or source) energy that supports the body's innate healing abilities. Practitioners seek to access this energy, allowing it to flow to the body and facilitate healing.

Although generally practiced as a form of self-care, Reiki can be received from someone else and may be offered in a variety of health care settings, including medical offices, hospitals, and clinics. It can be practiced on its own or along with other CAM therapies or conventional medical treatments.

In a Reiki session, the client lies down or sits comfortably, fully clothed. The practitioner's hands are placed lightly on or just above the client's body, palms down, using a series of 12 to 15 different hand positions. Each position is held for about 2 to 5 minutes, or until the practitioner feels that the flow of energy—experienced as sensations such as heat or tingling in the hands—has slowed or stopped. The number of sessions depends on the health needs of the client. Typically, the practitioner delivers at least four sessions of 30 to 90 minutes each. The duration of Reiki sessions may be shorter in certain health care settings (for example, during surgery).

Practitioners with appropriate training may perform Reiki from a distance, that is, on clients who are not physically present in the office or clinic.

Uses

According to the 2007 National Health Interview Survey, which included a comprehensive survey of CAM use by Americans, more than 1.2 million adults had used an energy healing therapy, such as Reiki, in the previous year. The survey also found that approximately 161,000 children had used an energy healing therapy in the previous year.

People use Reiki for relaxation, stress reduction, and symptom relief, in efforts to improve overall health and well-being. Reiki has been used by people with anxiety, chronic pain, HIV/AIDS [human immunodeficiency virus/acquired immunodeficiency syndrome], and other health conditions, as well as by people recovering from surgery or experiencing side effects from cancer treatments. Reiki has also been given to people who are dying (and to their families and caregivers) to help impart a sense of peace.

Effects and Safety

Clients may experience a deep state of relaxation during a Reiki session. They might also feel warm, tingly, sleepy, or refreshed.

Reiki appears to be generally safe, and no serious side effects have been reported.

Training, Licensing, and Certification

No special background or credentials are needed to receive training. However, Reiki must be learned from an experienced teacher or a Master; it cannot be self-taught. The specific techniques taught can vary greatly.

Training in traditional Reiki has three degrees (levels), each focusing on a different aspect of practice. Each degree includes one or more initiations (also called attunements or empowerments). Receiving an initiation is believed to activate the ability to access Reiki energy. Training for first- and second-degree practice is typically given in 8 to 12 class hours over about 2 days. In first-degree training, students learn to perform Reiki on themselves and on others. In second-degree training, students learn to perform Reiki on others from a distance. Some students seek master-level (third-degree) training. A Reiki Master can teach and initiate students. Becoming a Master can take years.

Reiki practitioners' training and expertise vary. Increasingly, many people who seek training are licensed health care professionals. However, no licensing or professional standards exist for the practice of Reiki.

If You Are Thinking about Using Reiki

- Do not use Reiki as a replacement for proven conventional care or to postpone seeing a doctor about a medical problem.
- Find out about the Reiki practitioner's background, including training and experience treating clients.
- Be aware that Reiki has not been well studied scientifically, but research on whether and how Reiki may work is under way.

Tell your health care providers about any complementary and alternative practices you use. Give them a full picture of what you do to manage your health. This will help ensure coordinated and safe care.

NCCAM-Funded Research

Some recent NCCAM-supported studies have been investigating the following areas:

- How Reiki might work

- Whether Reiki is effective and safe for treating the symptoms of fibromyalgia

- Reiki's possible impact on the well-being and quality of life in people with advanced AIDS

- The possible effects of Reiki on disease progression and/or anxiety in people with prostate cancer

- Whether Reiki can help reduce nerve pain and cardiovascular risk in people with type 2 diabetes

Chapter 70

Shiatsu

Are You Searching for the Answers to These Questions?

Is there a way to relieve my health problems with a gentle and non-invasive approach? Something nourishing for my body and soul? Something that I can look forward to receiving, which leaves me relaxed but energized? Something that addresses my health concerns in all these ways and is highly effective?

Shiatsu may be your answer.

What Is Shiatsu?

Shiatsu is a modern bodywork therapy with its origins in ancient Oriental medical philosophy. It is a form of acupressure, originating in Japan, that uses finger pressure to stimulate acupoints ("tsubos"), which are the same points used in acupuncture. It also uses the hands, fists, elbows, and feet to apply pressure to larger areas of the body. Shiatsu incorporates gentle assisted stretching and manipulation techniques to relax the joints.

Shiatsu works with the life force energy—called chi (or qi, ki)—encouraging it to flow more smoothly along the energy pathways, the

"Shiatsu," © Center for Integrative Health and Healing. Reprinted with permission. For additional information, visit www.cihh.net. The date of this document is unknown. The text that follows this document under the heading *"Health Reference Series* Medical Advisor's Notes and Updates" was provided to Omnigraphics, Inc. by David A. Cooke, MD, FACP, January 23, 2010. Dr. Cooke is not affiliated with the Center for Integrative Health and Healing.

meridians, of the body. Shiatsu stimulates the body's own healing systems and brings the body into balance, energetically and physically.

Benefits of Shiatsu

- Relieves pain, chronic and acute
- Releases stress and its effects
- Increases the circulation of blood and lymph
- Boosts the immune system
- Relaxes tight muscles
- Relieves headaches and migraines
- Eases and balances digestion
- Eases anxiety and depression
- Balances hormones
- Increases energy, vitality, stamina, and well-being

How Does Shiatsu Work?

Shiatsu uses the same Oriental medical philosophies that are used in acupuncture, but hands and fingers are used instead of needles, with gentle practitioner-assisted stretches and light massage incorporated into the session. While each therapist has his or her own style and emphasis, Shiatsu always involves acupressure work and stretching.

Oriental medical philosophy is based on the belief that life force energy called chi flows through the body along energy channels called meridians. As long as this energy is flowing smoothly, a person remains well. However, the flow of chi can become weak, sluggish, stagnant, or blocked due to stress, injury, poor diet and exercise habits, etc. An imbalance in the flow of chi can consequently contribute to pain, illness, and dysfunction.

The Shiatsu therapist evaluates the client in an in-depth interview and decides which meridians need attention to help address the problems that are present.

Case Studies

Osteoarthritis: A 57-year-old female presented with osteoarthritis in her knee, ankles, and toes. Four sessions of Shiatsu resulted in significant improvement of her medical condition allowing the client to awake without morning stiffness and to be significantly less dependent on medication.

Multiple sclerosis (MS): A 45-year-old female with MS presented with pain and weakness on one side of her body requiring the use of a cane to walk. Three weekly sessions of Shiatsu reduced dependency on the cane and lessened pain significantly.

What Is a Shiatsu Session Like?

Shiatsu sessions are done with the client dressed in comfortable clothing that will allow for the gentle stretching. The sessions are usually done with the client lying on a thick, comfortable mat on the floor, though it is fine to have the session done on a massage table if that is more comfortable for the client. The Shiatsu therapist does an in-depth interview to learn what the health problems are and to determine which meridians need addressing. The therapist then uses palm and finger pressure along the appropriate meridians and acupoints of the arms, legs and back. Gentle stretches and massage are interspersed throughout the session to help release restrictions in the joints that may hamper the flow of chi.

A shiatsu session lasts about an hour and leaves the client feeling very relaxed, yet energized at the same time.

History of Shiatsu

Shiatsu is a blend of ancient Eastern medical philosophy and modern Western science. China has always held high regard for the effectiveness of massage and acupressure for the treatment of a wide variety of health problems for over 2,000 years. Shiatsu has its roots in a traditional form of massage and acupressure called Anma Therapy. Anma Therapy originated in China hundreds of years ago and was then brought to Japan. It was used to treat pain and many common ailments as well as serious diseases and is still practiced today. Shiatsu is the culmination of Eastern and Western influence on this ancient healing art.

Shiatsu continues to evolve. In Japan, where there are currently over 87,000 registered Shiatsu practitioners, Shiatsu has been highly respected for its effectiveness in the treatment and prevention of disease for hundreds of years.

Health Reference Series *Medical Advisor's Notes and Updates*

The manner in which Shiatsu therapy may benefit patients remains subject to interpretation. Oriental medical philosophies provide one interpretation, but Western scientists have suggested other biological explanations for benefits. The subject can be viewed through more than one lens; perhaps the most important factor is whether the patient improves, whatever the mechanism.

Chapter 71

Therapeutic Touch

What is therapeutic touch?

Therapeutic touch is a form of healing that uses a practice called "laying on of hands" to correct or balance energy fields. The word "touch" is misleading because there is generally no direct physical touch involved. Instead, the hands are moved just over the body. Therapeutic touch is based on the theory that the body, mind, and emotions form a complex energy field. According to therapeutic touch, health is an indication of a balanced energy field, and illness represents imbalance. Studies suggest that therapeutic touch can help to heal wounds, reduce pain, and promote relaxation.

What is the energy field?

Although scientists differ on the nature and relevance of the human energy field, the concept of an energy field is also a part of other types of healing. In the ancient medical systems of India and China, the energy field is described as life energy. It is thought to exist throughout the body and is responsible for maintaining normal physiological, psychological, and spiritual functions. In Traditional Chinese Medicine, this energy is called qi (pronounced "chee"); in India's ayurvedic medicine it is called prana.

What is the history of therapeutic touch?

Dolores Krieger, a professor at New York University School of Nursing, and Dora Kunz, a natural healer, developed therapeutic touch in

---

the early 1970s. At first, Krieger and Kunz only taught the techniques to Krieger's graduate school nursing students, but Krieger's professional research and writing increased the popularity of the technique, particularly among nurses. The practice grew primarily through a grassroots effort of nurses throughout the United States. Today, therapeutic touch is taught at hospitals and health centers worldwide and is most commonly practiced by nurses.

How does therapeutic touch work?

Scientists are not certain how therapeutic touch works. There are few studies, and scientific investigators have so far not detected the human energy field discussed by Therapeutic Touch practitioners. Still, two theories have been put forward.

One theory is that the actual pain associated with a physically or emotionally painful experience (such as infection, injury, or a difficult relationship) remains in the body's cells. The pain stored in the cells is disruptive, and prevents some cells from working properly with other cells in the body. This results in disease. Therapeutic touch is thought to restore health by restoring communication between cells.

The other theory is based on the principles of quantum physics. As blood, which contains iron, circulates in our bodies an electromagnetic field is produced. According to this theory, at one time we could all easily see this field (called an aura), but now only certain individuals, such as those who practice therapeutic touch, develop this ability.

More generally, therapeutic touch is based on the idea that optimal health requires a balanced flow of life energy. Practitioners of therapeutic touch, by their own description, sense your energy through their hands and then send healthy energy back to you. When receiving therapeutic touch you usually feel such things as warmth, relaxation, and pain relief. The practitioner describes your energy as hot or cold, active or passive, blocked or free. There are eight general regions of the body above which energy is sensed—head, throat, heart, stomach, lower abdomen, sacral region, knees, and feet. Ultimately, you, the recipient of therapeutic touch are the healer. The practitioner simply allows your body's own healing mechanisms to emerge. The role of the practitioner is to facilitate this process.

What should I expect on my first visit?

Before the session begins, you will be asked to sit or lie down. No undressing is necessary. Sessions can be broken down into four steps:

- **(1) Centering**—The therapist becomes "centered" by using breathing, imagery, and meditation to achieve an altered state of consciousness for himself or herself.

- **(2) Assessment**—The therapist holds their hands 2–4 inches away from your body while moving from your head to your feet. This is done to assess the energy field surrounding your body. Therapists often describe feelings of warmth, coolness, static, and tingling over the areas of energy "congestion" or "blockage."

- **(3) Intervention**—Once a congested or blocked area is located, the therapist will move their hands in a rhythmic motion, starting at the top of the blocked area and moving down and away from your body. This action, known as unruffling, is repeated until the therapist no longer senses congestion or until you begin to sense relief. The therapist will also visualize and transmit life energy to specific areas of your body, also intended to correct imbalances.

- **(4) Evaluation/Closure**—Once you've had a few minutes to relax, the therapist will ask you how you feel. The therapist may recheck your energy field to be sure that no blockages were overlooked.

What is therapeutic touch good for?

Most studies indicate that therapeutic touch can relieve tension headaches and reduce pain, such as pain associated with burns, osteoarthritis, or following surgery. It may also speed the healing of wounds and improve function in those with arthritis.

Therapeutic touch also promotes relaxation. Cancer, heart disease, and burn patients have reported that therapeutic touch significantly lessens their anxiety. Generally, the deep relaxation associated with therapeutic touch reduces stress, lowers blood pressure, and improves breathing. Being relaxed may also lead to lower cholesterol levels and also may improve immune and bowel functions. Difficult pregnancies may also be made a little easier with the help of therapeutic touch.

Together with medical treatment, therapeutic touch can help with many additional conditions, including:

- fibromyalgia;
- sleep apnea;
- restless leg syndrome (a disorder that causes insomnia);
- allergies;
- bronchitis;
- addictions;
- lupus; and
- Alzheimer disease and, possibly, other forms of dementia.

481

Some people indicate that they experience emotional and spiritual changes after receiving therapeutic touch. These may include greater self-confidence, self-control, and self-understanding.

There is still controversy, however, as to whether the healing power of therapeutic touch has anything to do with the "laying on of hands." Critics suggest that the healing observed after therapeutic touch may be the result of the relaxing nature of the therapy itself and not the energy transfer that is believed to occur between the therapist's hands and the individual's body.

Is there anything I should watch out for?

You may feel thirsty, lightheaded, and a need to urinate. Light-headedness generally lasts only for 15 minutes after a session, but you may feel thirsty for days. According to some practitioners, if you were flooded with too much energy you might feel increased pain and be irritable, restless, anxious, or even nauseated. Therapeutic touch may also worsen fevers and active inflammation; therefore, it is best not to obtain therapeutic touch when you have either a fever or active inflammation (such as a swollen joint from arthritis).

Some therapeutic touch practitioners recommend that children, the elderly, and very sick people be treated for only a short time. Although there is no actual touching involved with therapeutic touch, talk with your practitioner about what to expect from a session, particularly if you have been physically or sexually abused in your past.

How can I find a qualified practitioner?

There is no formal certification program in the United States for therapeutic touch. Most therapeutic touch practitioners are in the nursing profession (although some massage therapists, physical therapists, chiropractors, acupuncturists, and others practice therapeutic touch as well). Nurse Healers-Professional Associates International (NH-PAI) recommends that people look for therapists who practice regularly (at least an average of two times per week), have at least 5 years of experience, and have completed at least 12 hours of therapeutic touch workshops. To locate a qualified practitioner near you, visit the NH-PAI web site, at www.therapeutic-touch.org.

What is the future of therapeutic touch?

While there seem to be many potential uses for therapeutic touch, particularly for chronically ill people, measuring the effectiveness of the technique is very difficult. Because of this, much of the research that exists has been criticized. Improved studies may lead to wider acceptance.

Chapter 72

Other Energy-Based Therapies

Chapter Contents

Section 72.1—Bioresonance Therapy 484

Section 72.2—Crystal and Gem Therapy 486

Section 72.3—Zero Balancing 487

Section 72.1

Bioresonance Therapy

"Turn off Allergies," by Nanci Bompey, *Asheville Citizen-Times*—
Asheville, NC. © 2009 Gannett Company, Inc. Reproduced with permission of the Gannett Company, via Copyright Clearance Center.

Julia Rosa has suffered from seasonal allergies and asthma her whole life, but after undergoing allergy desensitization at her naturopath's office, the Candler [North Carolina] resident said she hasn't sneezed this allergy season.

"Hands down, there really is no comparison," Rosa said.

Asheville naturopath Eric Lewis is one of the few practitioners in the region using electrodermal screening and acupressure to help desensitize patients to potential allergens.

"The goal of this is to change the way the body perceives a substance," Lewis said of the process. "The goal is to reverse sensitivity to these things so that a patient can tolerate these things in the future."

The technique, which is not approved by the Food and Drug Administration, first uses an electrodermal screening machine to determine what substances cause a person to have an allergic reaction.

During the process, the patient holds a rod containing the negative end of a circuit while Lewis uses another rod, the positive end, to touch different acupuncture points on the patient's body. These points correspond to different substances that could trigger an allergic reaction.

The machine then measures the electrical conductivity, or current, through the circuit that has been created. A drop in current flow indicates a resistance to electrical conductance, indicating a person's sensitivity to a particular substance, Lewis said.

"A change (in the energy flow) means that she is likely sensitive to that allergen," Lewis said as he demonstrated the technique on Rosa. "It shows her body's energy is reacting negatively to that substance. That's when we know that we have a problem."

Lewis said the machine he uses can screen for thousands of allergens that are environmental, like pollen, chemical, perfume or from food. He said because each substance has its own electromagnetic field, the machine is able to screen down to specific substances to determine if a person's sensitivity to dairy is from Cheddar cheese or cottage cheese.

While many people with allergies know what they are allergic to, Lewis said the machine can help those patients who have symptoms but don't know what causes them.

"It gives an objective reading," Lewis said. "It's a numerical presentation of what is going on."

The desensitization part of the process comes next. Once Lewis has determined what a patient is allergic to, he places a small vial containing water and alcohol into the machine, which imprints the electric signal from the substances that a person has sensitivity to into the mixture. Lewis calls this a remedy.

The patient then holds the remedy while Lewis presses on various acupressure points on the patient's back. The procedure simulates the person being in the presence of the allergen, Lewis said.

"The body is learning to not attack these allergens," he said.

Rosa has been through all four sessions for the allergy desensitization process, as has her 6-year-old son, Conor. She said the technique identified that her son was allergic to several foods, including dairy, which may have been causing his ear infections.

She said that since Conor had the desensitization procedure done, he hasn't had an ear infection.

"He has no excuse now to miss school," Rosa said.

Dr. Hal Jenkins, a doctor at Asheville's Regional Allergy, said he has not heard of the technique. He said that immunotherapy, or allergy shots, is the only proven way to build up a resistance to allergens.

"It is tried and true," he said. "None of the other modalities have been."

Section 72.2

Crystal and Gem Therapy

Reprinted with permission from the website of the John Moores University of California–San Diego Cancer Center, http://cancer.ucsd.edu. © 2002 University of California–San Diego. All rights reserved. Reviewed by David A. Cooke, MD, FACP, December 25, 2009.

This treatment modality is thought to promote wellness and optimize overall health. Crystal healing should be used with, not in place of, standard cancer therapy.

What does crystal healing involve?

Crystal healing is the belief that certain stones and crystals contain special healing energy that can be transferred into people to provide protection against illness and disease and provide spiritual guidance. This healing energy is transferred by touching, wearing, or placing the crystal on ailing parts of the body. Crystal healing also involves placing stones around the home, carrying them in a pocket, wearing them around the neck, and touching them as the need arises. A visit to a crystal healer involves the placement of various stones and crystals on acupoints or chakras, as identified by acupuncture and Ayurvedic medicine respectively, to restore vital energy within the patient.

How is crystal healing thought to promote wellness and optimize overall health?

Proponents of crystal healing believe that crystals and stones of different colors have different properties. These properties include the ability to purify the blood, calm the mind, and revive energy. The main value of crystals is the ability for those who believe in their healing powers to let go of negative emotions, reduce stress, and calm anxieties.

What has been proven about the benefit of crystal healing?

While formal research on the healing power of crystals has never been performed, there is no evidence or rationale that a crystal or stone can treat illness or aid healing. The placebo response may account for the benefits that do occur.

What is the potential risk or harm of crystal healing?

There is no intrinsic harm in using crystal healing to boost spirits and improve well-being.

How much does crystal healing cost?

Visits to crystal healers and the purchase of stones and crystals will vary with the practitioner and crystal shop owner, respectively.

Section 72.3

Zero Balancing

"About Zero Balancing," © 2009 Zero Balancing Health Association (www.zerobalancing.com). Reprinted with permission.

Zero Balancing (ZB) is an advanced studies program for the health care professional. It is a non-diagnostic system of healing which clarifies and coordinates energy fields in the body, and balances body energy with body structure. It is holistic in nature and is based on natural law. A typical session is done through clothing and lasts 30 to 45 minutes. A clear state of balancing helps to relive pain and suffering, provides a foundation for health and happiness, and brings a person closer to his or her true nature. Zero Balancing promotes this balanced state.

Zero Balancing is a hands-on body/mind therapy that combines the Western view of medicine and science with the Eastern view of energy and healing. It is based on the quantum physics notion that the particle and the wave are the two fundamental aspects that comprise our universe, and, in terms of the human being, comprise our structural and our energy bodies. Consciousness is the organizing principle that coordinates these foundations into one functioning whole and allows us to experience that process. Emotions are the vibratory frequencies that bring this process into awareness.

Zero Balancing uses energy as its working tool in the form of a fulcrum. A fulcrum is a field of tension which we create through touch. It serves as a catalyst to promote change. There are three, sometimes overlapping, classes of fulcrums: those that work as points of reference to promote balance and local change; those which work as fields to release weaker, or less organized vibration; and those which engage the client's own energy to promote change. The fulcrums in the first group are held stationary for brief periods; the second group utilizes the form of a curve or so-called half moon vector; and the third are moving foci of energy. In all cases the fulcrum is performed at interface of touch to ensure clear boundaries, and contacts both the energy body and the structural body of the person.

Zero Balancing teaches that the deepest currents of energy are in bone, that memory can be held in tissue, that energy fields in the body underlie mind, body, and emotions, and that imbalances in the field precede pathology.

Part Eight

Alternative Treatments for Specific Diseases and Conditions

Chapter 73

Arthritis and CAM

Rheumatoid Arthritis and CAM

Rheumatoid arthritis (RA) is a chronic disease that affects the joints, often those in a person's wrists, fingers, and feet. The common symptoms of RA are pain, stiffness, fatigue, sleep disturbances, and fever. There are treatments for RA in conventional medicine, but some people also try complementary and alternative medicine (CAM).

Scientific Research on CAM Treatments for RA

Botanical supplements and other dietary supplements: Overall, there is not much rigorous research available on the effectiveness and safety of botanical and other supplements that people try for RA. It is also important to know that while supplements are regulated by the U.S. Food and Drug Administration (FDA) as a category of foods, supplements made from plants and used for medicinal purposes (sometimes referred to as herbal medicines) can have effects as powerful as those of drugs. In fact, many conventional drugs first came from plants, such as digitalis (from the foxglove plant), used to treat heart failure and heart rhythm, and paclitaxel (from the yew tree), a cancer chemotherapy drug.

This chapter includes text excerpted from "Rheumatoid Arthritis and Complementary and Alternative Medicine," from the National Center for Complementary and Alternative Medicine (NCCAM, nccam.nih.gov), September 2005, and text from "Acupuncture Relieves Pain and Improves Function in Knee Osteoarthritis," by the NCCAM, December 20, 2004. Reviewed by David A. Cooke, MD, FACP, January 23, 2010.

It is important to be as informed as possible about the safety of any supplement you are considering or using. Some information already exists from a long history of botanical use outside conventional medicine. This knowledge is being strengthened as NCCAM supports rigorous studies on botanicals and other supplements that have shown promise in early studies to find out more about their molecular structure, their safety, how they may work, and for what diseases or conditions.

Thunder God vine: Thunder God vine (TGV for short; botanical name *Tripterygium wilfordii Hook F*) is a perennial vine native to China, Japan, and Korea. Preparations made from the skinned root of TGV have been used in traditional Chinese medicine to treat inflammatory and autoimmune diseases. Interestingly, TGV also has a history of use to kill insects in farm fields.

Some anti-inflammatory and immune-system-suppressing activity for TGV has been seen in laboratory and animal studies. The first clinical trial on TGV in the United States (the earlier ones were done in China) was carried out at the University of Texas Southwestern Medical Center and the National Institutes of Health (NIH). Its results were published in 2002. Twenty-one patients for whom conventional RA treatment had not worked completed the trial. Eighty percent of those who received a high-dose TGV extract and 40 percent of those who received a low-dose TGV extract experienced improvement in RA symptoms and physical functioning. No one in the placebo group improved. Longer and larger studies are needed to confirm these findings and to find out more about TGV.

Parts of the TGV plant are dangerous. The leaves, the flowers, the main stem, and the skin covering the root are poisonous, to a point that they could cause death. People should never try to make TGV medications themselves.

Currently, there are no consistent, high-quality TGV products being manufactured in the United States. Preparations of TGV made outside the United States (for example, in China) can sometimes be obtained, but it is not possible to verify whether they are safe and effective. An expert from the University of Texas/NIH study advises that consumers not use TGV until reliable TGV preparations become available.

If taken for a long time (according to one study, for more than 5 years), TGV may decrease the density of the minerals in women's bones, which would be of special concern for women who have osteoporosis or are at risk for it. If taken at high doses, TGV could suppress the immune system and increase the effects of immune-suppressing drugs.

The TGV extract made for the NIH study discussed in the previous text was well tolerated by study participants. However, side effects can occur and may include stomach upset, diarrhea, skin rash, changes in menstrual periods, and hair loss.

Gamma-linolenic acid (GLA): GLA is an omega-6 fatty acid that is found in the oils of some plant seeds, including evening primrose (*Oenothera biennis L.*), borage (*Borago officinalis L.*), and black currant (*Ribes nigrum L.*). GLA can be used by the body to make substances that reduce inflammation.

A 2000 Cochrane Collaboration review analyzed seven placebo-controlled studies of GLA (from evening primrose, borage, and black currant oils) for RA. The authors noted there were issues with these studies that made it difficult to draw conclusions. However, they thought the better studies indicated potential relief for RA pain, morning stiffness, and joint tenderness.

There are potential side effects and risks to know about with GLA. First, these plant seed oils may affect certain medical conditions and interact with prescription medications:

- Some borage seed oil preparations contain ingredients called PAs (for pyrrolizidine alkaloids) that can harm the liver or worsen liver disease. Only preparations that are certified and labeled as "PA-free" should be used.

- Borage oil and evening primrose oil might increase the risk of bleeding and bruising, especially in people taking blood-thinning drugs, such as aspirin, clopidogrel, NSAIDs, or warfarin.

- Evening primrose oil may cause problems for people taking a class of psychiatric drugs called phenothiazines, such as chlorpromazine or prochlorperazine.

- Side effects of these oils can include nausea, diarrhea, soft stool, intestinal gas, burping, and stomach bloating.

Fish oil: Fish oil contains high amounts of two omega-3 fatty acids: EPA (eicosapentaenoic acid) and DHA (docosahexaenoic acid). As with GLA, the body can use omega-3s to make substances that reduce inflammation.

There is some encouraging evidence from a number of laboratory studies, animal studies, and clinical trials about the potential usefulness of fish oil or omega-3 supplementation for various aspects of RA—such as the number of tender joints, morning stiffness, and the need for NSAIDs. However, more research is needed to definitively answer various questions, including what the most effective dosage or length of treatment would be, which patients would benefit most, and whether a placebo effect is at work.

In some people, the high amounts of omega-3s that are present in fish oil can increase the risk of bleeding or affect the time it takes blood to clot. If a person is taking drugs that affect bleeding or is going to have surgery, this is of special concern. Fish oil supplements interact with medicines for high blood pressure, so taking them together might lower a person's blood pressure too much.

Certain species of fish can contain high levels of contaminants, such as mercury, from the environment. Thus, their oils could pose a health risk, especially for pregnant or nursing women and for children. The fish that the federal government has found to have the highest levels of mercury are shark, swordfish, king mackerel, and tile fish. People who decide to use fish oil should look for products made from fish with lower mercury levels. Government information on this topic is available. You may have to contact the manufacturer to find out the type(s) of fish used in a product. Also, it is desirable to find out whether the manufacturer tests the product for contaminating substances and if the results of those tests are available.

Another point to note about safety is that a product called fish liver oil can contain more vitamin A than the recommended daily dosage, which could cause problems.

Generally, for low doses of fish oil supplements, the side effects are mild and can include a fishy aftertaste, belching, stomach disturbances, and nausea.

Valerian: The herb valerian has a history of use for sleep problems and anxiety disorders. Disrupted sleep has been called a common and often neglected symptom of arthritis. A large, nationally representative survey of people over 65 with arthritis in 2000 found that disruption of sleep, among all the disruptions of arthritis, was the main reason that people sought a variety of CAM, self-care, and conventional medical treatments. Valerian has also been taken for other reasons, such as the intent to relieve muscle and joint pain. The species of valerian most used in American supplements is *Valeriana officinalis*.

The evidence suggests that valerian has at least mild benefits for sleep problems in the general population, including insomnia. It has been theorized that valerian may have benefit for people with sleep problems from RA. However, research on valerian for RA specifically has not been done to answer this question.

There is not much evidence on how long it is safe to take valerian and which dose to use.

There is not enough reliable evidence to declare whether valerian is effective for muscle and joint pain, including pain from RA. There may be some biological basis for the theory that valerian could be beneficial for musculoskeletal pain.

Valerian is considered generally safe. However, it should not be taken with sedative drugs (for example, alcohol, benzodiazepines, or narcotics) or other sedative herbs (such as melatonin, SAMe [S-adenosyl-L-Methionine], or St. John's wort). Valerian will increase sedative effects. People who are taking antifungal drugs, statins, or certain anti-arrhythmia drugs should not take valerian. Valerian may not be safe for people who have a liver disorder or are at risk for one. After taking valerian, caution should be used in driving or using dangerous machinery. Side effects of valerian can include drowsiness in the morning, headache, stomach problems, excitability or anxiety, and sleeplessness.

Four other botanicals: Three of the other botanicals marketed with claims to benefit arthritis pain include the following:

- Ginger

- Curcumin (a component of the spice turmeric)

- Boswellia (also called Indian frankincense, made from the resin of a tree that grows in India)

These three botanicals have a history of use in Ayurveda to treat inflammatory conditions. Based on some early findings that may indicate promise, NCCAM is supporting studies at the University of Arizona on these three botanicals, to increase scientific knowledge about them and determine whether they are helpful for chronic inflammatory conditions such as arthritis and asthma.

A fourth botanical, feverfew, has been used in folk medicine with an intent to treat arthritis, migraine, and other conditions. One small published clinical trial was located for this report. It found no more benefit from feverfew than from the placebo. Overall, feverfew has not been proven to help RA symptoms.

Ginger's possible side effects include stomach upset, diarrhea, and irritation to the mouth and throat. Ginger is not recommended for people who have a bleeding disorder, a heart condition, or diabetes. Ginger may further slow blood clotting when combined with other herbs and drugs that slow blood clotting; add to the blood-pressure-lowering effects of drugs for high blood pressure and heart disease; and add to the blood-sugar-lowering effects of diabetes drugs.

Curcumin can have side effects of stomach problems, including nausea and diarrhea. Curcumin could add to the effects of other herbs and drugs that slow blood clotting. Curcumin can cause gallbladder contractions and should not be used by people with gallbladder disease or gallstones.

Boswellia can have side effects of stomach pain, stomach upset, nausea, and diarrhea. It is not known whether Boswellia interacts with any drugs, supplements, or diseases and conditions.

Feverfew appears to be safe for short-term use, but the safety of long-term use is not known. Feverfew can cause an allergic reaction, especially in people who are allergic to the daisy family. Side effects can include diarrhea and other stomach upsets. Chewing fresh leaves of feverfew may cause mouth irritation and sores. Feverfew might interact with medications broken down by the liver and increase the actions of drugs that slow blood clotting. Pregnant women should not take feverfew.

Glucosamine and chondroitin: Glucosamine sulfate (glucosamine for short) and chondroitin sulfate (chondroitin) are popular dietary supplements for arthritis. They are sold separately, in combination with each other, and in other combinations.

Glucosamine is a substance found in the fluid around the joints. It can also be obtained from the shells of shrimp, lobster, and crabs, or made in the laboratory. The body uses glucosamine to make and repair cartilage, a firm but flexible tissue that covers the ends of bones, keeps them from rubbing against each other, and absorbs the force of impact.

Chondroitin is a substance found in the cartilage around joints. As a supplement, it is obtained from sources such as sharks and cattle.

Both glucosamine and chondroitin have shown anti-inflammatory effects in animal studies. In humans, they have been studied only for osteoarthritis so far, not for RA. Osteoarthritis is a different form of arthritis than RA, with different causes, although the symptoms are similar (such as joint pain and problems with function). One cannot assume that if a treatment is helpful for one type of arthritis, it will also be helpful for another type. The studies of glucosamine and chondroitin for osteoarthritis mostly found a modest benefit. However, some design flaws have been noted in those studies. In sum, there is no evidence that glucosamine and chondroitin are helpful for RA.

Glucosamine appears to be safe for most people. However, it might worsen asthma through an allergic reaction. Also, glucosamine might cause higher blood sugar and insulin levels in people with diabetes, and those who decide to use it need to carefully monitor their blood sugar. Glucosamine could possibly decrease the effectiveness of certain medications—acetaminophen, some anticancer drugs, and antidiabetes drugs. Generally, side effects of glucosamine can include mild stomach problems and nausea; less commonly, there can be sleepiness, a skin reaction, or a headache. Some people who are allergic to shellfish are concerned about an allergic reaction to glucosamine. However, most shellfish allergies are to proteins in the meat, not to the shell material from which glucosamine supplements are made.

Chondroitin appears to be safe for most people. However, chondroitin may possibly worsen asthma (through an allergic response), blood clotting disorders, and prostate cancer. The side effects of chondroitin can include stomach pain and nausea; less commonly, diarrhea, constipation, swelling, and problems with heart rate.

Both supplements could affect the action of the drug warfarin, but this is not definite.

Special diets: Many people with RA are interested in whether certain foods can affect their symptoms. Examples of foods that are believed to possibly worsen the symptoms of arthritis (including RA) are the nightshade family of plants (white potatoes, tomatoes, eggplant, and peppers), dairy, citrus fruits, acidic foods, sweets, coffee, and animal protein. There are various theories about how foods may affect RA, including the following:

- The foods one eats and how the digestive system handles them are known to affect the immune system. Because RA is a disease of the immune system, a connection between diet and the disease has been proposed.

- Certain fats (mostly from animal sources, but also from corn and sunflower oils) break down in the body into substances that can cause inflammation.

- RA and/or medications to treat it may affect the way a person's digestive system handles foods.

- RA can affect a person's ability to prepare and eat food, leading to nutritional problems.

There is no strong, reproducible evidence that any foods or diets have a specific role in causing or treating RA.

It is important for people who have RA to eat a healthy, balanced diet. If one or more foods are eliminated from the diet, it is possible to miss key nutrients and not get enough calories. It is important to discuss any major dietary changes with your health care provider or a registered dietitian.

A true food allergy may exist in a small percentage of patients with RA. Many people think they have food allergies when they do not have them or when they have a different condition called food intolerance.

Acupuncture: Acupuncture is a practice that developed as a part of traditional Chinese medicine. Some people try acupuncture to treat RA pain or to treat the RA itself.

Good research studies have shown that acupuncture can help relieve pain associated with osteoarthritis. However, not much is known about its effectiveness for symptoms of RA. A handful of small studies have been conducted, and the findings do not clearly answer this question. Issues with the studies have included design problems, a small number of participants, variations in where acupuncture was given on the body, and how many treatments were given and for how long. More and better research is needed.

Acupuncture tends to have minimal side effects, if any. Relatively few complications from acupuncture have been reported to the FDA. If a person decides to use acupuncture, it is important to find a licensed and certified practitioner, as any complications have usually occurred from inadequate practitioner training and experience.

Magnets: Magnets are objects that produce a type of energy called magnetic fields. The term "magnets" is also used to refer to consumer products that contain magnets. Examples include shoe insoles, clothing, wraps for parts of the body, and mattress pads. These are of a type called static magnets, because their magnetic fields are unchanging.

The research so far does not firmly support claims that static magnets are effective for treating pain, including pain from RA. In those cases where some benefit was seen, it has not been proven why; many scientists think it may be due to a placebo effect. If someone does experience a benefit from a magnet, it will tend to occur quickly.

Static magnets should not be used by pregnant women; people who have a condition—such as an acute sprain, inflammation, infection, or wound—that could be affected by dilation of the blood vessels; and people who use a device such as a pacemaker, defibrillator, or insulin pump, or who use a medication patch.

The second type of magnets used for health purposes are called electromagnets (EMs), because they produce magnetic fields only when electric current flows through them. EMs are used in conventional medicine to treat bone fractures that have not healed well, and they are being studied in research settings for a number of other conditions (including cancer, epilepsy, RA, and mental disorders). Some consumer products using EMs are available.

EMs are being studied because there have been some encouraging early findings indicating the possibility of benefits for pain, physical function, and stiffness. However, it is too early to know for sure whether EMs are of benefit for patients with RA.

EMs should not be used by pregnant women; people who have a condition—such as an acute sprain, inflammation, infection, or wound—that could be affected by dilation of the blood vessels; and people who use a device such as a pacemaker, defibrillator, or insulin pump, or who use a medication patch. It may be advisable for people who have a history of cancer or seizure disorder to avoid using EMs until more is known about their effects on these medical conditions.

Hydrotherapy: Hydrotherapy is the use of water for therapeutic purposes. A few examples of hydrotherapy include bathing in heated water, as from hot springs or the sea; mineral baths; and water-jet massages. Another term used for hydrotherapy baths is balneotherapy.

Hydrotherapy dates back to ancient Greece and Rome. In recent centuries, it has been a popular treatment in Europe and Israel. Some forms of hydrotherapy are used in conventional medicine in the United States, such as whirlpool baths for athletic injuries and ice for sprains. As CAM, hydrotherapy is often combined with other treatments, such as exercises, massage, diets, herbs, and/or mud packs. It is used with the intent to benefit arthritis, circulation, and various other health issues, and to enhance feelings of relaxation and well-being. Some also claim that hydrotherapy "detoxifies" the body. In this report, the term hydrotherapy refers to external water treatments and not to internal treatments using water, such as colon irrigation or drinking specially treated water.

A small number of controlled studies have been done on hydrotherapy for RA, most based on sea-bath treatments given in Israel's Dead Sea area. Most of these studies reported benefit. However, there have been quality issues noted with these studies, and it is not considered proven that the hydrotherapy itself provided the benefits for RA claimed in these studies. Larger and better studies are needed to answer this question. Study authors have noted that there could be other reasons for any benefit, such as traveling to a spa, being removed from one's daily routine, relaxation, socializing, etc.

The safety of hydrotherapy has not been well studied. Overall, it appears to be a low-risk practice for most people if common-sense precautions are taken, such as not exposing the body to too much heat or cold or for too long a time, and being sure to drink enough fluid. However, hydrotherapy is riskier and could even be dangerous for certain people:

- Those who have a condition that could be worsened by exposure to extremes of heat or cold (for example, heart disease, lung disease, circulation disorder, Raynaud phenomenon, or chilblains) or by strong motions from water jets

- Those who have difficulty perceiving temperature (for example, from neuropathy, or damage to the nerves)

- Women who are pregnant

- People who have implanted medical devices such as pacemakers or pumps

Some people may get a skin irritation or infection from hydrotherapy water, either as a reaction to something in the water or if the water is not in sanitary condition.

Homeopathy: Homeopathy is a whole medical system that was developed in Germany and brought to the United States in the 19th century. Homeopathy involves giving very small doses of substances called remedies that would produce the same or similar symptoms of illness in healthy people when given in larger doses. This approach is called "like cures like." The remedies are diluted very highly, often to a point where not one molecule of the original substance remains.

Little rigorous research has been done on homeopathy for RA. The results have been mixed. It appears from some studies that homeopathy might be more effective than a placebo for rheumatic diseases and syndromes (including RA), but this evidence is not strong. Larger, better-designed studies are needed to resolve this question.

Homeopathic remedies are considered safe and unlikely to cause severe side effects. The FDA has learned of a few reports of illness associated with the use of these remedies, but determined that the remedies were not likely to be the cause. Homeopathic remedies are not known to interfere with conventional drugs.

Acupuncture Relieves Pain and Improves Function in Knee Osteoarthritis

Acupuncture provides pain relief and improves function for people with osteoarthritis of the knee and serves as an effective complement to standard care. This landmark study was funded by the National Center for Complementary and Alternative Medicine (NCCAM) and the National Institute of Arthritis and Musculoskeletal and Skin Diseases (NIAMS), both components of the National Institutes of Health. The findings of the study—the longest and largest randomized, controlled phase III clinical trial of acupuncture ever conducted—were published in the December 21, 2004, issue of the *Annals of Internal Medicine.*[1]

The multi-site study team, including rheumatologists and licensed acupuncturists, enrolled 570 patients, aged 50 or older with osteoarthritis of the knee. Participants had significant pain in their knee the month before joining the study, but had never experienced acupuncture, had not had knee surgery in the previous 6 months, and had not used steroid or similar injections. Participants were randomly assigned to receive one of three treatments: acupuncture, sham acupuncture, or participation in a control group that followed the Arthritis Foundation's self-help course for managing their condition. Patients continued to receive standard medical care from their primary physicians, including anti-inflammatory medications, such as COX-2 [cyclooxygenase-2] selective inhibitors, non-steroidal anti-inflammatory drugs, and opioid pain relievers.

"For the first time, a clinical trial with sufficient rigor, size, and duration has shown that acupuncture reduces the pain and functional impairment of osteoarthritis of the knee," said Stephen E. Straus, MD, NCCAM Director.

"These results also indicate that acupuncture can serve as an effective addition to a standard regimen of care and improve quality of life for knee osteoarthritis sufferers. NCCAM has been building a portfolio of basic and clinical research that is now revealing the power and promise of applying stringent research methods to ancient practices like acupuncture."

"More than 20 million Americans have osteoarthritis. This disease is one of the most frequent causes of physical disability among adults," said Stephen I. Katz, MD, PhD, NIAMS Director. "Thus, seeking an effective means of decreasing osteoarthritis pain and increasing function is of critical importance."

During the course of the study, led by Brian M. Berman, MD, Director of the Center for Integrative Medicine and Professor of Family Medicine at the University of Maryland School of Medicine, Baltimore, Maryland, 190 patients received true acupuncture and 191 patients received sham acupuncture for 24 treatment sessions over 26 weeks. Sham acupuncture is a procedure designed to prevent patients from being able to detect if needles are actually inserted at treatment points. In both the sham and true acupuncture procedures, a screen prevented patients from seeing the knee treatment area and learning which treatment they received. In the education control group, 189 participants attended six, 2-hour group sessions over 12 weeks based on the Arthritis Foundation's Arthritis Self-Help Course, a proven, effective model.

On joining the study, patients' pain and knee function were assessed using standard arthritis research survey instruments and measurement tools, such as the Western Ontario McMasters Osteoarthritis Index (WOMAC). Patients' progress was assessed at 4, 8, 14, and 26 weeks. By week 8, participants receiving acupuncture were showing a significant increase in function and by week 14 a significant decrease in pain, compared with the sham and control groups. These results, shown by declining scores on the WOMAC index, held through week 26.

Overall, those who received acupuncture had a 40 percent decrease in pain and a nearly 40 percent improvement in function compared to baseline assessments.

"This trial, which builds upon our previous NCCAM-funded research, establishes that acupuncture is an effective complement to conventional arthritis treatment and can be successfully employed as part of a multidisciplinary approach to treating the symptoms of osteoarthritis," said Dr. Berman.

Acupuncture—the practice of inserting thin needles into specific body points to improve health and well-being—originated in China more than 2,000 years ago. In 2002, acupuncture was used by an estimated 2.1 million U.S. adults, according to the Centers for Disease Control and Prevention's 2002 National Health Interview Survey.[2] The acupuncture technique that has been most studied scientifically involves penetrating the skin with thin, solid, metallic needles that are manipulated by the hands or by electrical stimulation. In recent years, scientific inquiry has begun to shed more light on acupuncture's possible mechanisms and potential benefits, especially in treating painful conditions such as arthritis.

References

1. Berman BM, Lao L, Langenberg P, Lee WL, Gilpin AMK, Hochberg MC. Effectiveness of Acupuncture as Adjunctive Therapy in Osteoarthritis of the Knee: A Randomized, Controlled Trial. *Annals of Internal Medicine.* 2004; 141(12):901–910.

2. Barnes P, Powell-Griner E, McFann K, Nahin R. *CDC Advance Data Report #343.* Complementary and Alternative Medicine Use Among Adults: United States, 2002. May 27, 2004.

Chapter 74

Asthma, Allergies, and CAM

What is alternative medicine?

Any unproven treatment for an illness or disease is considered an alternative medical approach by most American medical doctors. "Unproven" means there is not enough acceptable scientific evidence to show that the treatment works. The term alternative medicine refers to a wide variety of treatments considered outside "mainstream" or "usual" medical approaches in the United States today.

Many people turn to alternative medicine to help alleviate their asthma or allergy symptoms. These treatment approaches may include, but are not limited to, one or more of the following:

- Acupuncture

- Ayurvedic medicine

- Biofeedback; mental imaging; stress reduction; relaxation techniques

- Chiropractic spinal manipulation

- Diet, exercise, yoga, lifestyle changes

- Herbal medicine, vitamin supplements

- Folk medicine from various cultures

"Alternative Therapies," reprinted with permission from the Asthma and Allergy Foundation of America, © 2005. All rights reserved. Reviewed by David A. Cooke, MD, FACP, December 25, 2009.

- Laser therapy

- Massage

- Hypnosis

- Art or music therapy

Why do people use alternative medicine?

Recent statistics show that nearly 40 percent of Americans try some form of alternative medicine. Medical and scientific experts do believe that some remedies may be worth a try, providing they are not harmful. In some cases, specific alternative medical treatment may improve or relieve symptoms of a specific illness or disease. Risks should not outweigh the potential benefits.

If you believe a particular alternative medical approach might help reduce your asthma or allergy symptoms, talk with your doctor about it, and how you could integrate that treatment into your overall asthma/allergy management plan.

No one should use alternative medicine without first consulting a board-certified physician. Any alternative medical approach should be used in addition to your normal asthma or allergy management plan.

You should not substitute an alternative medical treatment for your regular medications or treatments. Be especially careful about use of alternative medicine on children. Approaches that are harmless for adults may not be harmless for children.

Does health insurance cover alternative medical treatment?

Health plans vary in what alternative medicine expenses they will pay. Many plans provide coverage for some but not all alternative therapies. If your doctor writes you a prescription for a specific treatment such as acupuncture or massage, you may be more likely to get partial or full reimbursement of the expense. Always check with your insurance provider before assuming the coverage is available.

What are cautions or considerations for people who use alternative medicine?

Beware the placebo effect. If you really want an alternative medical treatment to work, you may think it is working, even if it really isn't. This "placebo effect" often occurs for people using alternative medicine. Symptoms of asthma or allergy also may improve on their own as an illness (like a cold or flu) runs its course. If you use prescribed medications for your allergy or asthma symptoms, it may take time for them to "kick in." So you may simply be feeling better because your medications started working—not because the alternative medicine is working.

Read between the label lines. The federal government requires labels to state how an herb or vitamin may affect the body but labels are not required to carry health warnings. Labels also cannot claim any medical or health benefit. Products often are not properly labeled, especially those imported from other countries. Many people experience toxic—and sometimes deadly—effects from improperly using labeled herbs. Some products contain unnamed medicines such as steroids, anti-inflammatories, or sedatives that act to reduce your symptoms. Other "hidden ingredients" in various products can be dangerous or even lethal. Use products tested for safety and effectiveness.

Follow directions. Never increase the amount or frequency of a dose or use a treatment or device in a different way than recommended. Do not use herbs in combinations. Do not take herbs if you are pregnant or breast feeding.

Beware of developing allergy symptoms. Allergies to specific plants and other substances (such as latex or nickel) can build up over time. Products you've used for years may suddenly cause mild to serious allergy symptoms, especially if you already are allergic to something. Check to see if new herbs, foods, or other products you plan to use are in the same "family" as your known allergens.

Use quality products and services. Lack of quality standards is a serious problem for people who use various alternative medical treatments. Look for products that list the amount of the active ingredient(s). Make sure people giving you any kind of treatment are properly certified. Ask your pharmacist or health product store manager for recommendations. Research the product or service before you use it.

Consult with your physician before starting any new treatment. This point cannot be stressed enough. If you have symptoms of asthma or allergy, but you have not been diagnosed, consult a board-certified doctor for a proper diagnosis. Do not rely on health product store personnel to help treat undiagnosed symptoms. If you know you have asthma or allergies, again, talk with your doctor about the alternative medicine you want to use before you try it.

Are there useful alternative therapies for people who have asthma or allergies?

Keep in mind: Alternative therapy is medical treatment for which there is no conclusive, supporting scientific evidence. This does not necessarily mean the treatment is useless or ineffective. You simply must be careful in what you choose and how you use it.

Acupuncture: A technique that involves inserting needles into key points of the body. Evidence suggests that acupuncture may signal the brain to release endorphins. These are hormones made by the body. When released, endorphins can help reduce pain and create a sense of well-being. People with asthma or allergy may experience more relaxed or calmer breathing. Users should be aware of the risk of contaminated needles or punctured organs.

Biofeedback: A technique that helps people control involuntary physical responses. Results are mixed, with children and teenagers showing the greatest benefit.

Chiropractic spinal manipulation: A technique that emphasizes manipulation of the spine in order to help the body heal itself. There is no evidence that this treatment impairs the underlying disease or pulmonary function.

Hypnosis: An artificially induced dream state that leaves the person open to suggestion, hypnosis is a legitimate technique to help people manage various conditions. Hypnosis might give people with asthma or allergies more self-discipline to follow good health practices.

Laser treatment: A technique that uses high intensity light to shrink swollen tissue or unblock sinuses. Laser therapy may provide temporary relief, but it may also cause scarring or other long-term physical problems.

Massage, relaxation techniques, art/music therapy, yoga: Stress and anxiety may cause your airways to constrict more if you have asthma or allergies. Various techniques can help you relax, reduce anxiety, or control your breathing. The results may provide some benefit in helping you cope with asthma or allergy symptoms. However, evidence is not conclusive that these techniques improve lung function.

Chapter 75

Cancer and CAM

Cancer and CAM

What is complementary and alternative medicine?

Complementary and alternative medicine is a group of diverse medical and health care systems, practices, and products that are not presently considered to be part of conventional medicine. Conventional medicine is medicine as practiced by holders of MD (medical doctor) or DO (doctor of osteopathy) degrees and by their allied health professionals, such as physical therapists, psychologists, and registered nurses. Some health care providers practice both CAM and conventional medicine.

- Complementary medicine is used together with conventional medicine.

- Alternative medicine is used in place of conventional medicine.

This chapter includes text from "Cancer and CAM," by the National Center for Complementary and Alternative Medicine (NCCAM, nccam.nih.gov), part of the National Institutes of Health, June 2007. It also includes text from "PC-SPES," PDQ® Cancer Information Summary. National Cancer Institute; Bethesda, MD. PC-SPES (PDQ®): CAM—Patient. Updated 09/2007. Available at http://cancer. gov. Accessed January 12, 2010; and from "Selected Vegetables/Sun's Soup," PDQ® Cancer Information Summary. National Cancer Institute; Bethesda, MD. Selected Vegetables/Sun's Soup (PDQ®): CAM—Patient. Updated 02/2007. Available at http://cancer.gov. Accessed December 11, 2009.

- Integrative medicine combines treatments from conventional medicine and CAM for which there is some high-quality evidence of safety and effectiveness. It is also called integrated medicine.

Is CAM widely used?

According to a comprehensive survey on Americans' use of CAM, 36 percent of U.S. adults are using some form of CAM. When megavitamin therapy and prayer for health reasons are included in the definition of CAM, that percentage rises to 62 percent. These results are based on the 2002 National Health Interview Survey, which was supported by NCCAM and the National Center for Health Statistics (part of the Centers for Disease Control and Prevention). The survey found that rates of CAM use are especially high among patients with serious illnesses such as cancer.

Several smaller studies of CAM use by cancer patients have been conducted. A study of CAM use in patients with cancer in the July 2000 issue of the *Journal of Clinical Oncology* found that 69 percent of 453 cancer patients had used at least one CAM therapy as part of their cancer treatment. A study published in the December 2004 issue of the *Journal of Clinical Oncology* reported that 88 percent of 102 people with cancer who were enrolled in phase I clinical trials (research studies in people) at the Mayo Comprehensive Cancer Center had used at least one CAM therapy. Of those, 93 percent had used supplements (such as vitamins or minerals), 53 percent had used nonsupplement forms of CAM (such as prayer/spiritual practices or chiropractic care), and almost 47 percent had used both.

A review article in the March 2005 issue of the *Southern Medical Journal* reported that cancer patients take supplements to reduce side effects and organ toxicity, to protect and stimulate their immune systems, or to prevent further cancers or recurrences. Patients frequently see using supplements as a way to take control over their health and increase their quality of life.

Additional information about CAM use among cancer patients can be found in a review article published in *Seminars in Oncology* in December 2002.

How are CAM approaches evaluated?

The same rigorous scientific evaluation used to assess conventional cancer treatments should be used for CAM therapies. NCCAM is funding a number of clinical trials to evaluate CAM therapies for cancer.

Conventional cancer treatments are studied for safety and effectiveness through a rigorous scientific process that includes laboratory research and clinical trials with large numbers of patients. Less is known about the safety and effectiveness of complementary and alternative methods to treat cancer, although some CAM therapies have undergone rigorous evaluation.

A small number of CAM therapies, which were originally considered to be purely alternative approaches, are finding a place in cancer treatment—not as cures, but as complementary therapies that may help patients feel better and recover faster. One example is acupuncture. In 1997, a panel of experts at the National Institutes of Health (NIH) Consensus Conference found acupuncture to be effective in managing chemotherapy-associated nausea and vomiting and in controlling pain associated with surgery. In contrast, some approaches, such as the use of laetrile, have been studied and found ineffective or potentially harmful.

Is NCCAM sponsoring clinical trials on CAM for cancer?

NCCAM is sponsoring a number of clinical trials to study complementary and alternative treatments for cancer. Some of these trials study the effects of complementary approaches used in addition to conventional treatments, while others compare alternative therapies with conventional treatments. Recent trials include the following:

- Acupuncture to relieve neck and shoulder pain following surgery for head or neck cancer

- Ginger as a treatment for nausea and vomiting caused by chemotherapy

- Massage for the treatment of cancer pain

- Mistletoe extract combined with chemotherapy for the treatment of solid tumors

Patients who are interested in taking part in these or any other clinical trials should talk with their health care provider.

What should patients do when using or considering CAM therapies?

Cancer patients who are using or considering CAM should discuss this decision with their health care provider, as they would any therapy. Some complementary and alternative therapies may interfere with standard treatment or may be harmful when used along with standard treatment.

As with any medicine or treatment, it is a good idea to learn about the therapy, including whether the results of scientific studies support the claims that are made for it.

When considering CAM, what questions should patients ask their health care providers?

- What benefits can be expected from this therapy?
- What are the risks associated with this therapy?
- Do the known benefits outweigh the risks?
- What are the potential side effects?
- Will the therapy interfere with conventional treatment?
- Is this therapy part of a clinical trial? If so, who is sponsoring the trial?
- Will the therapy be covered by health insurance?

PC-SPES

What is PC-SPES?

PC-SPES is a mixture of herbs that was sold as a complementary and alternative medicine (CAM) treatment for prostate cancer. The mixture contains these eight herbs:

- Baikal skullcap (*Scutellaria baicalensis*)
- Licorice (*Glycyrrhiza glabra* or *Glycyrrhiza uralensis*)
- Reishi mushroom (*Ganoderma lucidum*)
- Isatis (*Isatis indigotica*)
- Ginseng (*Panax ginseng* or *Panax pseudoginseng var. notoginseng*)
- Chrysanthemum flowers (*Dendranthema morifolium*)
- Rabdosia rubescens (*Isodon rubescens*)
- Saw palmetto (*Serenoa repens*)

PC-SPES was taken off the market because some batches were found to contain prescription medicines in addition to the herbs.

Clinical trials of PC-SPES that were underway were stopped. There are products being sold now as substitutes for PC-SPES, but they are not the same mixture.

What is the history of the discovery and use of PC-SPES as a complementary and alternative treatment for cancer?

Most of the herbs in PC-SPES have been used in traditional Chinese medicine (TCM) for many health problems, including prostate problems, for hundreds of years. A chemist in New York and a doctor/herbalist in China worked together to create the mixture.

In 1997, a company was formed to make PC-SPES and sell it in the United States without a prescription. Interest in PC-SPES grew, and researchers began looking at it. Tests found that some batches of PC-SPES contained one or more of the following drugs, which are not found in nature:

- DES [diethylstilbestrol], a type of estrogen made in a lab

- Warfarin (Coumadin), a blood thinner

- Indomethacin, a drug used to decrease inflammation

Because these drugs are to be used only by prescription and could be harmful to some people, PC-SPES was taken off the market in 2002. The company that made PC-SPES has closed.

What is the theory behind the claim that PC-SPES is useful in treating cancer?

In lab tests, each herb used in PC-SPES has been reported to help keep cancer cells from growing or to help prevent cell damage that can lead to cancer and other diseases.

PC-SPES was reported to slow the growth of prostate cancer but did not cure it. It is not known how PC-SPES works in the body. Some of the herbs in the mixture contain phytoestrogens, which are estrogen-like substances found in plants. Estrogen can cause the testicles to stop making testosterone, which makes some prostate cancers grow. Patients' responses to PC-SPES were similar to responses to estrogen therapy using DES. The DES found in some batches of PC-SPES, however, may not have been enough to cause all of the estrogen-like effects that were seen in users of the mixture. There is some evidence that the mixture works in a different way than DES does, and that PC-SPES alone (without DES in it) may fight prostate cancer.

PC-SPES has also shown anticancer effects on prostate cancers that do not depend on testosterone and on other types of cancer. This suggests that PC-SPES may have anticancer qualities other than its estrogen-like effects.

How is PC-SPES administered?

PC-SPES is taken by mouth in capsules.

Have any preclinical (laboratory or animal) studies been conducted using PC-SPES?

Studies of PC-SPES in test tubes and using rats showed that it might keep cancer cells from growing. These studies were done, however, before it became known that some batches of the product contained unlisted prescription medicines. Also, the product was not standardized (different batches of PC-SPES were found to contain different strengths of the herbal ingredients). For these reasons, the results of the lab tests and animal studies are not considered to be good evidence.

The National Center for Complementary and Alternative Medicine (NCCAM) is doing three laboratory studies using existing PC-SPES supplies. The studies are being done to see how the herbs in PC-SPES might act in the body.

Have any clinical trials (research studies with people) of PC-SPES been conducted?

Clinical trials of PC-SPES had begun before the product was taken off the market. In these trials, PC-SPES was reported to improve quality of life, reduce pain, and lower PSA (prostate specific antigen) levels in patients with prostate cancer. Rising PSA levels can be a sign that prostate cancer is growing.

After it was learned that some batches of PC-SPES contained prescription medicines, ongoing studies were stopped and previous study results came into question. The responses reported in the studies may have been caused by the prescription medicines that were in the PC-SPES, as well as by the herbal ingredients. Also, since different batches of PC-SPES contained different ingredients, the studies cannot easily be compared.

NCCAM plans to do clinical trials of PC-SPES once a standard product is available.

Have any side effects or risks been reported from PC-SPES?

Common side effects were the same as those reported with estrogen therapy:

- Breast swelling and tenderness
- Loss of sex drive
- Impotence (inability to have an erection)

There were other, less common, side effects:

- Blood clots in the legs
- Diarrhea

PC-SPES may also change the way drugs, including anticancer drugs, work in the body. It may cause drugs to be more or less effective, or cause effects on the body that are not expected.

Is PC-SPES approved by the U.S. Food and Drug Administration (FDA) for use as a cancer treatment in the United States?

The U.S. Food and Drug Administration has not approved PC-SPES for use in cancer treatment. It is not legally sold in the United States.

Selected Vegetables/Sun's Soup

What is Selected Vegetables/Sun's Soup?

"Selected Vegetables" and " Sun's Soup " are names given to several different mixtures of vegetables and herbs that are being studied as treatments for cancer and other medical conditions, including acquired immunodeficiency syndrome (AIDS). The following versions have been used:

- Original Mixture: Shiitake mushroom; mung beans; *Hedyotis diffusa*; *Scutellaria barbata* (barbat skullcap). This mixture is not sold in the United States.

- Freeze-dried Selected Vegetables (DSV): A freeze-dried mixture of vegetables and herbs sold in the United States as a dietary supplement. DSV is reported to contain the following ingredients:

  - Soybean
  - Shiitake mushroom
  - Mung bean
  - Red date
  - Scallion
  - Garlic

  - Leek
  - Lentils
  - Hawthorn fruit
  - Onion
  - Ginseng
  - Angelica root

  - Licorice
  - Dandelion root
  - Senega root
  - Ginger
  - Olive
  - Sesame seed
  - Parsley

513

- Frozen Selected Vegetables (FSV): A frozen mixture of fresh vegetables and herbs, sold in the United States as a dietary supplement. It contains the same vegetables and herbs as in DSV.

What is the history of the discovery and use of Selected Vegetables/Sun's Soup as a complementary and alternative treatment for cancer?

The vegetable and herb mixture now called Selected Vegetables/Sun's Soup was created by Dr. Alexander Sun to treat cancer.

- In the mid-1980s, Sun created the mixture to treat a relative who was diagnosed with stage IV non-small cell lung cancer and not helped by standard treatment. The mixture contained shiitake mushroom, mung bean, and the herbs *Hedyotis diffusa* and *barbat skullcap*. Sun believed these ingredients contain substances that may block the growth of cancer cells and/or help the body's immune system attack cancer cells. The relative was reported to be alive and free of cancer more than 13 years later. Three more patients with advanced cancer were treated with a combination of shiitake mushroom and mung bean. These patients were also reported to benefit from the treatment.

- In 1992, Sun applied for a patent for Selected Vegetables/Sun's Soup as an herbal treatment of cancer. He reported on animal studies done in mice. Sun then began doing clinical trials to test Selected Vegetables/Sun's Soup in cancer patients.

- In 1995, Sun was awarded a patent for Selected Vegetables/Sun's Soup.

- In 1998, Sun reported at a scientific meeting that patients with different types of cancer had been helped by treatment with Selected Vegetables/Sun's Soup.

Many of the vegetables and herbs in Selected Vegetables/Sun's Soup were chosen because previous research and traditional Chinese medicine suggest they contain anticancer phytochemicals (substances found in plants that may have effects on the body). These include substances such as protease inhibitors, plant sterols, and isoflavones. These ingredients may block the growth of cancer cells and/or improve the way the body's immune system attacks cancer cells.

What is the theory behind the claim that Selected Vegetables/ Sun's Soup is useful in treating cancer?

The theory is that certain ingredients in Selected Vegetables/Sun's Soup may contain phytochemicals that have significant anticancer effects in humans. One of these ingredients is shiitake mushroom. Lentinan, which is taken from shiitake mushroom, has been used in Japan to treat stomach and colon cancer after surgery. Treatment with lentinan is reported to help patients with stomach cancer live longer and have a better quality of life. Lentinan may not be easily absorbed by the body from food, so it is usually given by injection. Other substances in shiitake mushroom that are more easily used by the body from food have shown anticancer activity in animal tests.

How is Selected Vegetables/Sun's Soup administered?

Selected Vegetables/Sun's Soup is eaten as part of the diet. Daily doses of either 1 ounce of the DSV (mixed with water or other soup) or 10 ounces of the FSV were used in clinical trials.

Have any preclinical (laboratory or animal) studies been conducted using Selected Vegetables/Sun's Soup?

Few preclinical studies have been done with Selected Vegetables/ Sun's Soup. Research in a laboratory or using animals is done to find out if a drug, procedure, or treatment is likely to be useful in humans. Preclinical studies are done before clinical trials (in humans) are begun.

A small number of mice were injected with tumor cells and fed either standard food or food mixed with one or more ingredients from Selected Vegetables/Sun's Soup. The researchers reported that the growth of tumors was slower in the mice that were fed the Selected Vegetables/Sun's Soup ingredients, compared to the mice that ate standard food. The tumor growth was slowest when the mice were fed both mung bean and shiitake mushroom.

Have any clinical trials (research studies with people) of Selected Vegetables/Sun's Soup been conducted?

Clinical trials using Selected Vegetables/Sun's Soup to treat cancer have been done with small numbers of patients. These patients received other types of treatment, either before or during treatment with Selected Vegetables/Sun's Soup, and different vegetable mixtures were used in the different studies.

515

The results of these trials were compared with published information on similar patients who did not receive Selected Vegetables/Sun's Soup. Most patients receiving the vegetable mixtures lived longer, were better able to carry out their daily activities, and either gained weight or did not lose weight. In some patients who ate Selected Vegetables/Sun's Soup, tumor growth slowed or the tumor completely went away. Because patients in these trials received other treatments, it is not known if their responses were caused by Selected Vegetables/Sun's Soup, the other treatments, or both. None of the trials were randomized or controlled. Randomized clinical trials give the highest level of evidence. In randomized trials, volunteers are put randomly (by chance) into one of two or more groups that compare different treatments. In a controlled trial, one group (called the control group) does not receive the new treatment being studied. The control group is then compared to the groups that receive the new treatment, to see if the new treatment works. Randomized controlled trials, enrolling larger numbers of people, are needed to confirm the results of studies done so far on Selected Vegetables/Sun's Soup.

One randomized clinical trial of patients with stage IIIB or stage IV non-small cell lung cancer is now being conducted. The trial is comparing the survival of patients receiving Selected Vegetables/Sun's Soup with patients receiving a placebo (inactive substance). Both groups are receiving treatment with supportive care, such as radiation therapy, surgery, or palliative care.

Have any side effects or risks been reported from Selected Vegetables/Sun's Soup?

No harmful side effects or risks have been reported in the use of Selected Vegetables/Sun's Soup. Some patients felt full or bloated after eating the dry form, but patients who ate the frozen mixture did not report this.

Is Selected Vegetables/Sun's Soup approved by the U.S. Food and Drug Administration (FDA) for use as a cancer treatment in the United States?

The FDA has not approved any form of Selected Vegetables/Sun's Soup for the treatment of cancer or any other medical condition. Well-designed clinical trials that test identical mixtures of vegetables and herbs are needed to prove whether Selected Vegetables/Sun's Soup is useful in treating cancer.

Chapter 76

Cognitive Decline and CAM

Grape Seed Extract May Help Prevent and Treat Alzheimer Disease

According to the National Institute on Aging (NIA), Alzheimer disease affects nearly 4.5 million Americans and is the most common form of dementia in the elderly. Alzheimer disease is an incurable disease with a slow progression beginning with mild memory loss and ending with severe brain damage and death.

While no treatment is proven to stop Alzheimer disease, some conventional drugs may limit symptoms for a short period of time in the early stages of the disease. Emerging research shows a correlation between red wine consumption and reduced risk of Alzheimer disease-type cognitive decline. Authors of a new NCCAM-funded study in mice found that grape seed-derived polyphenolics—similar to that in red wine—significantly reduced Alzheimer disease-type cognitive deterioration.

This chapter contains text from "Grape Seed Extract May Help Prevent and Treat Alzheimer's," by the National Center for Complementary and Alternative Medicine (NCCAM, nccam.nih.gov), part of the National Institutes of Health, June 2008; "Pilot Study Provides New Insight on Effect of Ginkgo Extract on Dementia in the Elderly," by the NCCAM, 2008; and "Study Suggests Coenzyme Q10 Slows Functional Decline in Parkinson Disease," by the National Institute of Neurological Disorders and Stroke (NINDS, www.ninds.nih.gov), part of the National Institutes of Health, October 14, 2002. Reviewed and revised by David A. Cooke, MD, FACP, January 23, 2010.

Researchers from Mount Sinai School of Medicine conducted experiments in mice with Alzheimer disease to see if a highly purified 100 percent water-soluble polyphenolic extract from Vitis vinifera (cabernet sauvignon) grape seeds, could affect Alzheimer disease-type cognitive deterioration. The mice received 5 months of either water containing grape seed extract or water alone as a placebo treatment. The mice were then given behavioral maze tests to determine cognitive function and brain tissue samples were tested to determine evidence of disease.

The researchers found that mice treated with grape seed extract had significantly reduced Alzheimer disease-type cognitive deterioration compared to the control mice. This is due to the prevention of a molecule called amyloid forming in the brain that has been shown to cause Alzheimer disease-type cognitive impairment.

Reference: Wang J, Ho L, Zhao W, et al. Grape-Derived Polyphenolics Prevent A-Beta Oligomerization and Attenuate Cognitive Deterioration in a Mouse Model of Alzheimer's Disease. *The Journal of Neuroscience.* June 18, 2008. 28(25);6388–6392.

Pilot Study Provides New Insight on Effect of Ginkgo Extract on Dementia in the Elderly

Overall, in a pilot study of a ginkgo biloba extract for delaying the onset of dementia in the elderly, researchers did not find a reduction in progression to dementia in those using ginkgo versus those using placebo. However, when the researchers took into account participants' adherence to taking the compound, the group that took ginkgo did appear to have a reduced risk of progression and a smaller decline in memory.

This small study funded by the National Institute on Aging and NCCAM and led by Hiroko Dodge, PhD, and colleagues at the Oregon Health & Science University and the Oregon State University, followed 118 volunteers age 85 or older over the course of 42 months. The double-blind, randomized, and placebo-controlled study used 80 mg of ginkgo extract taken three times per day. The participants were tested on entering the trial for memory function and other measures of health and were seen every 6 months to assess changes. Overall, both groups had similar reports of adverse events; however, the ginkgo group had more incidences of stroke, but there were no deaths due to stroke.

The study focused on those 85+ years, as more than half of individuals with dementia in developed countries are in their 80s or are older, according to the authors. In addition, with an estimated 8 to 15 percent of those in the same age group progressing to dementia yearly, it is important to find safe treatments that can slow this process. The authors conclude that there are limitations to the study and the suggestive results of a possible benefit from ginkgo need to be confirmed by larger prevention clinical trials.

Reference: Dodge HH, Zitzelberger T, Oken BS, et al. A Randomized Placebo-Controlled Trial of Ginkgo Biloba for the Prevention of Cognitive Decline. *Neurology*. February 2008.

Study Suggests Coenzyme Q10 Slows Functional Decline in Parkinson Disease

Results of the first placebo-controlled, multicenter clinical trial of the compound coenzyme Q10 suggest that it can slow disease progression in patients with early-stage Parkinson disease (PD). While the results must be confirmed in a larger study, they provide hope that this compound may ultimately provide a way of treating PD.

The phase II study, led by Clifford Shults, MD, of the University of California, San Diego (UCSD) School of Medicine, looked at a total of 80 PD patients at 10 centers across the country to determine if coenzyme Q10 is safe and if it can slow the rate of functional decline. The study was funded by the National Institute of Neurological Disorders and Stroke (NINDS) and appears in the October 15, 2002, issue of the *Archives of Neurology*.

"This trial suggested that coenzyme Q10 can slow the rate of deterioration in Parkinson disease," says Dr. Shults. "However, before the compound is used widely, the results need to be confirmed in a larger group of patients."

PD is a chronic, progressive neurological disease that affects about 500,000 people in the United States. It results from the loss of brain cells that produce the neurotransmitter dopamine and causes tremor, stiffness of the limbs and trunk, impaired balance and coordination, and slowing of movements. Patients also sometimes develop other symptoms, including difficulty swallowing, disturbed sleep, and emotional problems. PD usually affects people over the age of 50, but it can affect younger people as well. While levodopa and other drugs can ease the symptoms of PD, none of the current treatments has been shown to slow the course of the disease.

The investigators believe coenzyme Q10 works by improving the function of mitochondria, the "powerhouses" that produce energy in cells. Coenzyme Q10 is an important link in the chain of chemical reactions that produces this energy. It also is a potent antioxidant— a chemical that "mops up" potentially harmful chemicals generated during normal metabolism. Previous studies carried out by Dr. Shults, Richard Haas, MD, of UCSD and Flint Beal, MD, of Cornell University have shown that coenzyme Q10 levels in mitochondria from PD patients are reduced and that mitochondrial function in these patients is impaired. Animal studies have shown that coenzyme Q10 can protect the area of the brain that is damaged in PD. Dr. Shults and colleagues also conducted a pilot study with PD patients that showed that consumption of up to 800 mg/day of coenzyme Q10 was well-tolerated and significantly increased the level of coenzyme Q10 in the blood.

All of the patients who took part in the new study had the three primary features of PD—tremor, stiffness, and slowed movements—and had been diagnosed with the disease within 5 years of the time they were enrolled. After an initial screening and baseline blood tests, the patients were randomly divided into four groups. Three of the groups received coenzyme Q10 at three different doses (300 mg/day, 600 mg/day, and 1,200 mg/day), along with vitamin E, while a fourth group received a matching placebo that contained vitamin E alone. Each participant received a clinical evaluation 1 month later and every 4 months for a total of 16 months or until the investigator determined that the patient needed treatment with levodopa. None of the participants or the study investigators knew which treatment each patient had received until the study ended.

The investigators found that most side effects of coenzyme Q10 were mild, and none of the patients required a reduction of their dose. The percentage of people receiving coenzyme Q10 who reported side effects was not significantly different from that of the placebo group. During the study period, the group that received the largest dose of coenzyme Q10 (1,200 mg/day) had 44 percent less decline in mental function, motor (movement) function, and ability to carry out activities of daily living, such as feeding or dressing themselves. The greatest effect was on activities of daily living. The groups that received 300 mg/day and 600 mg/day developed slightly less disability than the placebo group, but the effects were less than those in the group that received the highest dosage of coenzyme Q10.

The groups that received coenzyme Q10 also had significant increases in the level of coenzyme Q10 in their blood and a significant increase in energy-producing reactions within their mitochondria. The results of this study suggest that doses of coenzyme Q10 as high as 1,200 mg/day are safe and may be more effective than lower doses, says Dr. Shults. The findings are consistent with those of a published study of patients with early Huntington disease—another degenerative neurological disorder—that showed slightly less functional decline in groups that received 600 mg/day of coenzyme Q10.

The new study also used an efficient phase II clinical trial design—developed by biostatistician David Oakes, PhD, of the University of Rochester, and other study investigators—which should be useful for testing other drugs that might slow the progression of PD, says Dr. Shults. The design allowed the researchers to study the effects of three doses plus a placebo in less than 3 years, and to obtain useful data about the compound's effectiveness. Dr. Shults and his colleagues strongly caution patients against taking coenzyme Q10 until a larger, definitive trial can be conducted. Because coenzyme Q10 is classified as a dietary supplement, it is not regulated by the U.S. Food and Drug Administration. The versions of the supplement sold in stores may differ, they may not contain potentially beneficial amounts of the compound, and taking coenzyme Q10 over a number of years may be costly, says Dr. Shults. In addition, the current study included only a small number of patients, and the findings may not extend to people in later stages of PD or to those who are at risk but have not been diagnosed with the disorder, he notes. Finally, if many people begin taking coenzyme Q10 because of these early results, it might make it impossible for investigators to find enough patients to carry out definitive studies of the compound's effectiveness and the proper dosages, since patients must not be taking any treatments in order to be considered for enrollment in a definitive trial.

The investigators are now planning a larger clinical trial that will examine the effects of 1,200 mg/day of coenzyme Q10 , and possibly a higher dose as well, in a larger number of patients.

Source: Shults CW, Oakes D, Kieburtz K, Beal F, Haas R, Plumb S, Juncos JL, Nutt J, Shoulson I, Carter J, Kompoliti K, Perlmutter JS, Reich S, Stern M, Watts RL, Kurlan R, Molho E, Harrison M, Lew M, and the Parkinson Study Group. "Effects of coenzyme Q10 in early Parkinson disease: evidence of slowing of the functional decline." *Archives of Neurology,* October 2002, Vol. 59, No. 10, pp. 1541–1550.

Editor's Note: Additional studies of coenzyme Q10 therapy for Parkinson disease since the above study have shown positive results in some, but not all, cases. Additional research is needed, particularly regarding high-dose coenzyme Q10 therapy, as many of the studies performed to date have used lower doses of the drug. The overall place, if any, of coenzyme Q10 therapy in treatment of Parkinson disease remains uncertain.

Chapter 77

Diabetes and CAM

Diabetes is a chronic condition affecting millions of Americans. Conventional medical treatments are available to control diabetes and its complications. However, some people also try complementary and alternative medicine (CAM) therapies, including dietary supplements.

About Diabetes

Diabetes encompasses a group of diseases. Type 2 diabetes accounts for 90 to 95 percent of all diagnosed cases and occurs more frequently in older people. Type 1 diabetes, which accounts for 5 to 10 percent of cases, usually strikes children and young adults. A third form, gestational diabetes, develops in some women during pregnancy.

In all forms of diabetes, the body's ability to convert food into energy is impaired. After a meal, the body breaks down most food into glucose (a kind of sugar), the main source of fuel for cells. In people with diabetes, the body does not make enough insulin—a hormone that helps glucose enter cells—or the cells do not respond to insulin properly. Often, both insulin production and insulin action are impaired. Without treatment, glucose builds up in the blood instead of moving into the cells, where it can be converted into energy. Over time, the high blood glucose levels caused by diabetes can damage many parts of the body,

Excerpted from "CAM and Diabetes: A Focus on Dietary Supplements," by the National Center for Complementary and Alternative Medicine (NCCAM, nccam .nih.gov), part of the National Institutes of Health, June 2009.

including the heart and blood vessels, eyes, kidneys, nerves, feet, and skin. Such complications can be prevented or delayed by controlling blood glucose, blood pressure, and cholesterol levels.

Type 2 diabetes, the focus of this text, most often is associated with older age (although it is increasingly being diagnosed in children), obesity (about 80 percent of people with type 2 diabetes are overweight), a family history of diabetes, and physical inactivity. Certain minority population groups are at greater risk, as are women who have had gestational diabetes. Type 2 diabetes usually begins as insulin resistance, a disorder in which cells do not use insulin properly. Symptoms develop gradually and may include fatigue, frequent urination, excessive thirst and hunger, weight loss, blurred vision, and slow-healing wounds or sores. However, it is possible to have type 2 diabetes without experiencing any symptoms.

People with diabetes should try to keep their blood glucose in a healthy range. The basic tools for managing type 2 diabetes are healthy eating, physical activity, and blood glucose monitoring. Many people also need to take prescription pills, insulin, or both.

Dietary Supplements and Type 2 Diabetes

Some people with diabetes use CAM therapies for their health condition. For example, they may try acupuncture or biofeedback to help with painful symptoms. Some use dietary supplements in efforts to improve their blood glucose control, manage symptoms, and lessen the risk of developing serious complications such as heart problems.

This portion of text addresses what is known about a few of the many supplements used for diabetes, with a focus on some that have been studied in clinical trials, such as alpha-lipoic acid, chromium, omega-3 fatty acids, and polyphenols.

Alpha-lipoic acid (ALA, also known as lipoic acid or thioctic acid) is an antioxidant—a substance that protects against cell damage. ALA is found in certain foods, such as liver, spinach, broccoli, and potatoes. Some people with type 2 diabetes take ALA supplements in the hope of lowering blood glucose levels by improving the body's ability to use insulin; others use ALA to prevent or treat diabetic neuropathy (a nerve disorder). Supplements are marketed as tablets or capsules.

- ALA has been researched for its effect on insulin sensitivity, glucose metabolism, and diabetic neuropathy. Some studies have found benefits, but more research is needed. (There are some studies, reported from outside the United States, of ALA delivered intravenously; however, this research is outside the scope of this text.)

- Because ALA might lower blood sugar too much, people with diabetes who take it must monitor their blood sugar levels very carefully.

Chromium is an essential trace mineral—that is, the body requires small amounts of it to function properly. Some people with diabetes take chromium in an effort to improve their blood glucose control. Chromium is found in many foods, but usually only in small amounts; relatively good sources include meat, whole grain products, and some fruits, vegetables, and spices. In supplement form (capsules and tablets), it is sold as chromium picolinate, chromium chloride, and chromium nicotinate.

- Chromium supplementation has been researched for its effect on glucose control in people with diabetes. Study results have been mixed. Some researchers have found benefits, but many of the studies have not been well designed. Additional, high-quality research is needed.

- At low doses, short-term use of chromium appears to be safe for most adults. However, people with diabetes should be aware that chromium might cause blood sugar levels to go too low. High doses can cause serious side effects, including kidney problems—an issue of special concern to people with diabetes.

Omega-3 fatty acids are polyunsaturated fatty acids that come from foods such as fish, fish oil, vegetable oil (primarily canola and soybean), walnuts, and wheat germ. Omega-3 supplements are available as capsules or oils (such as fish oil). Omega-3s are important in a number of bodily functions, including the movement of calcium and other substances in and out of cells, the relaxation and contraction of muscles, blood clotting, digestion, fertility, cell division, and growth. In addition, omega-3s are thought to protect against heart disease, reduce inflammation, and lower triglyceride levels.

- Omega-3 fatty acids have been researched for their effect on controlling glucose and reducing heart disease risk in people with type 2 diabetes. Studies show that omega-3 fatty acids lower triglycerides, but do not affect blood glucose control, total cholesterol, or HDL (high-density lipoprotein, or good) cholesterol in people with diabetes. In some studies, omega-3 fatty acids also raised LDL (low-density lipoprotein, or bad) cholesterol. Additional research, particularly long-term studies that look specifically at heart disease in people with diabetes, is needed.

- Omega-3s appear to be safe for most adults at low-to-moderate doses. Safety questions have been raised about fish oil supplements, because some species of fish can be contaminated by substances such as mercury, pesticides, or PCBs [polychlorinated biphenyls]. In high doses, fish oil can interact with certain medications, including blood thinners and drugs used for high blood pressure.

Polyphenols—antioxidants found in tea and dark chocolate, among other dietary sources—are being studied for possible effects on vascular health (including blood pressure) and on the body's ability to use insulin.

- Laboratory studies suggest that EGCG [(-)-epigallocatechin-3-gallate], a polyphenol found in green tea, may protect against cardiovascular disease and have a beneficial effect on insulin activity and glucose control. However, a few small clinical trials studying EGCG and green tea in people with diabetes have not shown such effects.

- No adverse effects of EGCG or green tea were discussed in these studies. Green tea is safe for most adults when used in moderate amounts. However, green tea contains caffeine, which can cause, in some people, insomnia, anxiety, or irritability, among other effects. Green tea also has small amounts of vitamin K, which can make anticoagulant drugs, such as warfarin, less effective.

Other supplements are also being studied for diabetes-related effects.

- Preliminary research has explored the use of garlic for lowering blood glucose levels, but findings have not been consistent.

- Studies of the effects of magnesium supplementation on blood glucose control have had mixed results, although researchers have found that eating a diet high in magnesium may lower the risk of diabetes.

- There is not enough evidence to evaluate the effectiveness of coenzyme Q10 supplementation as a CAM therapy for diabetes; studies of its ability to affect glucose control have had conflicting findings.

- Researchers are studying whether the herb ginseng and the trace mineral vanadium might help control glucose levels.

- Some people with diabetes may also try botanicals such as prickly pear cactus, gurmar, *Coccinia indica,* aloe vera, fenugreek, and bitter melon to control their glucose levels. However, there is limited research on the effectiveness of these botanicals for diabetes.

If You Have Diabetes and Are Thinking about Using a Dietary Supplement

Tell your health care providers about any complementary and alternative practices you use. Give them a full picture of what you do to manage your health. This will help ensure coordinated and safe care. Medicines for diabetes and other health conditions may need to be adjusted if a person is also using a dietary supplement.

- Women who are pregnant or nursing, or people who are thinking of using supplements to treat a child, should consult their health care provider before using any dietary supplement.

- Do not replace scientifically proven treatments for diabetes with CAM treatments that are unproven. The consequences of not following one's prescribed medical regimen for diabetes can be very serious.

- Be aware that the label on a dietary supplement bottle may not accurately reflect what is inside. For example, some tests of dietary supplements have found that the contents did not match the dose on the label, and some herbal supplements have been found to be contaminated.

Chapter 78

Fibromyalgia and CAM

People with chronic health conditions such as fibromyalgia often turn to some form of complementary and alternative medicine (CAM)— a group of diverse medical and health care systems, practices, and products that are not generally considered part of conventional medicine. If you are considering a CAM therapy for fibromyalgia, this information can help you talk to your health care provider about it.

About Fibromyalgia

Fibromyalgia is a disorder that causes muscle pain and fatigue. People with fibromyalgia have chronic widespread pain, as well as "tender points" on the neck, shoulders, back, hips, arms, and legs, which hurt when slight pressure (about 9 pounds) is applied.

People with fibromyalgia may also have other symptoms, such as the following:

- Trouble sleeping

- Morning stiffness

- Headaches

- Problems with thinking and memory (sometimes called "fibro fog")

- Irritable bowel syndrome

Excerpted from "CAM and Fibromyalgia: At a Glance," by the National Center for Complementary and Alternative Medicine (NCCAM, nccam.nih.gov), part of the National Institutes of Health, July 2009.

Women with fibromyalgia may also have painful menstrual periods. Fibromyalgia may also be associated with depression.

The causes of fibromyalgia are unknown, but problems with the nervous system could be involved. It is estimated that fibromyalgia affects as many as one in 50 Americans. Most people with fibromyalgia are women, and most are diagnosed during middle age. However, men and children also can have the disorder.

CAM Practices Used for Fibromyalgia

Conventional therapies for fibromyalgia are limited, and research shows that about 90 percent of people with fibromyalgia use some form of CAM. CAM practices used by people with fibromyalgia include the following:

- Acupuncture
- Biofeedback
- Chiropractic care
- Hypnosis
- Magnesium supplements
- Magnet therapy
- Massage therapy
- SAMe (S-Adenosyl-L-Methionine)
- Tai chi

What the Science Says about CAM and Fibromyalgia

According to reviewers who have assessed the research on CAM and fibromyalgia, much of the research is still preliminary, and evidence of effectiveness for the various therapies used is limited.

- Research on acupuncture—stimulation of anatomical points with thin metallic needles—for fibromyalgia has produced mixed results. One review article notes that three studies found some evidence to support the use of electroacupuncture (in which the needles are pulsed with electric current). However, the effects of electroacupuncture in these studies were mostly short lived, and two studies of traditional acupuncture had negative results.

- Some researchers believe that low levels of magnesium may contribute to fibromyalgia. However, there is no conclusive scientific evidence that magnesium supplements relieve fibromyalgia symptoms. Two small studies had conflicting results.

- A review of the research on massage therapy for fibromyalgia notes only modest, preliminary support. Two studies had some positive findings, but two others found either no benefits or only short-term improvements.

- Supplements containing the amino acid derivative SAMe are used for a variety of conditions. Although several small studies of SAMe for fibromyalgia have had mixed results, there is some evidence of a benefit. Reviewers conclude that more research is needed.

- Finally, according to reviewers, research evidence is insufficient to draw conclusions about the effectiveness of other CAM treatments—biofeedback, chiropractic care, hypnosis, and magnet therapy—used for fibromyalgia.

NCCAM Research on Fibromyalgia

The National Center for Complementary and Alternative Medicine (NCCAM) funds clinical trials that look at CAM for fibromyalgia, including the following:

- The effects of tai chi on fibromyalgia patients' musculoskeletal pain, fatigue, sleep quality, psychological distress, physical performance, and health status

- Brain-imaging techniques for determining whether acupuncture relieves pain due to fibromyalgia

- The effectiveness of a form of electroencephalograph (EEG) biofeedback in treating fibromyalgia

If You Are Considering CAM for Fibromyalgia

Talk to your health care providers. Tell them about the therapy you are considering and ask any questions you may have. They may know about the therapy and be able to advise you on its safety, use, and likely effectiveness in relieving your fibromyalgia symptoms.

If you are considering a practitioner-provided CAM therapy such as acupuncture, check with your insurer to see if the services will be covered, and ask a trusted source (such as your fibromyalgia doctor or a nearby hospital or medical school) to recommend a practitioner.

Although acupuncture treatment is generally safe, complications can result if needles are not adequately sterilized or if the treatment is not properly delivered.

If you are considering dietary supplements, keep in mind that they can act in the same way as drugs. They can cause medical problems if not used correctly or if used in large amounts, and some may interact with medications you may take. The health care providers you see about your fibromyalgia can advise you.

Tell all your health care providers about any complementary and alternative practices you use. Give them a full picture of what you do to manage your health. This will help ensure coordinated and safe care.

Chapter 79

Headache and CAM

Acupuncture

This form of treatment originated in China some 3,000 years ago. Although widely used in Europe since early in this century and universally acclaimed for its pain-relieving qualities, it has been of interest in the United States for a much shorter time.

Physicians in the United States have not embraced acupuncture mainly because it has lacked documented scientific validity and has been taught as a practice based on Taoist philosophy passed down through the centuries with relatively little change.

A small but increasing number of U.S. physicians have found acupuncture to be a useful part of their practice, despite the inability to explain in terms acceptable to their colleagues how they obtained favorable results by this method of treatment. Thus every day in the United States and elsewhere, thousands of patients are being treated with acupuncture for a variety of issues and reporting favorable results. Family physicians are with increasing frequency being asked about acupuncture if established medical treatments have not relieved the pain.

This chapter includes text from: "Acupuncture," © 2009 National Headache Foundation (www.headaches.org). Reprinted with permission; "Biofeedback," © 2009 National Headache Foundation (www.headaches.org). Reprinted with permission; "Chiropractors," © 2009 National Headache Foundation (www.headaches.org). Reprinted with permission; and "Feverfew (*Tanacetum Parthenium*)," © 2009 National Headache Foundation (www.headaches.org). Reprinted with permission.

While traditional acupuncturists select from some 400 or more points located on hypothetical meridians, the modern acupuncturist uses a smaller number of points. Work from Albert Einstein Medical School has pointed out that many of the most effective acupuncture points coincide with the motor points commonly used in electromyography and, indeed, it has seemed that these may be the only points that need stimulation. In the treatment of pain, motor points are selected from within the same neural segment adjacent to the area of pain. Other points are selected from the extremities where the largest number of muscles is located. One of the most effective and widely used acupuncture points, Ho Ku, is located at the base of the thumb. The thumb, of all the digits and limb segments, has the largest cortical representation.

Gaining scientific support is the theory that, in part, acupuncture works through the release of brain neurotransmitters. Some evidence indicates that acupuncture induces a release of endorphins in the human brain. Electrical stimulation has been found more effective than needle twirling. Stimulation must be sufficiently above the threshold of medium-sized fibers. Too strong a stimulus, however, serves to intensify pain.

Treatment with acupuncture needles inserted deeply into muscle, as with electroacupuncture, is the most commonly used technique. With this the changes produced in the central nervous system seem to be sufficient to continue the beneficial effect long after the stimulation has ceased. However, traditional acupuncturists may utilize other forms of treatment such as moxibustion (a form of heat therapy) and a variety of massage and movement techniques.

Biofeedback

Biofeedback can be an effective non-medicinal modality utilized in managing headache (both migraine and tension-type). It is a way that sufferers can learn to control body functions that were previously thought to be involuntary. The patient becomes integrally involved in his or her own headache treatment.

A person must be amenable to this type of therapy and willing to practice and make a commitment. Relaxation techniques, through warming of the hands and muscle relaxation, are practiced with the aid of instruments such as a finger thermometer or computer for measuring temperature or muscle tension. Some biofeedback techniques monitor brain wave activity. After repeated exercise, the patient gradually learns physiological sensations or body cues that eventually allow the elimination of the measuring instruments. Thus, biofeedback can be utilized at any time or any place when needed.

Depending on the patient, biofeedback can be utilized alone or in combination with medication to prevent attacks or reverse attacks once started.

Chiropractors

Chiropractors are health care professionals that utilize manual therapy as a component of their treatments.

Chiropractic manipulation can be of help in relaxing muscles in cases where there is muscle spasm present. Sometimes a chiropractor may refer to the vertebrae of the neck or back being out of alignment. This does not represent a serious structural defect such as would occur if a vertebra were dislocated. It is believed to be used in reference to the visual changes seen on x-rays of the back associated with postural and mechanical abnormalities of the back including muscle spasm. Other manual techniques such as massage and heat also can be soothing.

The U.S. Headache Guidelines Consortium did not find evidence to recommend manual therapy including chiropractic manipulation as a treatment for migraine headache. There is no consistent evidence for manual therapy being effective in tension-type headache.

There are several different methods of applying manual treatments to the back and neck. They vary in the amounts of rotation and force used. Rarely manipulative treatment of the neck has been associated with serious injury.

Chiropractors are not allowed to prescribe medications.

Feverfew (Tanacetum Parthenium)

Feverfew is *Tanacetum parthenium,* a member of the daisy family. However, it is sometimes obtained under the name of "Chrysanthemum parthenium." It is easy to confuse the medicinal variety of feverfew with chrysanthemum or even other varieties of feverfew—though none of these are toxic, so a mistake would not be injurious.

Drs. Johnson, Hylands, and Hylands (1983) did several studies on the use of feverfew for headache. One of these was a double-blind study on 20 patients who had eaten fresh leaves of feverfew daily as a migraine preventative for at least 3 months prior to the study. They had a history of common or classical migraine for at least 2 years' duration with no more than eight attacks a month at the time of the test. No subjects were used who had taken certain medications within 1 month before the test.

The average dosage for patients prior to the test was around 60 mg/day. During the test, the fixed dose was 25 mg per capsule of freeze-dried feverfew leaf. The freeze-dried herb was chosen because it is most like fresh leaves. Preparations like powdered extract or air-dried herb may be too old or have been heated to 100 degrees Celsius, possibly making it inactive.

The result of this test was that the patients now receiving the placebo had "significant increase in the frequency and severity of headache, nausea, and vomiting" while the feverfew group "showed no change in frequency or severity of symptoms of migraine." Johnson, et al. (1985) concluded that feverfew does in fact prevent migraine attacks. Most people need to take feverfew for many months before fully realizing the beneficial effects.

A low starting dose of 50 mg a day is recommended because the potential for side effects is then reduced. One problem is that freeze-dried feverfew capsules are not standardized in manufacture and different preparations may vary in the active ingredients.

Feverfew is currently receiving a great deal of interest in the United States although most headache experts still regard its use as experimental. The recent reports of research indicate that continually taking feverfew extracts may decrease the symptoms of migraine headaches.

Recently there has been a commercial product developed that utilizes a standardized dose of feverfew based on the activity of the purported active agent, along with therapeutic amounts of vitamin B-2 and Magnesium. This may be a more suitable formulation than others of feverfew.

Used with permission of the National Headache Foundation. For more information on headache causes and treatments visit www.headaches.org.

Chapter 80

Heart Disease and Chelation Therapy

What is coronary artery disease?

Coronary artery disease (CAD) is the most common form of heart disease. In CAD the coronary arteries, the vessels that bring oxygen-rich blood to the tissues of the heart, become blocked by deposits of a fatty substance called plaque. As plaque builds, the arteries become narrower and less oxygen and nutrients are transported to the heart. This condition can lead to serious problems, such as angina (pain caused by not enough oxygen-carrying blood reaching the heart) and heart attack. In a heart attack, or myocardial infarction, there is such poor oxygen supply to the heart that part of the heart muscle dies. If a sufficiently large portion of the heart is affected, it may no longer be able to pump blood efficiently to the rest of the body, resulting in death or chronic heart failure.

Approximately 7 million Americans suffer from CAD. It is the leading cause of death among American men and women; more than 500,000 Americans die of CAD-related heart attacks each year.

There are several factors that can each increase the risk of developing CAD:

Excerpted from "Questions and Answers: The NIH Trial of EDTA Chelation Therapy for Coronary Artery Disease," by the National Center for Complementary and Alternative Medicine (NCCAM, nccam.nih.gov), part of the National Institutes of Health, June 2004. Reviewed and revised by David A. Cooke, MD, FACP, January 23, 2010.

- High blood pressure
- High cholesterol levels
- Smoking
- Obesity
- Physical inactivity

- Diabetes
- Family history of CAD
- Gender
- Age

A person with CAD may or may not have symptoms. Symptoms can include chest pain from angina, shortness of breath, lightheadedness, cold sweats, or nausea.

How is CAD diagnosed and treated?

Because the severity of CAD and its symptoms can vary from person to person, the way the disease is diagnosed and treated can also vary. CAD is often diagnosed through a series of tests that can include blood tests to see if protein has been released into the bloodstream from damaged heart tissues, electrocardiograms (EKG) to check the heart's electrical activity, stress tests to record the heartbeat during exercise, nuclear scanning to check for damaged areas of the heart, and angiography to see how blood flows.

Treatment of CAD depends on many factors, such as the patient's age, heart function, and overall health. Often, treatment begins with focusing on lifestyle—stopping smoking for patients who smoke, reducing fat in the diet, and engaging in a prescribed exercise program. Medications may also be prescribed, such as aspirin to prevent additional heart attacks, medications that decrease the workload on the heart, or medicines to reduce high blood cholesterol levels or high blood pressure. If these efforts are not effective, a patient may need to have the narrowed or blocked arteries reopened through a procedure called balloon angioplasty, or bypassed through surgery. Balloon angioplasty involves threading a thin tube into the artery and expanding a balloon-like apparatus as a way to increase the size of the artery so more blood can flow. Bypass surgery is used to treat severe blockages by using veins or arteries from other areas of the body to divert blood flow around the blocked coronary arteries.

What is EDTA (ethylene diamine tetra-acetic acid) chelation therapy?

Chelation is a chemical process in which a substance is used to bind molecules, such as metals or minerals, and hold them tightly so that they can be removed from a system, such as the body. In medicine, chelation has been scientifically proven to rid the body of excess or toxic metals. For example, a person who has lead poisoning may be given chelation therapy in order to bind and remove excess lead from the body before it can cause damage.

In the case of EDTA chelation therapy, the substance that binds and removes metals and minerals are the salts of EDTA (ethylene diamine tetra-acetic acid), a synthetic, or man-made, amino acid that is delivered intravenously (through the veins). EDTA was first used in the 1940s for the treatment of heavy metal poisoning. Calcium disodium EDTA chelation removes heavy metals and minerals from the blood, such as lead, iron, copper, and calcium, and is approved by the U.S. Food and Drug Administration (FDA) for use in treating lead poisoning and toxicity from other heavy metals. In order to discover the safety and efficacy of chelation therapy for people with coronary artery disease, the National Institutes of Health have launched the Trial to Assess Chelation Therapy (TACT). Rather than testing calcium disodium EDTA, TACT uses another salt, disodium EDTA, under an FDA license as an investigational new drug (IND). Although disodium EDTA it is not approved by the FDA to treat CAD, some physicians and alternative medicine practitioners have recommended disodium EDTA chelation as a way to treat this disorder.

Does EDTA chelation therapy have side effects?

The most common side effect is a burning sensation at the site where the EDTA is delivered into the vein. Rare side effects can include fever, headache, nausea, and vomiting. Even more rare are serious and potentially fatal side effects that can include heart failure, a sudden drop in blood pressure, abnormally low calcium levels in the blood, permanent kidney damage, and bone marrow depression (meaning that blood cell counts fall). Reversible injury to the kidneys, although infrequent, has been reported with EDTA chelation therapy. Other serious side effects can occur if EDTA is not administered by a trained health professional.

How might EDTA chelation therapy work to clear blocked arteries?

Several theories have been suggested by those who recommend this form of treatment. One theory suggests that EDTA chelation might work by directly removing calcium found in fatty plaques that block the arteries, causing the plaques to break up. Another is that the process of chelation may stimulate the release of a hormone that in turn causes calcium to be removed from the plaques or causes a lowering of cholesterol levels. A third theory is that EDTA chelation therapy may work by reducing the damaging effects of oxygen ions (oxidative stress) on the walls of the blood vessels. Reducing oxidative stress could reduce inflammation in the arteries and improve blood vessel function. None of these theories has been well tested in scientific studies.

Is there evidence that EDTA chelation therapy works for CAD?

There is a lack of adequate prior research to verify EDTA chelation therapy's safety and effectiveness for CAD. The bulk of the evidence supporting the use of EDTA chelation therapy is in the form of case reports and case series. Some patients who have undergone chelation therapy and the physicians who prescribed it claim improvement in CAD. In addition, there are approximately 12 published descriptive studies and five randomized controlled clinical trials regarding the use of EDTA chelation for CAD. Although each descriptive study did report a reduction in angina, they were uncontrolled clinical observations or retrospective data, typically with a small number of participants. Of the five clinical trials in which patients were randomly selected to receive chelation therapy or a placebo (a dummy solution), the most rigorous way of assessing a new treatment, three trials involved so few people that only a dramatic improvement could have been detected. Studies need a larger number of participants to detect more mild benefits of a treatment. The fourth study was never published in final form, so its conclusions are uncertain. Finally, the fifth study reported that EDTA chelation was associated with an improvement in ability to exercise, but it had only 10 participants. [Editor's Note: Additional studies and analyses performed since this article was written have failed to prove benefit or safety of chelation therapy for CAD. Other studies have found no benefits of chelation therapy for peripheral arterial disease, a condition that has many relationships with coronary artery disease. The possibility of benefit in CAD has not been fully excluded, but there is little positive evidence to support its use at this time. The results of the NIH study discussed in this article are expected to be published in 2010.]

How frequently is EDTA chelation therapy used?

It is estimated by the American College for Advancement in Medicine, a professional association that supports the use of chelation therapy, that more than 800,000 visits for chelation therapy were made in the United States in 1997 alone.

Chapter 81

Hepatitis C and CAM

Hepatitis C, a liver disease caused by a virus, is usually chronic (long-lasting), with symptoms ranging from mild (or even none) to severe. Conventional medical treatments are available for hepatitis C; however, some people also try complementary and alternative medicine (CAM) therapies, especially herbal supplements.

About Hepatitis C

Hepatitis C, a communicable (contagious) disease of the liver, is caused by the hepatitis C virus (HCV). The term "hepatitis" means inflammation of the liver; HCV is one of several viruses in the hepatitis family. If the liver becomes inflamed, it cannot function properly and remove harmful material from the blood or convert food into energy.

Hepatitis C is transmitted primarily through contact with infected blood. It is not spread through sneezing, coughing, food or water, or casual contact. There is no vaccine for hepatitis C; the only way to prevent it is to avoid exposure.

People who are newly infected have what is called acute hepatitis C. Most people with acute hepatitis C develop chronic hepatitis C, which can injure the liver over time. Many people with hepatitis C show no symptoms for many years; others experience mild or more serious symptoms.

Excerpted from "CAM and Hepatitis C: A Focus on Herbal Supplements," by the National Center for Complementary and Alternative Medicine (NCCAM, nccam.nih.gov), October 2008.

People with more serious hepatitis C may need medication—interferon, alone or combined with ribavirin. However, not everyone with hepatitis C responds to drug therapy, and the drugs have side effects that can be difficult to tolerate.

Use of Herbal Supplements for Hepatitis C

A number of herbal products claim to be beneficial for the liver, and hepatitis C patients who do not respond to conventional drug therapy, cannot tolerate its side effects, or simply want to support their body's fight against the disease may try these products. For example, a recent survey of 1,145 participants in the HALT-C (Hepatitis C Antiviral Long-Term Treatment Against Cirrhosis) trial, a study supported by the National Institutes of Health (NIH), found that 23 percent were using herbal products at the time of enrollment. Although participants reported using many different herbal products, silymarin (milk thistle) was by far the most common.

What the Science Says

A review of the scientific evidence on CAM and hepatitis C found the following:

- No CAM treatment has been scientifically proven to successfully treat hepatitis C.

- A 2003 analysis of results from 13 clinical trials testing the effects of various medicinal herbs on hepatitis C concluded that there is not enough evidence to support using herbs to treat the disease.

- Two other reviews that covered a variety of CAM modalities for hepatitis C concluded that conventional therapies are the only scientifically proven treatments for the disease.

- In a 2002 NIH consensus statement on the management of hepatitis C, a panel of medical and scientific experts concluded that "alternative and nontraditional medicines" should be studied. Participants in a 2001 NIH research workshop on the benefits and risks of CAM therapies for chronic liver disease recommended research support for related laboratory and clinical studies.

The following text summarizes what is known about the safety and effectiveness of milk thistle and some of the other CAM products that people with hepatitis C use.

Milk thistle (scientific name *Silybum marianum*) is a plant from the aster family. Silymarin, the active extract of milk thistle, is believed to be responsible for the herb's medicinal qualities. Milk thistle has been used in Europe as a treatment for liver disease and jaundice since the 16th century. In the United States, silymarin is the most popular CAM product taken by people with liver disease.

Laboratory studies suggest that milk thistle may benefit the liver by protecting and promoting the growth of liver cells, fighting oxidation (a chemical process that can damage cells), and inhibiting inflammation. Study results from small clinical trials on milk thistle for liver diseases have been mixed; however, most of these studies have not been rigorously designed, or they have looked at various types of liver diseases—not just hepatitis C. High-quality, well-designed clinical trials have not proven that milk thistle or silymarin is beneficial for treating hepatitis C. The HALT-C study mentioned above found that silymarin use by hepatitis C patients was associated with fewer and milder symptoms of liver disease and somewhat better quality of life, but there was no change in virus activity or liver inflammation. The researchers emphasize that this was a retrospective study, not a controlled clinical trial. More research on milk thistle for hepatitis C is needed before a recommendation can be made.

Milk thistle is generally well tolerated and has shown few side effects in clinical trials involving patients with liver disease. It may cause a laxative effect, nausea, diarrhea, abdominal bloating, fullness, and pain, and it can produce allergic reactions (especially among people who are allergic to plants in the same family, such as ragweed, chrysanthemum, marigold, and daisy).

Other supplements are also being studied for hepatitis C.

- Ginseng has shown some beneficial effects on the liver in laboratory studies but has not yet shown effects in people.

- Thymus extract and colloidal silver are sometimes marketed for the treatment of hepatitis C, but there is currently no research to support their use for this purpose. Colloidal silver products can cause serious side effects.

- People with chronic liver disease sometimes use licorice root or its extract glycyrrhizin. Some studies, reported from outside the United States, have looked at glycyrrhizin administered intravenously for hepatitis C. Preliminary evidence from these studies suggests that glycyrrhizin may have beneficial effects against hepatitis C. However, additional research is needed before reaching any conclusions.

- Preliminary studies conducted primarily outside the United States have examined the potential of the following herbal products for treating chronic hepatitis C: lactoferrin, TJ-108 (a mixture of herbs used in Japanese Kampo medicine), schisandra, and oxymatrine (an extract from the Sophora root). More research is needed before the safety and effectiveness of these products can be fully evaluated.

If You Have Hepatitis C and Are Thinking about Using an Herbal Supplement

- Do not replace proven conventional treatments for hepatitis C with CAM treatments that are unproven.

- Be aware that some herbal products may damage the liver. For example, the herbs kava and comfrey have been linked to serious liver damage.

- Also be aware that the label on a supplement bottle may not accurately reflect what is inside. For example, some tests of dietary supplements have found that the contents did not match the dosage on the label, and some herbal supplements have been found to be contaminated.

- Tell your health care providers about any complementary and alternative practices you use. Give them a full picture of what you do to manage your health. This will help ensure coordinated and safe care. If you are pregnant or nursing a child, or if you are considering giving a child a dietary supplement, it is especially important to consult your health care provider. Supplements can act like drugs, and many have not been tested in pregnant women, nursing mothers, or children.

NCCAM-Funded Research

Recent NCCAM-supported research includes projects studying the effectiveness of the following:

- Silymarin for preventing and reversing complications of chronic hepatitis C

- Silymarin for the treatment of chronic hepatitis C in people who did not respond to conventional antiviral therapy, and in people with nonalcoholic steatohepatitis (a type of fatty liver disease)

- Commonly used herbal remedies for the treatment of hepatitis C in methadone-maintained patients

- Arginine (an amino acid) in reducing liver injury in individuals with alcohol-related hepatitis

Also, NCCAM has supported studies that test the safety and tolerability of different dosages of silymarin in people with hepatitis C.

Chapter 82

Hormones, CAM, and Aging

People are living longer. In 1970, the average life expectancy at birth was 70.8 years; in 2000, it was 76.9 years; and by 2030 it is estimated that the "oldest-old," age 85 and older, could grow to 10 million people.

Views on aging are also changing. It no longer necessarily means physical decline and illness—in the last two decades, the rate of disability among older people has declined dramatically.

The National Institute on Aging (NIA), part of the federal government's National Institutes of Health (NIH), investigates ways to support healthy aging and prevent or delay the onset of diseases that disproportionately affect us as we age. These studies not only may increase what is known as "active life expectancy"—the time of advancing years free of disability—but also may promote longevity. NIA's research includes hormone and dietary approaches, including calorie restriction.

Results from NIA-sponsored studies and others are likely to improve our understanding of the benefits and risks of hormone supplements, calorie restriction, and other interventions to promote healthy aging. This text provides an overview of what we know about hormone supplements and calorie restriction and the research needed to learn more. Until we have a better understanding, it is a good idea to be skeptical of claims that hormone or other supplements can solve your age-related problems. Instead, focus on what is known to help promote healthy aging: healthy eating and physical activity.

From "Can We Prevent Aging?" by the National Institute on Aging (NIA, nia.nih.gov), part of the National Institutes of Health, February 19, 2009.

What Is a Hormone?

The word "hormone" comes from the Greek word, hormo, meaning to set in motion. Hormones are chemical messengers that set in motion different processes to keep our bodies working properly. For example, they are involved in our metabolism, immune function, sexual reproduction, and growth. Hormones are made by specialized groups of cells within the body's glands. The glands—such as the pituitary, thyroid, adrenals, ovaries, and testes—release hormones into the body as needed to stimulate, regulate, and control the function of other various tissues and organs involved in biological processes.

We cannot survive without hormones. As children, hormones help us "grow up." In teenagers, they drive puberty. As we get older, some of our hormone levels naturally decline. But what does that mean? Scientists do not know exactly. In order to know more, NIA investigates how replenishing hormones in older people affects frailty and function. Many of these studies focus on hormones that decline with age, including:

- Growth hormone

- Melatonin

- Dehydroepiandrosterone (DHEA)

- Testosterone

- Estrogen and progesterone (as part of menopausal hormone therapy)

How Hormones Work

Most hormones are typically found in very low concentrations in the bloodstream. But a hormone's concentration will fluctuate depending on the body's activity. Like a key that unlocks a door, a hormone molecule is released by a gland and travels through the blood until it finds a cell with the right fit, a "receptor." The hormone latches onto a cell's receptor and a signal is sent into the cell. These signals may instruct the cell to multiply, make proteins or enzymes, or perform other vital tasks. Some hormones can even cause a cell to release other hormones.

One hormone may fit with many types of cells but may not affect all cells in the same way. For example, one hormone may stimulate one cell to perform a task but it might also turn off a different cell. Additionally, how a cell responds to a hormone may change throughout life.

Hormone Supplements

Levels of some hormones change naturally over the lifespan. Some hormones increase with age, like parathyroid hormone that helps regulate the amount of calcium in the blood and bone. Some tend to decrease over time, such as testosterone in men and estrogen in women. When the body fails to make enough of a hormone because of a disease or disorder, a doctor may prescribe hormone supplements. As opposed to hormones produced naturally by the body, hormone supplements come in many forms such as pills, shots, topical (rub-on) gels, and medicated skin patches.

You may have read magazine articles or seen television segments suggesting that hormone supplements can make people feel young again or can slow or prevent aging. That's because finding a "fountain of youth" is an attractive story that captivates us all. The truth is no research to date has shown that hormone supplements add years to life or prevent age-related frailty. And, while some supplements have real health benefits for people with clinical hormone deficiencies due to a disease or disorder, they also can cause harmful side effects. That's why people who have a diagnosed hormone deficiency should still only take hormone supplements under a doctor's supervision.

In some cases, the U.S. Food and Drug Administration (FDA) may have approved a hormone supplement for one purpose, but it is prescribed by physicians for another. This "off-label" use may occur when physicians believe that research, such as clinical studies done on other groups of people, demonstrates a supplement's usefulness for another condition. While this is the normal process for evaluating drugs already approved by the FDA, consumers should be aware that a particular off-label use of a drug may not have been tested and verified to the same degree as the original use of the drug.

Dangers of Hormone Supplements

Higher concentrations of hormones in your body are not necessarily better. The body maintains a delicate balance between how much hormone it produces and how much it needs to function properly. Natural hormone production fluctuates throughout the day. That means that the amount of hormone in your blood when you wake up may be different 2, 12, or 20 hours later.

If you take hormone supplements, especially without medical supervision, you can adversely affect this tightly controlled, regulated system. Hormone supplements cannot replicate your body's natural variation. Because hormonal balance is so intricate, too much of a hormone in your system may actually cause the opposite of your intended effect. For example, taking a hormone supplement can cause your own hormone regulation to stop working. Or, your body may process the supplements differently than the naturally produced hormone, causing an alternate, undesired effect. It is also possible that a supplement could amplify negative side effects of the hormone naturally produced by the body. Scientists may not know the consequences.

Some hormone-like products are sold over-the-counter without a prescription. Self-medicating with them can be dangerous. Products that are marketed as dietary supplements are not regulated by the FDA. This means that companies making dietary supplements do not need to get FDA approval or provide any proof that their products are safe and effective before selling them. There is no guarantee that the "recommended" dosage is safe, that there is the same amount of active ingredients in every bottle, or that the substance is what the company claims. Because there are no standards, the hormone-like dietary supplements sold over-the-counter may not have been thoroughly studied and potential negative side effects may not be understood or defined. In addition, these over-the-counter products may interfere with your other medications. NIA does not recommend taking any supplement touted as an "anti-aging" remedy because there is no proof of effectiveness and the health risks of short- and long-term use are unknown.

Human Growth Hormone

Human growth hormone (hGH) is important for normal growth and development, as well as for maintaining tissues and organs. It is made by the pituitary gland, a pea-sized structure located at the base of the brain.

Research supports supplemental use of hGH injections in certain circumstances. For instance, hGH injections can improve the growth of children who do not produce enough hGH. Sometimes hGH injections may be prescribed for young adults whose obesity is the result of having had their pituitary gland surgically removed. These uses are different from taking hGH as an anti-aging strategy. As with other hormones, hGH levels often decline with age, but this decrease is not necessarily bad. At least one epidemiological study suggests that people who have high levels of hGH are more apt to die at younger ages than those with lower levels of the hormone. Researchers have also studied animals with genetic disorders that suppress growth hormone production and secretion and found reduced growth hormone secretion may actually promote longevity in those species that have been tested.

Although there is no conclusive evidence that hGH can prevent aging or halt age-related physical decline, some clinics market hGH for that purpose and some people spend a great deal of money on such supplements. Shots can cost more than $15,000 a year. These shots are only available by prescription and should be administered by a doctor. But, because of the unknown risks, it is hard to find a doctor who will prescribe hGH shots. Over-the-counter dietary supplements, known as human growth hormone releasers, are currently being marketed as low-cost alternatives to hGH shots. But claims of their anti-aging effects, like all those regarding hGH, are unsubstantiated.

Research is starting to paint a fuller picture of the effects of hGH supplements, but there is still much to learn. For instance, study findings indicate that supplemental hGH can increase muscle mass; however, it seems to have little impact on muscle strength or function. Questions about potential side effects, such as diabetes, joint pain, and fluid buildup leading to high blood pressure or heart failure remain unanswered, too. A recent report that children who were treated with pituitary growth hormone have an increased risk of cancer created a heightened concern about the dangers of hGH injections. Whether older people treated with hGH for extended periods have an increased risk of cancer is unknown. To date, only small, short-term studies have looked specifically at hGH as an anti-aging therapy for older people. Before supporting the use of hGH as an anti-aging therapy, the potential benefits and risks should be assessed through additional research.

Melatonin

Melatonin is a hormone involved with our daily sleep/wake cycle. It is made by the pineal gland located in the brain. Despite some claims to the contrary, melatonin production and release does not necessarily decrease with age. Instead, a number of factors, including light exposure and use of some common medications can affect melatonin secretion in people of any age.

As with other hormones, melatonin is marketed as a dietary supplement. Consumers should look with caution at claims about melatonin supplements' effects.

One claim for melatonin supplements is that they are an anti-aging remedy, but research on the anti-aging effects has been very limited and focused on animals, not humans. There are also claims that melatonin helps with sleep. Research findings have shown that melatonin supplements, in amounts ranging from 0.1 to 0.5 milligrams, can improve sleep in some cases; however, if taken at the wrong time, melatonin can actually disrupt the sleep/wake cycle. And, melatonin's benefits as an antioxidant have been touted. Antioxidants protect the body from the harmful effects of by-products, known as free radicals, made when the body changes oxygen and food into energy. Early test-tube studies suggested that, in large doses, melatonin might be an effective antioxidant. More research is needed to know if using melatonin supplements as an antioxidant will decrease the amount of antioxidants cells produce naturally.

Side effects of melatonin supplements may include confusion, drowsiness, and headache. Animal studies suggest that melatonin may cause some blood vessels to constrict, a condition that could be dangerous for people with high blood pressure or other cardiovascular problems.

The usual dose of melatonin sold without a prescription in stores is 3 milligrams. This dose is much larger than the 0.1 to 0.5 milligrams of melatonin researchers used to study its effects on sleep. People who take these supplements may have a 10- to 40-times higher blood concentration of melatonin than normal. Long-term effects of such high concentrations of melatonin on the body are still unknown. Use caution when considering taking these supplements until researchers learn more.

DHEA

Dehydroepiandrosterone, or DHEA, is made from cholesterol by the adrenal glands, which sit on top of each kidney. It is converted by the body into two other important hormones: testosterone and estrogen.

For most people, DHEA production peaks in the mid-20s and then gradually declines with age. The effects of this decline including its role in the aging process are unclear. Even so, some proponents claim that over-the-counter DHEA supplements can improve energy and strength and boost immunity. Claims are also made that supplements increase muscle and decrease fat. To date, there is no conclusive scientific evidence that DHEA supplements have any of these benefits.

The conversion of naturally produced DHEA into a different amount of estrogen and testosterone is highly individualized. There is no way to predict whose body will make more and whose will make less of these hormones. Having an excess of testosterone and estrogen in your body can be risky.

Scientists do not yet know the effects of long-term use (over 1 year) of DHEA supplements. Early indications are that these supplements, even when taken briefly, may have several detrimental effects on the body, including liver damage. But the picture is not clear. Two short-term studies showed that taking DHEA supplements has no harmful effects on blood, prostate, or liver function. However, these studies were too small to lead to conclusions about the safety or efficacy of DHEA supplementation.

Researchers are working to find more definite answers about DHEA's effects on aging, muscles, and the immune system. In the meantime, if you are thinking about taking DHEA supplements, be aware that the effects are not fully known and might turn out to cause more harm than good.

Testosterone

Most people know testosterone as the hormone that transforms a boy into a man and is somehow associated with sex drive. That may be why some men are concerned about a possible decrease in testosterone production as they age.

Testosterone is a vital sex hormone that plays an important role in puberty. In men, testosterone not only regulates sex drive (libido), it also helps regulate bone mass, fat distribution, muscle mass and strength, and the production of red blood cells and sperm. But testosterone isn't exclusively a male hormone—women produce small amounts, as well. In men, testosterone is produced in the testes, the reproductive glands that also produce sperm. The amount of testosterone produced in the testes is regulated by the hypothalamus and the pituitary gland.

As men age, their testes often produce somewhat less testosterone, especially when compared to years of peak testosterone production during adolescence and early adulthood. Normal testosterone production ranges widely, and it is unclear what amount of decline or how low a level of testosterone will cause adverse effects.

In recent years, the popular press has reported frequently about male menopause, a condition supposedly caused by diminishing testosterone levels in aging men. There is scant scientific evidence that this condition, also known as andropause or viropause, exists. And the likelihood that an aging man will experience a major shutdown of testosterone production similar to a woman's menopause is very remote. In fact, many of the changes that take place in older men often are incorrectly attributed to decreasing testosterone levels. For instance, some men experiencing erectile difficulty (impotence) may be tempted to blame it on lowered testosterone, when in many cases erectile problems are due to circulatory problems.

In certain cases, such as in men whose bodies make very little or no testosterone, testosterone supplementation may offer benefits. FDA-approved testosterone supplements come in different forms, including patches, injections, and topical gels. Men whose testes have been damaged or whose pituitary glands have been harmed or destroyed by trauma, infections, or tumors may be prescribed testosterone. Supplements can also help men with exceptionally low testosterone levels maintain strong muscles and bones and increase their sex drive. It is unclear if men who are at the lower end of the normal range for testosterone production would benefit from supplementation.

More research is needed to learn what effects testosterone replacement may have in healthy older men without these extreme deficiencies. NIA is investigating the role of testosterone therapy in delaying or preventing frailty and helping with other age-related health issues. Results from preliminary studies involving small groups of men have been inconclusive. Specifically, it remains unclear to what degree testosterone supplements can help men maintain strong muscles and sturdy bones, sustain robust sexual activity, or sharpen memory.

There are also concerns about the long-term harmful effects that supplemental testosterone might have on the aging body. Some epidemiologic studies suggest that higher natural levels of testosterone are not associated with a higher incidence of prostate cancer—the second leading cause of cancer death among men. However, scientists do not know if taking supplemental testosterone increases men's risk for developing prostate cancer or promoting the growth of an existing tumor. There is also concern about a potential increased risk for stroke based on studies that suggest that testosterone supplementation might trigger excessive red blood cell production, which thickens the blood.

The bottom line: Although some older men who use testosterone therapy may report feeling more energetic or younger, there is no scientific proof that testosterone therapy in healthy men will help them age better. Until more scientifically rigorous studies are conducted, it is not known if the possible benefits of testosterone therapy outweigh any of its potential risks. NIA continues to conduct research to gather more evidence about the effects of testosterone supplements in aging men.

Hormones in Women

Estrogen and progesterone are two hormones that play an important part in women's menstrual cycle and pregnancy. Estrogen also helps maintain bone strength and might prevent heart disease and protect memory before menopause. Both estrogen and progesterone are produced naturally by the ovaries. However, after menopause, the ovaries stop making these hormones. For more than 60 years, millions of women have used estrogen supplements to control for menopausal symptoms, especially hot flashes and vaginal dryness. Women also take it to prevent or treat osteoporosis—loss of bone strength—that often happens after menopause. The use of estrogen (by women whose uterus has been removed) or estrogen with progesterone or a progestin, a synthetic form of progesterone (by women with a uterus), to treat the symptoms of menopause is called menopausal hormone therapy (MHT), formerly known as hormone replacement therapy (HRT).

There is a rich research base investigating estrogen. Many large, reliable long-term studies of estrogen and its effects on the body have been conducted. Yet, much remains unknown. In fact, the history of estrogen research demonstrates why it is important to examine both the benefits and risks of a hormone before it becomes widely used. Here's what scientists know:

- **Endometrial problems**—While estrogen helps some women with symptom management during and after menopause, it can raise the risk of certain problems. Estrogen may cause a thickening of the lining of the uterus (endometrium) and a slightly increased risk of endometrial cancer. To lessen these risks, doctors now prescribe progestin to women with a uterus to protect the lining.

- **Heart disease**—The role of estrogen in heart disease is complex. Early studies suggested MHT could lower postmenopausal women's risk for heart disease—the number one killer of women in the United States. But results from the Women's Health Initiative (WHI), a study of MHT by the NIH, suggest that using estrogen with or without a progestin after menopause does not protect women from heart disease and may even increase their risk. In 2002, WHI scientists reported that using estrogen plus progestin actually elevates some postmenopausal women's chance of developing heart disease, stroke, blood clots, and breast cancer, but women also experienced fewer hip fractures and cases of colorectal cancer. In 2004, WHI scientists published another report, this time on postmenopausal women who used estrogen alone, which had some similar findings: Women had an increased risk of stroke and blood clots, but fewer hip fractures. Then, in 2007, a closer analysis of the WHI results indicated that younger women, ages 50 to 59 at the start of the trial, who used estrogen alone had significantly less plaque in their coronary arteries than women not using estrogen. Increased plaque in coronary arteries is a risk factor for heart attacks. Scientists also determined that the risk of heart attack might not be increased in women who started MHT less than 10 years after menopause, but that there is increasing risk in women who begin MHT more than 10 years after menopause.

- **Dementia**—Some studies suggest that estrogen may protect against Alzheimer disease. However, this has not yet been proven. In 2003, researchers in a sub-study of the WHI, called the WHI Memory Study (WHIMS), reported that women age 65 and older who take a combination of estrogen and progestin were at twice the risk for developing dementia than women who do not take any hormones. In 2004, these WHIMS scientists reported that using estrogen alone could also increase the risk of developing dementia in women age 65 and older compared to women not taking any hormones.

For all the research findings, there are still many unknowns about the risks of MHT. For instance, scientists have not yet determined if risks differ between women who have menopausal symptoms and those who don't. Also, because women in their early 50s were only a small part of the WHI, scientists do not yet know if certain risks are applicable to younger women who use estrogen to control symptoms during the menopausal transition.

You may also have heard about a relatively new approach to hormone therapy for women—bioidentical hormones. These are man-made hormones (from plants such as soy or yams) that have the same chemical structure as hormones produced by the human body. The term "bioidentical hormones" is now also being applied to the practice of compounding or combining hormones such as estrogen and progesterone, theoretically based on a woman's individual hormonal needs. Large clinical trials of these compound hormones have not been done, and many bioidentical hormones that are available without a prescription are not regulated or approved for safety and efficacy by the FDA. FDA-regulated bioidentical hormones, such as estradiol and progesterone, are available by prescription for women considering MHT.

For middle age and older women, the decision to take hormones is far more complex and difficult than ever before. Questions about menopausal hormone therapy remain: Would using a different estrogen and/or progestin or different dose change the risks? Would the results be different if the hormones were given as a patch or cream, rather than a pill? Would taking the progestin less often be as effective and safe? Does starting menopausal hormone therapy around the time of menopause compared to years later change the risks? Can we predict which women will benefit or be harmed by using menopausal hormone therapy? As these and other questions are addressed by research, women should re-review the pros and cons of menopausal hormone therapy with their doctors, assess the personal risks and benefits, and then make an informed decision about whether or not this therapy is for them.

Calorie Restriction, Intermittent Fasting, and Resveratrol

Scientists are discovering that what you eat, how frequently, and how much may have an effect on quality and years of life. Of particular interest has been calorie restriction, a diet comprised by generally 25 to 40 percent fewer calories than normal but including all needed nutrients. Research in animals has shown calorie restriction to have an impressive effect on disease and markers of aging. It has been found to extend the life of protozoa (very small, one-celled organisms), yeast, fruit flies, mice, and rats. Recent calorie restriction studies with humans and other primates, such as monkeys, are ongoing. However, early findings of the Comprehensive Assessment of Long-term Effects of Reducing Intake of Energy (CALERIE) study, show that adults who cut their calorie consumption by 25 percent lowered their fasting insulin levels and core body temperature, both of which correlate with increased longevity in animal models. In other studies with non-human primates, researchers have found that calorie restriction reduced incidence of heart disease and cancer.

Scientists do not know if long-term calorie restriction is safe for humans. It is unclear whether or not a calorie-restricted diet will ever be recommended for people. However, studying calorie restriction may offer new insights into the aging process and biological mechanisms that could influence healthy aging. This research may also provide clues about how to prevent or delay diseases that become more prevalent with age.

Other ongoing studies focus on identifying chemicals that mimic calorie restriction's benefits. Resveratrol, found naturally in very small amounts in grapes and nuts, is one of the compounds being studied. Scientists compared two groups of overweight mice on a high fat diet. One group was given a high dose of resveratrol. The overweight mice receiving resveratrol were healthier and lived longer than the other overweight group. In a follow-up study, scientists found that, when started at middle age, resveratrol slowed age-related health problems in mice on a standard diet but did not increase longevity. More research is needed before scientists know if resveratrol is safe for people or even if it has the same effects as it has in mice.

Scientists are also studying the effect of intermittent fasting or reduced meal frequency. In animal models, like mice, reduced meal frequency appears to have a protective effect on the brain and may also help with heart function and regulating sugar in the blood. However, the influence of intermittent fasting on human health and longevity is currently unclear.

While research into calorie restriction and intermittent fasting continues, there is already plenty of research supporting the value of a healthy, balanced diet and physical activity to help delay or prevent age-related health problems.

Many Questions, Seeking Answers

NIA supports research that seeks to tell us more about aging and the risks and benefits of potential interventions such as hormone therapies, supplements, and calorie restriction. One goal is to determine whether DHEA, melatonin, and other hormonal supplements improve the health of older people, have no effect, or are harmful. Researchers are also trying to determine if calorie restriction is safe for humans and if there are any compounds that could replicate in humans the benefits of calorie restriction seen in animals.

These studies will take some time. Research on supplements and calorie restriction is ongoing and a great deal of basic animal and clinical research is yet to be done. Don't be surprised if these studies open the door to more questions as well as answers. Research is an incremental process; results can move knowledge forward, but can also take you back to basics.

Until more is known about DHEA, melatonin, hGH, and resveratrol, consumers should view these types of supplements with a good deal of caution and doubt. Despite what advertisements and media, like television and magazines, may claim, there are no specific therapies proven to "prevent" aging. Some harmful side effects already have been discovered and additional research may uncover others.

People with genuine deficiencies of hormones should consult with their doctors about supplements. Talk to your doctor if you are interested in any form of hormone supplementation or "anti-aging" approaches beyond healthy diet and physical activity. Meanwhile, people who choose to take any hormone supplement without a doctor's supervision should be aware that these supplements appear to have few clear-cut benefits for healthy individuals and no proven influence on the aging process.

Chapter 83

Infertility and CAM

Chapter Contents

Section 83.1—Herbal Remedies for Infertility 560

Section 83.2—Infertility and CAM... 561

Section 83.1

Herbal Remedies for Infertility

"Treating Infertility with Herbal Medications," © 2006 American Pregnancy Association (www.americanpregnancy.org). Reprinted with permission.

Chinese herbs have been used for approximately 2,500 years to treat a wide array of health problems. Herbal medicines may enhance fertility by supporting the natural functions of the ovulation and fertility process.

Herbs are not regulated by the FDA [U.S. Food and Drug Administration], but are they safe?

In general, herbs are safe to use. However, there are herbs that should not be taken during pregnancy, so it is always important to discuss with your healthcare provider which herbs are safe to take. When using herbs to enhance fertility, it is recommended that you consult a healthcare provider who is familiar with which herbs affect different aspects of your fertility.

When should herbs not be taken?

One of the purposes of prescribing herbal medicines is to increase ovarian function. Therefore, individuals who are taking birth control pills, Antigon/Cetrotide, or Lupron should not take herbs. These medications are used to impede or lessen ovarian function; in other words they have the opposite desired effect of herbs.

How long should I take herbs?

The effects of herbal medicines are generally cumulative, and the clinical effect, at least from the perspective of treating the infertile couple, is usually seen after 60–120 days. Herbs are also cycle-dependent, meaning they need the entire menstrual cycle and work best with multiple cycles. In other words, if a woman is going to have an IVF [in vitro fertilization] transfer in 1 week, herbs would not be prescribed.

560

What types of infertility can herbal medicines treat?

In general, all types of infertility conditions are appropriate for herbal medicines. Whether it is advanced maternal age, luteal-phase-defect, premature ovarian failure, male factor, or unexplained, herbs have positive potential. Clinical observation has seen impressive results when mixing herbs with gonadotropins during IUI [intrauterine insemination] and IVF cycles. The herbs seem to enhance the effects of the gonadotropins, and they do not pose the risk of OHSS (ovarian hyper stimulation syndrome).

Is herbal medicine a licensed profession?

Herbal medicine is not a licensed profession; however, there is Board certification which some practitioners acquire. It is recommended that you consult with a healthcare provider who is educated on the benefits and use of herbs for treatment of infertility. The recommendation is to locate a healthcare provider who is Board certified to prescribe herbal medicines.

Section 83.2

Infertility and CAM

"Acupuncture Shows Promise in Improving Rates of Pregnancy Following IVF," by the National Center for Complementary and Alternative Medicine (NCCAM, nccam.nih.gov), part of the National Institutes of Health, February 2008.

A review of seven clinical trials of acupuncture given with embryo transfer in women undergoing in vitro fertilization (IVF) suggests that acupuncture may improve rates of pregnancy. An estimated 10 to 15 percent of couples experience reproductive difficulty and seek specialist fertility treatments, such as IVF. IVF, which involves retrieving a woman's egg, fertilizing it in the laboratory, and then transferring the embryo back into the woman's womb is an expensive, lengthy, and stressful process. Identifying a complementary approach that can improve success would be welcome to patients and providers.

According to Eric Manheimer of the University of Maryland School of Medicine's Center for Integrative Medicine and colleagues who conducted the systematic review, acupuncture has been used in China for centuries to regulate the female reproductive system. With this in mind, the reviewers analyzed results from seven clinical trials of acupuncture in women who underwent IVF to see if rates of pregnancy were improved with acupuncture. The studies encompassed data on over 1,366 women and compared acupuncture, given within 1 day of embryo transfer, with sham acupuncture, or no additional treatment.

The reviewers found that acupuncture given as a complement to IVF increased the odds of achieving pregnancy. According to the researchers, the results indicate that 10 women undergoing IVF would need to be treated with acupuncture to bring about one additional pregnancy. The results, considered preliminary, point to a potential complementary treatment that may improve the success of IVF and the need to conduct additional clinical trials to confirm these findings.

References

Manheimer E, Zhang G, Udoff L, et al. Effect of acupuncture on rates of pregnancy and live birth among women undergoing in vitro fertilization: systematic review and meta-analysis. *British Medical Journal.* Published online, February 2008.

Chapter 84

Low Back Pain and CAM

Low-back pain is a common condition that can be difficult to treat. Spinal manipulation is among the treatment options used by people with low-back pain in attempts to relieve pain and improve functioning. It is performed by chiropractors and other health care professionals such as physical therapists, osteopaths, and some conventional medical doctors.

About Low-Back Pain

Each year, up to one quarter of U.S. adults experience low-back pain. Most people have significant back pain at least once in their lives; often, the cause is unknown. Back pain varies widely. For many people, it lasts only a few weeks, no matter what treatment is used. But for others, the pain can become chronic and even debilitating. Low-back pain is a challenging condition to diagnose, treat, and study.

Spinal Manipulation and Low-Back Pain

Spinal manipulation—sometimes called "spinal manipulative therapy"—is practiced by health care professionals such as chiropractors, physical therapists, osteopaths, and some conventional medical doctors. Practitioners perform spinal manipulation by using their

From "Spinal Manipulation for Low-Back Pain," from the National Center for Complementary and Alternative Medicine (NCCAM, nccam.nih.gov), part of the National Institutes of Health, April 2009.

hands or a device to apply a controlled force to a joint of the spine, moving it beyond its passive range of motion. The amount of force applied depends on the form of manipulation used. The goal of the treatment is to relieve pain and improve physical functioning.

In the United States, spinal manipulation is often performed as part of chiropractic care. Chiropractic is a health care approach that focuses on the relationship between the body's structure—mainly the spine—and its functioning. In chiropractic, spinal manipulation is sometimes called "adjustment." Back problems are the most common reason people seek chiropractic care.

What the Science Says

Study Findings to Date

Overall, studies have shown that spinal manipulation can provide mild-to-moderate relief from low-back pain and appears to be as effective as conventional medical treatments. In 2007 guidelines, the American College of Physicians and the American Pain Society include spinal manipulation as one of several treatment options for practitioners to consider using when pain does not improve with self-care.

Research is under way to determine whether the effects of spinal manipulation depend on the duration and frequency of treatment. Recent studies have found that spinal manipulation provides relief from low-back pain at least over the short term (i.e., up to 3 months), and that pain-relieving effects may continue for up to 1 year. In one study funded by the National Center for Complementary and Alternative Medicine (NCCAM) that examines long-term effects in more than 600 people with low-back pain, results to date suggest that chiropractic care involving spinal manipulation is at least as effective as conventional medical care for up to 18 months. However, less than 20 percent of participants in this study were pain free at 18 months, regardless of the type of treatment used.

Challenges Facing Researchers

When considering the evidence on spinal manipulation for low-back pain, it is important to know about the research behind the evidence. Although many clinical trials have been conducted, earlier trials tended to be small and poorly designed, making their findings less reliable. Moreover, studies have differed in focus (the specific type of back pain treated and form of manipulation used) and design (comparisons with other treatments vs. placebos). It can be difficult to clearly interpret findings when what is being measured varies widely from one study to the next. Recent research has begun to address these issues.

Side Effects and Risks

Common Side Effects

Reviews have concluded that spinal manipulation is relatively safe when performed by a trained and licensed practitioner. The most common side effects are generally minor and include temporary discomfort in the treated area, headache, or tiredness. These effects usually go away in 1 to 2 days.

Serious Complications

The rate of serious complications from spinal manipulation, although not definitely known, appears to be very low overall. A potential complication from low-back manipulation is cauda equina syndrome, a condition in which nerves in the lower part of the spinal cord become compressed, resulting in pain, weakness, and loss of feeling in one or both legs. Other functions—such as bowel or bladder control—may also be affected. Reports indicate that cauda equina syndrome is an extremely rare complication. In people whose pain is caused by a herniated disc, manipulation of the low back also appears to have a very low chance of either causing or worsening cauda equina syndrome.

NCCAM Research

Projects supported by NCCAM to study spinal manipulation for low-back pain include studies of the following:

- The optimal number and frequency of treatments and the duration of care

- Estimated use, costs, and outcomes of chiropractic care for recurrent back pain

- What happens in the body during manipulation of the low back

Chapter 85

Menopausal Symptoms and CAM

Menopause is the permanent end of a woman's menstrual periods. Menopause can occur naturally or be caused by surgery, chemotherapy, or radiation. Many women use complementary and alternative medicine (CAM) for menopausal symptoms.

This text is based on findings from a 2005 National Institutes of Health (NIH) State-of-the-Science conference on the management of menopause-related symptoms.

About Menopause

A woman is said to have completed natural menopause when she has not had a period for 12 consecutive months. For American women, this typically happens at around age 51 or 52. Menopause occurs immediately if the uterus or both ovaries are surgically removed, or if the ovaries are damaged in cancer treatment with radiation therapy or certain drugs.

Common Symptoms during the Menopausal Transition

Some symptoms that women experience are related to menopause and decreased activity of the ovaries. Others may be related to aging in general.

From "Menopausal Symptoms and CAM," by the National Center for Complementary and Alternative Medicine (NCCAM, nccam.nih.gov), part of the National Institutes of Health, January 2008.

Scientific evidence of a link to menopause is strongest for the following symptoms:

- Hot flashes and night sweats (also called vasomotor symptoms, because they involve the expansion of the blood vessels)

- Sleep difficulties

- Vaginal dryness, which can lead to painful intercourse and other sexual problems

It is not certain whether the following symptoms are due to menopause, other factors that can come with aging, or a combination of menopause and these factors:

- Problems in thinking or in remembering things

- Urinary incontinence

- Physical complaints, such as tiredness and stiff or painful joints

- Changes in mood, such as depression, anxiety, and/or irritability

The expert panel assembled for the NIH State-of-the-Science conference noted that menopause is a normal part of women's aging and advised that menopause should not be "medicalized" (or viewed as a disease).

Hormone Replacement for Menopausal Symptoms

For decades, hormone replacement therapy (HRT)—more recently known as menopausal hormone therapy (MHT)—was conventional medicine's main treatment for menopausal symptoms. In 2002, findings from a large study called the Women's Health Initiative raised serious concerns about the long-term safety of MHT. These concerns are one reason that many women are turning to CAM therapies.

What the Science Says about CAM Therapies for Menopausal Symptoms

The NIH State-of-the-Science conference panel discussed the evidence on several CAM therapies:

- Six botanicals—black cohosh, dong quai root, ginseng, kava, red clover, and soy

- DHEA (dehydroepiandrosterone), a dietary supplement

Very little well-designed research has been done on CAM therapies for menopausal symptoms. A small number of studies have been published, but they have had limitations (such as the way the research was done or treatment periods that may not have been long enough). As a result, the findings from these studies are not strong enough for scientists to draw any conclusions. Also, many studies of botanicals have not used a standardized product (i.e., one that is chemically consistent). The National Center for Complementary and Alternative Medicine (NCCAM) is sponsoring a number of studies on botanicals using products that are both well characterized (i.e., their ingredients have been carefully studied) and well standardized and on other CAM therapies that have shown possible promise for reducing menopausal symptoms.

Because CAM products used for menopausal symptoms can have side effects and can interact with other botanicals or supplements or with drugs, research in this area is addressing safety as well as efficacy. Some findings from this research are highlighted in the following text.

Botanicals

Black cohosh (*Actaea racemosa, Cimicifuga racemosa*): This herb has received more scientific attention for its possible effects on menopausal symptoms than have other botanicals. Studies of its effectiveness in reducing hot flashes have had mixed results. A study funded by NCCAM and the National Institute on Aging found that black cohosh, whether used alone or with other botanicals, failed to relieve hot flashes and night sweats in postmenopausal women or those approaching menopause. Other research suggests that black cohosh does not act like estrogen, as once was thought.

United States Pharmacopeia experts suggest women should discontinue use of black cohosh and consult a health care practitioner if they have a liver disorder or develop symptoms of liver trouble, such as abdominal pain, dark urine, or jaundice. There have been several case reports of hepatitis (inflammation of the liver), as well as liver failure, in women who were taking black cohosh. It is not known if black cohosh was responsible for these problems. Although these cases are very rare and the evidence is not definitive, scientists are concerned about the possible effects of black cohosh on the liver.

Dong quai (*Angelica sinensis*): Only one randomized clinical study of dong quai has been done. The researchers did not find it to be useful in reducing hot flashes. Dong quai is known to interact with, and increase the activity in the body of, the blood-thinning medicine warfarin. This can lead to bleeding complications in women who take this medicine.

Ginseng (*Panax ginseng* or *Panax quinquefolius*): The panel concluded that ginseng may help with some menopausal symptoms, such as mood symptoms and sleep disturbances, and with one's overall sense of well-being. However, it has not been found helpful for hot flashes.

Kava (*Piper methysticum*): Kava may decrease anxiety, but there is no evidence that it decreases hot flashes. It is important to note that kava has been associated with liver disease. The FDA [U.S. Food and Drug Administration] has issued a warning to patients and providers about kava because of its potential to damage the liver.

Red clover (*Trifolium pratense*): The panel reported that five controlled studies found no consistent or conclusive evidence that red clover leaf extract reduces hot flashes. Clinical studies in women report few side effects, and no serious health problems have been discussed in the literature. However, there are some cautions. Some studies have raised concerns that red clover, which contains phytoestrogens, might have harmful effects on hormone-sensitive tissue (for example, in the breast and uterus).

Soy: The scientific literature includes both positive and negative results on soy extracts for hot flashes. When taken for short periods of time, soy extracts appear to have few if any serious side effects. However, long-term use of soy extracts has been associated with thickening of the lining of the uterus.

About phytoestrogens: Some botanical products, such as soy and red clover, contain estrogen-like compounds called phytoestrogens. Plants rich in phytoestrogens may help relieve some symptoms of menopause. However, it is uncertain whether this relief comes from phytoestrogens or from other compounds in the plant. Much remains to be learned about these plant products, including exactly how they work in the human body. Doctors caution that certain women need to be particularly careful about using phytoestrogens, especially:

- women who have had or are at increased risk for diseases or conditions that are affected by hormones, such as breast, uterine, or ovarian cancer; endometriosis; or uterine fibroids; or

- women who are taking drugs that increase estrogen levels in the body, such as birth control pills; MHT; or a type of cancer drug called selective estrogen receptor modulators (SERMs), such as tamoxifen.

DHEA [Dehydroepiandrosterone]

DHEA is a naturally occurring substance that is changed in the body to the hormones estrogen and testosterone. It is also manufactured and sold as a dietary supplement. A few small studies have suggested that DHEA might possibly have some benefit for hot flashes and decreased sexual arousal, although small randomized controlled trials have shown no benefit. Because levels of natural DHEA in the body decline with age, some people believe that taking a DHEA supplement can help treat or prevent conditions related to aging; however, there is no good scientific evidence to support this notion.

Concerns have been raised about whether DHEA is safe and effective. Its long-term effects, risks, and benefits have not been well studied, and scientists are not certain whether it might increase the risk for breast or prostate cancer. Before using DHEA for any purpose, people should talk to their health care provider about potential benefits and risks.

If You Are Considering CAM for Menopausal Symptoms

Although there is very little scientific evidence to support the effectiveness of CAM therapies for menopausal symptoms, it is possible that some CAM therapies may provide some relief to women during the menopausal transition. Here a few important points to keep in mind if you are considering these therapies:

- Tell your health care providers about any complementary and alternative practices you use. Give them a full picture of what you do to manage your health. This will help ensure coordinated and safe care.

- Keep in mind that although many dietary supplements (and some prescription drugs) come from natural sources, "natural" does not always mean "safe." For example, the herbs comfrey and kava can cause serious harm to the liver. Also, a manufacturer's use of the term "standardized" (or "verified" or "certified") does not necessarily guarantee product quality or consistency.

- Be aware that an herbal supplement may contain dozens of compounds and that its active ingredients may not be known.

Researchers are studying many of these products in an effort to identify active ingredients and understand their effects in the body. Also consider the possibility that what's on the label may not be what's in the bottle. Analyses of dietary supplements sometimes find differences between labeled and actual ingredients.

Women who are looking for alternatives to MHT should be aware that CAM therapies are not their only option. Certain lifestyle changes can contribute to healthy aging, including during the menopausal transition. For example, quitting smoking, eating a healthy diet, and exercising regularly have been shown to reduce the risks of heart disease and osteoporosis.

NCCAM Research on CAM for Menopausal Symptoms

NCCAM supports a number of studies on CAM treatments (such as botanicals and mind-body practices) for menopausal symptoms, as do some of the other institutes and centers at NIH. Recent examples of NCCAM-funded projects include the following:

- An initiative to improve measures of hot flashes, which is expected to add to the understanding of hot flashes and to aid future clinical studies

- A study of whether black cohosh can help with the anxiety that may be experienced as a symptom of menopause

- A study to identify botanicals from Central America that have been used by the native population for menopausal symptoms and to develop and test standardized extracts from these plants

- Several studies looking at the effect of acupuncture on the recurrence and severity of hot flashes in postmenopausal women and others who may suffer from hot flashes, such as men being treated for prostate cancer

- A study to determine the effects of mindfulness-based stress reduction (a type of meditation) on hot flashes in menopausal women

- A study to understand how soy supplements might affect hot flashes and night sweats

In addition, NCCAM and other NIH components are cofunding an initiative to establish a network of research centers looking at potential new treatments for menopausal symptoms.

Chapter 86

Mental Health Care and CAM

Chapter Contents

Section 86.1—Overview of CAM Used in Mental
      Health Care 574

Section 86.2—Alcohol Addiction and
      Electroacupuncture 579

Section 86.3—Attention Deficit Hyperactivity
      Disorder (ADHD) and CAM 580

Section 86.4—Anxiety and Self-Hypnosis 582

Section 86.5—Posttraumatic Stress Disorder
      and Acupuncture 583

Section 86.1

Overview of CAM Used in Mental Health Care

From "Alternative Approaches to Mental Health Care," by the Substance Abuse and Mental Health Services Administration (SAMHSA, mentalhealth.samhsa.gov), part of the U.S. Department of Health and Human Services, April 2003. Reviewed and revised by David A. Cooke, MD, FACP, January 23, 2010.

What Are Alternative Approaches to Mental Health Care?

An alternative approach to mental health care is one that emphasizes the interrelationship between mind, body, and spirit. Although some alternative approaches have a long history, many remain controversial. The National Center for Complementary and Alternative Medicine at the National Institutes of Health was created in 1992 to help evaluate alternative methods of treatment and to integrate those that are effective into mainstream health care practice. It is crucial, however, to consult with your health care providers about the approaches you are using to achieve mental wellness.

Self-Help

Many people with mental illnesses find that self-help groups are an invaluable resource for recovery and for empowerment. Self-help generally refers to groups or meetings that have the following characteristics:

- Involve people who have similar needs

- Are facilitated by a consumer, survivor, or other layperson

- Assist people to deal with a "life-disrupting" event, such as a death, abuse, serious accident, addiction, or diagnosis of a physical, emotional, or mental disability, for oneself or a relative

- Are operated on an informal, free-of-charge, and nonprofit basis

- Provide support and education

- Are voluntary, anonymous, and confidential

Diet and Nutrition

Adjusting both diet and nutrition may help some people with mental illnesses manage their symptoms and promote recovery. For example, research suggests that eliminating milk and wheat products can reduce the severity of symptoms for some people who have schizophrenia and some children with autism. Similarly, some holistic/natural physicians use herbal treatments, B-complex vitamins, riboflavin, magnesium, and thiamine to treat anxiety, autism, depression, drug-induced psychoses, and hyperactivity. [Editor's Note: Due to a lack of good-quality research, it is unclear whether improvements in the above listed disorders are due to these interventions, as opposed to other factors. Many of these conditions have significant natural variation, and it is difficult to accurately measure change.]

Pastoral Counseling

Some people prefer to seek help for mental health problems from their pastor, rabbi, or priest, rather than from therapists who are not affiliated with a religious community. Counselors working within traditional faith communities increasingly are recognizing the need to incorporate psychotherapy and/or medication, along with prayer and spirituality, to effectively help some people with mental disorders.

Animal-Assisted Therapies

Working with an animal (or animals) under the guidance of a health care professional may benefit some people with mental illness by facilitating positive changes, such as increased empathy and enhanced socialization skills. Animals can be used as part of group therapy programs to encourage communication and increase the ability to focus. Developing self-esteem and reducing loneliness and anxiety are just some potential benefits of individual-animal therapy.

Expressive Therapies

Art therapy: Drawing, painting, and sculpting help many people to reconcile inner conflicts, release deeply repressed emotions, and foster self-awareness, as well as personal growth. Some mental health providers use art therapy as both a diagnostic tool and as a way to help treat disorders such as depression, abuse-related trauma, and schizophrenia. You may be able to find a therapist in your area who has received special training and certification in art therapy.

Dance/movement therapy: Some people find that their spirits soar when they let their feet fly. Others—particularly those who prefer more structure or who feel they have "two left feet"—gain the same sense of release and inner peace from the Eastern martial arts, such as Aikido and Tai Chi. Those who are recovering from physical, sexual, or emotional abuse may find these techniques especially helpful for gaining a sense of ease with their own bodies. The underlying premise to dance/movement therapy is that it can help a person integrate the emotional, physical, and cognitive facets of "self."

Music/sound therapy: It is no coincidence that many people turn on soothing music to relax or fast tunes to help feel upbeat. Research suggests that music stimulates the body's natural "feel good" chemicals (opiates and endorphins). This stimulation results in improved blood flow, blood pressure, pulse rate, breathing, and posture changes. Music or sound therapy has been used to treat disorders such as stress, grief, depression, schizophrenia, and autism in children, and to diagnose mental health needs.

Culturally Based Healing Arts

Traditional Oriental medicine (such as acupuncture, shiatsu, and Reiki), Indian systems of health care (such as Ayurveda and yoga), and Native American healing practices (such as the Sweat Lodge and Talking Circles) all incorporate the following beliefs:

- Wellness is a state of balance between the spiritual, physical, and mental/emotional "selves."

- An imbalance of forces within the body is the cause of illness.

- Herbal/natural remedies, combined with sound nutrition, exercise, and meditation/prayer, will correct this imbalance.

Acupuncture: The Chinese practice of inserting needles into the body at specific points manipulates the body's flow of energy to balance the endocrine system. This manipulation regulates functions such as heart rate, body temperature, and respiration, as well as sleep patterns and emotional changes. Acupuncture has been used in clinics to assist people with substance abuse disorders through detoxification; to relieve stress and anxiety; to treat attention deficit and hyperactivity disorder in children; to reduce symptoms of depression; and to help people with physical ailments.

Ayurveda: Ayurvedic medicine is described as "knowledge of how to live." It incorporates an individualized regimen—such as diet, meditation, herbal preparations, or other techniques—to treat a variety of conditions, including depression, to facilitate lifestyle changes, and to teach people how to release stress and tension through yoga or transcendental meditation.

Yoga/meditation: Practitioners of this ancient Indian system of health care use breathing exercises, posture, stretches, and meditation to balance the body's energy centers. Yoga is used in combination with other treatment for depression, anxiety, and stress-related disorders.

Native American traditional practices: Ceremonial dances, chants, and cleansing rituals are part of Indian Health Service programs to heal depression, stress, trauma (including those related to physical and sexual abuse), and substance abuse.

Cuentos: Based on folktales, this form of therapy originated in Puerto Rico. The stories used contain healing themes and models of behavior such as self-transformation and endurance through adversity. Cuentos is used primarily to help Hispanic children recover from depression and other mental health problems related to leaving one's homeland and living in a foreign culture.

Relaxation and Stress Reduction Techniques

Biofeedback: Learning to control muscle tension and "involuntary" body functioning, such as heart rate and skin temperature, can be a path to mastering one's fears. It is used in combination with, or as an alternative to, medication to treat disorders such as anxiety, panic, and phobias. For example, a person can learn to "retrain" his or her breathing habits in stressful situations to induce relaxation and decrease hyperventilation. Some preliminary research indicates it may offer an additional tool for treating schizophrenia and depression.

Guided imagery or visualization: This process involves going into a state of deep relaxation and creating a mental image of recovery and wellness. Physicians, nurses, and mental health providers occasionally use this approach to treat alcohol and drug addictions, depression, panic disorders, phobias, and stress.

Massage therapy: The underlying principle of this approach is that rubbing, kneading, brushing, and tapping a person's muscles can help release tension and pent-up emotions. It has been used to treat trauma-related depression and stress. A highly unregulated industry, certification for massage therapy varies widely from state to state. Some states have strict guidelines, while others have none.

Technology-Based Applications

The boom in electronic tools at home and in the office makes access to mental health information just a telephone call or a mouse click away. Technology is also making treatment more widely available in once-isolated areas.

Telemedicine: Plugging into video and computer technology is a relatively new innovation in health care. It allows both consumers and providers in remote or rural areas to gain access to mental health or specialty expertise. Telemedicine can enable consulting providers to speak to and observe patients directly. It also can be used in education and training programs for generalist clinicians.

Telephone counseling: Active listening skills are a hallmark of telephone counselors. These also provide information and referral to interested callers. For many people telephone counseling often is a first step to receiving in-depth mental health care. Research shows that such counseling from specially trained mental health providers reaches many people who otherwise might not get the help they need. Before calling, be sure to check the telephone number for service fees; a 900 area code means you will be billed for the call, an 800 or 888 area code means the call is toll-free.

Electronic communications: Technologies such as the internet, bulletin boards, and electronic mail lists provide access directly to consumers and the public on a wide range of information. Online consumer groups can exchange information, experiences, and views on mental health, treatment systems, alternative medicine, and other related topics.

Radio psychiatry: Another relative newcomer to therapy, radio psychiatry was first introduced in the United States in 1976. Radio psychiatrists and psychologists provide advice, information, and referrals in response to a variety of mental health questions from callers.

The American Psychiatric Association and the American Psychological Association have issued ethical guidelines for the role of psychiatrists and psychologists on radio shows.

This text does not cover every alternative approach to mental health. A range of other alternative approaches—psychodrama, hypnotherapy, recreational, and Outward Bound-type nature programs—offer opportunities to explore mental wellness. Before jumping into any alternative therapy, learn as much as you can about it. In addition to talking with your health care practitioner, you may want to visit your local library, book store, health food store, or holistic health care clinic for more information. Also, before receiving services, check to be sure the provider is properly certified by an appropriate accrediting agency.

Section 86.2

Alcohol Addiction and Electroacupuncture

From "Electroacupuncture May Help Alcohol Addiction," by the National Center for Complementary and Alternative Medicine (NCCAM, nccam.nih .gov), part of the National Institutes of Health, October 2008.

Alcohol and drug addiction pose serious medical, social, and economic problems in the United States. However, finding effective treatments for addiction is challenging. Many people relapse due to intense cravings and/or painful withdrawal symptoms. Electroacupuncture (acupuncture combined with electrical stimulation) is currently being studied as a possible treatment option, and preliminary evidence suggests that electroacupuncture can counteract addiction by affecting related chemicals (opiates) in the brain.

In a study funded through a research center program jointly sponsored by NCCAM and the National Institute on Alcohol Abuse and Alcoholism (NIAAA), researchers examined the effects of electroacupuncture on alcohol intake by alcohol-preferring rats. After being trained to drink alcohol voluntarily and then subjected to alcohol deprivation, the rats received either electroacupuncture or sham electroacupuncture, and their alcohol intake was monitored after the intervention. Some rats were also pretreated with naltrexone (a drug that blocks the effects of opiates), so researchers could look for evidence that opiate mechanisms are involved in electroacupuncture's effects.

The results showed that electroacupuncture reduced the rats' alcohol intake. The researchers also found that injecting the rats with naltrexone blocked the effect of electroacupuncture on alcohol intake—an indication that this effect may be through the brain's opiate system. On the basis of their findings, the researchers recommend rigorous clinical trials to study the effects of electroacupuncture in alcohol-addicted people. They also recommend further investigation of how electroacupuncture affects the brain.

Reference

Overstreet DH, Cui C-L, Ma Y-Y, et al. Electroacupuncture reduces voluntary alcohol intake in alcohol-preferring rats via an opiate-sensitive mechanism. *Neurochemical Research*. 2008;33(10):2166–2170.

Section 86.3

Attention Deficit Hyperactivity Disorder (ADHD) and CAM

From "St. John's Wort Shows No Impact on the Symptoms of ADHD," by the National Center for Complementary and Alternative Medicine (NCCAM, nccam.nih.gov), part of the National Institutes of Health (NIH), 2008.

According to the National Institute of Mental Health (NIMH)at NIH, attention deficit hyperactivity disorder (ADHD) affects 3 to 5 percent of children in the United States and it is one of the most common mental disorders that develop in children. NIMH states that children with ADHD have impaired functioning in multiple settings, including home, school, and in relationships with peers. Children with chronic conditions like ADHD are reported to have higher rates of complementary and alternative medicine use and may turn to dietary and herbal supplements such as St. John's wort. However, according to authors of an NCCAM-funded study, St. John's wort does not appear to have an impact on the symptoms of ADHD in children and adolescents.

Researchers at Bastyr University conducted an 8-week randomized, placebo-controlled, double-blind trial of St. John's wort among a volunteer sample of 54 children aged 6 to 17 years with ADHD. Participants were randomly assigned to receive 300 mg of *Hypericum perforatum* (St. John's wort) standardized to 0.3 percent hypericin—an active ingredient in St. John's wort—or placebo three times daily for 8 weeks. The participants were evaluated for changes in inattentiveness and hyperactivity from baseline at weeks 1, 2, 4, 6, and 8.

While symptom improvement was noted in both the treatment and the placebo groups, the data suggest that St. John's wort had no additional benefit beyond that of placebo for treating symptoms of ADHD.

This study used a preparation of St. John's wort with a standardized hypericin content. However the researchers note that studies involving St. John's wort also standardized to hyperforin—another active ingredient in St. John's wort—could be beneficial. Hyperforin is believed to inhibit reuptake of key brain chemicals—serotonin, dopamine, and norepinephrine. The authors note that hyperforin is highly unstable and can become inactive quickly. The researchers believe that if a St. John's wort product with a higher and more stable hyperforin content became available, it would be worthy of further investigation in ADHD.

Reference

Weber W, Vander Stoep A, McCarty RL, et al. Hypericum perforatum (St. John's Wort) for Attention-Deficit/Hyperactivity Disorder in Children and Adolescents. *JAMA*. 2008;299(22):2633–2641.

Section 86.4

Anxiety and Self-Hypnosis

From "Self-Hypnosis Beneficial for Women Undergoing Breast Biopsy," by the National Center for Complementary and Alternative Medicine (NC-CAM, nccam.nih.gov), part of the National Institutes of Health, December 2006.

An NCCAM-funded trial found that women who used self-hypnosis during a type of core needle breast biopsy experienced anxiety relief and reduced pain when compared with standard care.

A large core needle breast biopsy is usually an outpatient procedure that limits the use of anesthetic. Women having this procedure often experience anxiety because of the possibility of a cancer diagnosis in addition to the anxiety that patients typically experience during a medical procedure. In this randomized, controlled trial researchers at Beth Israel Deaconess Medical Center in Boston recruited 236 women who were randomly assigned to receive standard care, structured empathic attention from a research assistant, or guided self-hypnotic relaxation during the biopsy.

The study found that both self-hypnosis and empathic attention reduced pain and anxiety during the procedure. Self-hypnosis provided greater anxiety relief than empathic attention. Neither intervention increased procedure time or significantly increased cost. As a result, the researchers suggest that self-hypnosis appears attractive for outpatient pain management.

Reference

Elvira V. Lang, Kevin S. Berbaum, Salomao Faintuch, et al. Adjunctive self-hypnotic relaxation for outpatient medical procedures: A prospective randomized trial with women undergoing large core breast biopsy. *Pain,* December 2006.

Section 86.5

Posttraumatic Stress Disorder and Acupuncture

From "Acupuncture May Help Symptoms of Posttraumatic Stress Disorder," by the National Center for Complementary and Alternative Medicine (NC-CAM, nccam.nih.gov), part of the National Institutes of Health, June 2007.

A pilot study shows that acupuncture may help people with posttraumatic stress disorder. Posttraumatic stress disorder (PTSD) is an anxiety disorder that can develop after exposure to a terrifying event or ordeal in which grave physical harm occurred or was threatened. Traumatic events that may trigger PTSD include violent personal assaults, natural or human-caused disasters, accidents, or military combat.

Michael Hollifield, MD, and colleagues conducted a clinical trial examining the effect of acupuncture on the symptoms of PTSD. The researchers analyzed depression, anxiety, and impairment in 73 people with a diagnosis of PTSD. The participants were assigned to receive either acupuncture or group cognitive-behavioral therapy over 12 weeks, or were assigned to a wait-list as part of the control group. The people in the control group were offered treatment or referral for treatment at the end of their participation.

The researchers found that acupuncture provided treatment effects similar to group cognitive-behavioral therapy; both interventions were superior to the control group. Additionally, treatment effects of both the acupuncture and the group therapy were maintained for 3 months after the end of treatment.

The limitations of the study are consistent with preliminary research. For example, this study had a small group of participants that lacked diversity, and the results do not account for outside factors that may have affected the treatments' results.

Reference

Michael Hollifield, Nityamo Sinclair-Lian, Teddy D. Warner, and Richard Hammerschlag. Acupuncture for Posttraumatic Stress Disorder: A

Randomized Controlled Pilot Trial. *The Journal of Nervous and Mental Disease,* June 2007.

Chapter 87

Sleep Disorders and CAM

A good night's sleep is more than a luxury. Sleep is as important to survival as food and water. On too little, we humans don't function well—for example, we run a higher risk of accidents, we sometimes perform poorly at work or school, and our moods can turn sour.

A sleepless night or two isn't a medical emergency. However, if difficulties persist, a sleep disorder may be involved. People with sleep disorders may have difficulty falling or staying asleep or waking up in the morning, fall asleep at inappropriate times, sleep too much, or show unusual behaviors during sleep. Important new research, including studies supported by the National Institutes of Health (NIH), has linked lack of sleep with obesity, diabetes, and other related conditions. The National Center for Complementary and Alternative Medicine (NCCAM) is supporting a number of research studies on potential treatment options for sleep disorders using complementary and alternative medicine (CAM).

"Sleep disorders are an important public health issue that is receiving serious attention from NCCAM and several other components of NIH," said NCCAM Director Stephen E. Straus, MD.

As many as 70 million Americans—about one quarter of the population—experience sleep disorders; half of this group have chronic sleep problems. Conventional therapies are available for most sleep disorders, but for some people they don't work well, cause unwanted side effects, or cost too much. As a result, many people turn to CAM therapies.

From "Can't Sleep? Science Is Seeking New Answers," by the National Institutes of Health (NIH, www.nih.gov), Summer 2005.

According to the 2002 National Health Interview Survey, 2.2 percent of all adults in the survey who used CAM did so for sleep problems. This represents approximately 1.6 million U.S. adults. CAM therapies commonly used for sleep problems include dietary supplements (such as melatonin and valerian); approaches that emphasize the interaction between the mind and the body (such as meditation); and therapies that are part of non-Western traditional medical systems (such as acupuncture and yoga).

"While some CAM products used to treat sleep disorders are already available to consumers, in most cases they have not been proven to be efficacious through rigorous research," explained Nancy J. Pearson, PhD, NCCAM Program Officer and member of the Trans-NIH Sleep Research Coordinating Committee. "There is very little knowledge about whether CAM therapies for sleep disorders work, and, if so, how they work. NCCAM is supporting research to help answer these questions."

Types and Causes of Sleep Disorders

Sleep problems can start with a sudden event. For example, a job loss can lead to nighttime worries, which in turn can lead to trouble sleeping. When a sleep problem occurs without another identified disease or condition, it is referred to as a primary sleep disorder. However, in many cases, sleep disorders are associated with other causes. Some circumstances and illnesses that can lead to sleep problems are as follows:

- Because of lifestyles or work schedules, sleep just isn't a priority for some people. Stress from hectic schedules can make it difficult to relax and fall asleep.

- The body's internal clock programs people to feel sleepy during the nighttime and to be active during daylight hours. When that clock goes off-kilter, sleep becomes difficult. For example, travelers who fly across multiple time zones quickly get "jet lag" because they cannot maintain a regular sleep-wake schedule.

- People who work at night and try to sleep during the day are constantly fighting their internal clocks. This puts them at risk for disturbed sleep. Without adequate rest, they are more likely to make errors or have accidents at work.

- Sleep disorders often occur in people who have a chronic disease that involves pain or infection, a neurological or psychiatric disorder, or an alcohol or substance abuse disorder. (These are sometimes called secondary sleep disorders.) For these individuals, sleep becomes difficult, potentially worsening the other medical condition, and affecting the person's health and safety, mood and behavior, and quality of life.

Sleep problems can arise during any period of life:

- In children, inadequate sleep may lead to daytime sleepiness, which can interfere with a child's ability to learn in school and perform well in other activities. Sleep-deprived children may also tend to fall or have other accidents that lead to injury. Many children who are chronically deprived of sleep may not seem sleepy and may even appear to be overactive. Chronic sleep loss in these children may be overlooked or mistakenly attributed to hyperactivity or other behavior disorders.

- Teenagers are notorious for getting too little sleep as they burn the midnight oil to study for exams or socialize late into the night. Body clocks actually shift during these years, so teens often stay up late and sleep beyond the morning hours. This tendency, when combined with an increased need for sleep in adolescence and an early first bell at most high schools, can put teenagers at risk for sleep disorders.

- Women going through the menopausal transition are more likely to experience sleep problems than are other women.

- Older adults' sleep is often easily disturbed by noise and other environmental factors. Older people are also more likely to have chronic health conditions or pain that make it more difficult for them to get into the deep, restful stages of sleep.

- Certain medical conditions, such as rheumatoid arthritis, Parkinson disease, or chronic pain, may contribute to sleep problems.

NCCAM Research

NCCAM supports studies on whether certain CAM therapies might be helpful for sleep disorders. Some examples include the following:

- University of Washington researchers are testing the herb valerian in healthy older adults who experience sleep disturbances. At Emory University, valerian is being studied in people with

Parkinson disease, and at the University of Virginia, it is being studied in people with rheumatoid arthritis.

- Researchers at Brigham and Women's Hospital in Boston are studying a program of yoga and relaxation exercises as a treatment for insomnia.

- University of Chicago researchers are studying the mechanism of action of hops, an herb that has been used both alone and in combination with valerian for sleep problems.

- A preliminary study at Brigham and Women's Hospital will determine the mechanism of action of vitamin B_{12} as a treatment for a form of delayed sleep phase syndrome that affects more than half of blind individuals and is also common in sighted individuals. In delayed sleep phase syndrome, a person's internal body clock is out of sync, causing difficulty falling asleep until very late at night and difficult waking up in the morning.

- Researchers at the University of Pennsylvania are comparing the effects of a low-dose melatonin supplement, a high-dose melatonin supplement, and a placebo in elderly people who have insomnia and a low level of natural melatonin in the body.

- At the University of North Carolina, researchers are investigating whether high-intensity light, installed in common areas in a nursing home, could lessen the problems of sleep/wake disorders, depressive symptoms, and agitation—all frequent, difficult issues for people with Alzheimer disease. At Harvard University, researchers are studying the effects of blue light therapy on sleep cycles.

- At the University of Arizona, researchers are examining the impact of two different homeopathic remedies on sleep patterns in adults.

Along with supporting studies, NCCAM also participates in other activities to improve the state of scientific knowledge about treatments for sleep disorders. First, NCCAM is part of the Trans-NIH Sleep Research Coordinating Committee, which coordinates research efforts across NIH and issues a report each year. NCCAM is supporting—along with 12 other NIH institutes, centers, and offices—an initiative to stimulate research on sleep and sleep disorders.

Second, NCCAM cosponsors conferences and workshops on areas related to sleep disorders. In 2004, NCCAM cosponsored a conference on the biology of the brain's pineal gland, which produces melatonin.

In June 2005, NCCAM was one of several sponsors of the State-of-the-Science Conference on insomnia at NIH. At that conference, the invited panel of experts called for further research on commonly used CAM treatments for insomnia, including supplements like melatonin and valerian, and mind-body practices such as tai chi and yoga. Acupuncture and light therapy were also mentioned as treatments that call for additional evaluation.

Because the use of melatonin supplements by the public for sleep problems is widespread, NCCAM requested and funded a report published by the Agency for Healthcare Research and Quality that analyzed the existing scientific evidence on this topic. The authors found that melatonin appears safe for short-term use, but that it may not be effective for treating most primary sleep disorders, such as jet lag. It may offer some benefit for delayed sleep phase syndrome. How melatonin works in humans is not well understood, and more research is needed to answer many questions about this therapy.

"Many people struggle with getting enough sleep or the right kind of sleep," said Dr. Pearson. "Better sleep improves our quality of life. NCCAM, on its own and in collaboration with other institutes and centers at NIH, is committed to supporting research to uncover potential new options from CAM for those with sleep problems."

Tips for Better Sleep

- Follow a regular sleep schedule. It is helpful to go to sleep and wake up at the same times as much as possible, even on weekends.

- Exercise at a regular time each day, at least 3 hours before bedtime.

- Get some natural, outdoor light each day.

- Avoid caffeine late in the day.

- Don't drink alcohol to help you sleep.

- Avoid smoking.

- Create a safe and comfortable place to sleep (quiet, dark, and well ventilated).

- Develop a nighttime routine that helps you slow down and relax.

- If you're having trouble falling asleep after about 15 minutes, get up, do a quiet activity, and return to bed when you are sleepy.

- Try these tips and record your sleep and sleep-related activities in a sleep diary. If problems continue, discuss the sleep diary with your doctor.

Source for tips: National Institute on Aging, with credit also to the National Sleep Foundation.

Part Nine

Additional Help and Information

Chapter 88

Glossary of Terms Related to Alternative and Complementary Medicine

acupuncture: A family of procedures that originated in traditional Chinese medicine. Acupuncture is the stimulation of specific points on the body by a variety of techniques, including the insertion of thin metal needles through the skin. It is intended to remove blockages in the flow of qi and restore and maintain health.[1]

aromatherapy: Aromatherapy is the use of essential oils from plants to support and balance the mind, body, and spirit. Aromatherapy may be combined with other complementary treatments like massage therapy and acupuncture, as well as with standard treatments.[2]

Ayurvedic medicine: Ayurvedic medicine (also called Ayurveda) is one of the world's oldest medical systems. It originated in India and has evolved there over thousands of years. In the United States, Ayurvedic medicine is considered complementary and alternative medicine. The aim of Ayurvedic medicine is to integrate and balance the body, mind, and spirit. This is believed to help prevent illness and promote wellness.[1]

biofeedback: A method of learning to voluntarily control certain body functions such as heartbeat, blood pressure, and muscle tension with the help of a special machine. This method can help control pain.[2]

Definitions in this chapter were compiled from documents published by several public domain sources. Terms marked 1 are from publications by the National Center for Complementary and Alternative Medicine (nccam.nih.gov); terms marked 2 are from the National Cancer Institute (cancer.gov); terms marked 3 are from the Office of Dietary Supplements (ods.od.nih.gov); and terms marked 4 are from the Office on Women's Health (womenshealth.gov).

biologically based therapy: This area of CAM includes, but is not limited to, botanicals, animal-derived extracts, vitamins, minerals, fatty acids, amino acids, proteins, prebiotics and probiotics, whole diets, and functional foods.[1]

botanical: A plant or plant part valued for its medicinal or therapeutic properties, flavor, and/or scent. Herbs are a subset of botanicals. Products made from botanicals that are used to maintain or improve health may be called herbal products, botanical products, or phytomedicines.[3]

chelation therapy: Chelation therapy is an investigational therapy using a man-made amino acid, called EDTA (ethylene-diamine-tetra-acetic acid). It is added to the blood through a vein. Disodium EDTA has been in widespread use since the 1970s for disease of the heart and arteries.[1]

chiropractic: A whole medical system that focuses on the relationship between the body's structure—mainly the spine—and function. Practitioners perform adjustments (also called manipulation) with the goal of correcting structural alignment problems to assist the body in healing.[1]

clinical trial: A type of research study that uses volunteers to test the safety and efficacy (the ability to produce a beneficial effect) of new methods of screening (checking for disease when there are no symptoms), prevention, diagnosis, or treatment of a disease. Also called a clinical study.[3]

complementary and alternative medicine: A group of diverse medical and health care systems, practices, and products that are not presently considered to be part of conventional medicine. Complementary medicine is used together with conventional medicine, and alternative medicine is used in place of conventional medicine.[1]

conventional medicine: Medicine as practiced by holders of MD (medical doctor) or DO (doctor of osteopathy) degrees and by their allied health professionals such as physical therapists, psychologists, and registered nurses.[1]

Daily Value (DV): A term used on a food or dietary supplement product label to describe the recommended levels of intake of a nutrient. The percent Daily Value (% DV) represents how much of a nutrient is provided in one serving of the food or dietary supplement. For example, the DV for calcium is 1,000 mg (milligrams); a food that has

200 mg of calcium per serving would state on the label that the % DV for calcium is 20%.[3]

dietary supplement: A product that is intended to supplement the diet; contains one or more dietary ingredients (including vitamins, minerals, herbs or other botanicals, amino acids, and certain other substances) or their constituents; and is intended to be taken by mouth, in forms such as tablet, capsule, powder, softgel, gelcap, or liquid.[1]

energy medicine: Energy medicine is a domain in CAM that deals with energy fields of two types: veritable, which can be measured, and putative, which have yet to be measured. Practitioners of energy medicine believe that illness results from disturbances of these subtle energies (the biofield).[1]

guided imagery: A type of CAM that encourages imagining a pleasant scene to take your mind off your pain or anxiety.[4]

herbal supplements: One type of dietary supplement. An herb is a plant or plant part (such as leaves, flowers, or seeds) that is used for its flavor, scent, and/or therapeutic properties. Botanical is often used as a synonym for herb. An herbal supplement may contain a single herb or mixtures of herbs.[1]

homeopathy: A whole medical system that originated in Europe. Homeopathy seeks to stimulate the body's ability to heal itself by giving very small doses of highly diluted substances that in larger doses would produce illness or symptoms (an approach called "like cures like").[1]

hypnosis: A trance-like state in which a person becomes more aware and focused and is more open to suggestion.[2]

magnet therapy: A magnet produces a measurable force called a magnetic field. Magnets are used for many different types of pain, including foot pain and back pain from conditions such as arthritis and fibromyalgia. Magnets in products such as magnetic patches and disks, shoe insoles, bracelets, and mattress pads are used for pain in the foot, wrist, back, and other parts of the body.[1]

manipulation: The application of controlled force to a joint, moving it beyond the normal range of motion in an effort to aid in restoring health. Manipulation may be performed as a part of other therapies or whole medical systems, including chiropractic medicine, massage, and naturopathy.[1]

manipulative and body-based practices: A group of CAM interventions and therapies that include chiropractic and osteopathic manipulation, massage therapy, Tui Na, reflexology, Rolfing, Bowen technique, Trager bodywork, Alexander technique, Feldenkrais method, and a host of others.[1]

massage: Pressing, rubbing, and moving muscles and other soft tissues of the body, primarily by using the hands and fingers. The aim is to increase the flow of blood and oxygen to the massaged area.[1]

meditation: Refers to a variety of techniques or practices intended to focus or control attention. Most of them are rooted in Eastern religious or spiritual traditions. These techniques have been used by many different cultures throughout the world for thousands of years.[1]

mind-body medicine: Medicine that focuses on the interactions among the brain, mind, body, and behavior, and the powerful ways in which emotional, mental, social, spiritual, and behavioral factors can directly affect health. It regards as fundamental an approach that respects and enhances each person's capacity for self-knowledge and self-care, and it emphasizes techniques that are grounded in this approach.[1]

mineral: In nutrition, an inorganic substance found in the earth that is required to maintain health.[3]

naturopathy: A whole medical system that originated in Europe. Naturopathy aims to support the body's ability to heal itself through the use of dietary and lifestyle changes together with CAM therapies such as herbs, massage, and joint manipulation.[1]

omega-3 fatty acids: Polyunsaturated fatty acids that come from foods such as fish, fish oil, vegetable oil (primarily canola and soybean), walnuts, and wheat germ. Omega-3s are important in a number of bodily functions, including the movement of calcium and other substances in and out of cells, the relaxation and contraction of muscles, blood clotting, digestion, fertility, cell division, and growth. In addition, omega-3s are thought to protect against heart disease, reduce inflammation, and lower triglyceride levels.[1]

probiotics: Live microorganisms (in most cases, bacteria) that are similar to beneficial microorganisms found in the human gut. They are also called friendly bacteria or good bacteria. Probiotics are available to consumers mainly in the form of dietary supplements and foods.[1]

qi: In traditional Chinese medicine, the vital energy or life force proposed to regulate a person's spiritual, emotional, mental, and physical health and to be influenced by the opposing forces of yin and yang.[1]

reflexology: A type of massage, which applies pressure to the feet (or sometimes the hands or ears), to promote relaxation or healing in other parts of the body.[1]

Reiki: A healing practice that originated in Japan. Reiki practitioners place their hands lightly on or just above the person receiving treatment, with the goal of facilitating the person's own healing response.[1]

spirituality: Spirituality may be defined as an individual's sense of peace, purpose, and connection to others, and beliefs about the meaning of life. Spirituality may be found and expressed through an organized religion or in other ways.[2]

tai chi: Tai chi, which originated in China as a martial art, is a mind-body practice in complementary and alternative medicine. Tai chi is sometimes referred to as moving meditation—practitioners move their bodies slowly, gently, and with awareness, while breathing deeply.[1]

traditional Chinese medicine: A whole medical system that originated in China. It is based on the concept that disease results from disruption in the flow of qi and imbalance in the forces of yin and yang. Practices such as herbs, meditation, massage, and acupuncture seek to aid healing by restoring the yin-yang balance and the flow of qi.[1]

vegan: A person who does not eat any foods that come from animals, including meat, eggs, and dairy products.[2]

vegetarian: A person who eats a diet free of meat. Lacto-vegetarians consume milk and milk products along with plant-based foods. They do not eat eggs. Lacto-ovo vegetarians eat eggs and milk and milk products, in addition to plant-based foods.[4]

vitamin: A nutrient that the body needs in small amounts to function and maintain health. Examples are vitamins A, C, and E.[3]

whole medical system: A complete system of theory and practice that has evolved over time in different cultures and apart from conventional medicine. Examples of whole medical systems include traditional Chinese medicine, Ayurvedic medicine, homeopathy, and naturopathy.[1]

yin and yang: The concept of two opposing yet complementary forces described in traditional Chinese medicine. Yin represents cold, slow, or passive aspects of the person, while yang represents hot, excited, or active aspects. A major theory is that health is achieved through balancing yin and yang and disease is caused by an imbalance leading to a blockage in the flow of qi.[1]

yoga: A mind-body practice in complementary and alternative medicine with origins in ancient Indian philosophy. The various styles of yoga that people use for health purposes typically combine physical postures, breathing techniques, and meditation or relaxation.[1]

Chapter 89

Directory of Organizations That Provide Information about Alternative and Complementary Medicine

Government Agencies That Provide Information about Alternative and Complementary Medicine

Agency for Healthcare Research and Quality
Office of Communications and Knowledge Transfer
540 Gaither Road, Second Floor
Rockville, MD 20850
Phone: 301-427-1364
Fax: 301-427-1873
Website: www.ahrq.gov

Centers for Disease Control and Prevention
1600 Clifton Road
Atlanta, GA 30333
Toll-Free: 800-CDC-INFO (232-4636)
Phone: 404-639-3311
Website: www.cdc.gov
E-mail: cdcinfo@cdc.gov

Healthfinder®
National Health Information Center
P.O. Box 1133
Washington, DC 20013-1133
Toll-Free: 800-336-4797
Phone: 301-565-4167
Fax: 301-984-4256
Website: www.healthfinder.gov
E-mail: healthfinder@nhic.org

National Cancer Institute
6116 Executive Blvd. Rm 3036A
Bethesda, MD 20892-8322
Toll-Free: 800-4-CANCER (422-6237)
TTY Toll-Free: 800-332-8615
Website: www.cancer.gov
E-mail: cancergovstaff@mail.nih.gov

Resources in this chapter were compiled from several sources deemed reliable; all contact information was verified and updated in January 2010.

National Center for Complementary and Alternative Medicine

National Institutes of Health
NCCAM Clearinghouse
P.O. 7923
Gaithersburg, MD 20898-7923
Toll-Free: 888-644-6226
TTY: 866-464-3615
Fax: 866-464-3616
Website: nccam.nih.gov
E-mail: info@nccam.nih.gov

National Institute of Arthritis and Musculoskeletal and Skin Diseases

National Institutes of Health
1 AMS Circle
Bethesda, MD 20892-3675
Toll Free: 877-22-NIAMS
(226-4267)
TTY: 301-5652966
Phone: 301-495-4484
Fax: 301-718-6366
Website: www.niams.nih.gov
E-mail: NIAMSinfo@mail.nih.gov

National Institute of Diabetes, Digestive and Kidney Diseases

Building 31, Rm. 9A06
31 Center Drive, MSC 2560
Bethesda, MD 20892-2560
Phone: 301-496-3583
Website: www.niddk.nih.gov

National Institute of Neurological Disorders and Stroke

NIH Neurological Institute
P.O. Box 5801
Bethesda, MD 20824
Toll-Free: 800-352-9424
Phone: 301-496-5751
TTY: 301-468-5981
Website: www.ninds.nih.gov
E-mail: braininfo@ninds.nih.gov

National Institutes of Health

9000 Rockville Pike
Bethesda, MD 20892
Phone: 301-496-4000
TTY: 301-402-9612
Website: www.nih.gov
E-mail: NIHinfo@od.nih.gov

National Institute on Aging

Building 31, Room 5C27
31 Center Drive, MSC 2292
Bethesda, MD 20892
Phone: 301-496-1752
Fax: 301-496-1072
Website: www.nia.nih.gov

Office of Dietary Supplements

Suite 3B01
6100 Executive Boulevard
Bethesda, MD 20892-7517
Phone: 301-435-2920
Fax: 301-480-1845
Website: dietary-supplements
.info.nih.gov
E-mail: ods@nih.gov

Substance Abuse and Mental Health Services Administration

SAMHSA's Health Information Network
P.O. Box 2345
Rockville, MD 20847-2345
Phone: 877-SAMHSA-7 (726-4727)
TTY: 800-487-4889
Fax: 240-221-4292
Website: www.samhsa.gov
E-mail: SHIN@samhsa.hhs.gov

U.S. Department of Health and Human Services

200 Independent Avenue, SW
Washington, DC 20201
Toll-Free: 877-696-6775
Website: www.hhs.gov

U.S. Food and Drug Administration

10903 New Hampshire Avenue
Silver Spring, MD 20903
Toll-Free: 888-463-6332
Website: www.fda.gov

U.S. National Library of Medicine

8600 Rockville Pike
Bethesda, MD 20894
Toll-Free: 888-FIND-NLM (346-3656)
Phone: 301-594-5983
TDD: 800-735-2258
Fax: 301-402-1384
Website: www.nlm.nih.gov
E-mail: custserv@nlm.nih.gov

Private Agencies That Provide Information about Alternative and Complementary Medicine

Academy for Guided Imagery

10780 Santa Monica Boulevard, Suite 290
Los Angeles, CA 90025
Toll-Free: 800-726-2070
Fax: 800-727-2070
Website: www. academyforguidedimagery.com

Acupressure Institute

Website: www.acupressure.com
E-mail: info@acupressure.com

Alexander Technique International

1692 Massachusetts Ave., 3rd Fl.
Cambridge, MA 02138
Toll-Free: 888-668-8996
Phone: 617-497-5151
Fax: 617-497-2615
Website: www.ati-net.com

Alternative Medicine Foundation, Inc.

P.O. Box 60016
Potomac, MD 20859
Website: www.amfoundation.org

American Academy of Anti-Aging Medicine

301 Yamato Road, Suite 2199
Boca Raton, FL 33431
Toll-Free: 888-997-0112
Fax: 561-997-0287
Website: www.worldhealth.net
E-mail: info@a4m.com

American Academy of Family Physicians
11400 Tomahawk Creek Parkway
Leawood, KS 66211-2680
Toll-Free: 800-274-2237
Fax: 913-906-6075
Website: www.aafp.org

American Academy of Medical Acupuncture
1970 E. Grand Ave, Suite 330
El Segundo, CA 90245
Phone: 310-364-0193
Website: www.medicalacupuncture.org
E-mail: administrator@medicalacupuncture.org

American Apitherapy Society
500 Arthur Street
Centerport, NY 11721
Phone: 631-470-9446
Website: www.apitherapy.org

American Art Therapy Association
225 North Fairfax Street
Alexandria, VA 22314
Toll-Free: 888-290-0878
Phone: 703-548-5860
Fax: 703-783-8468
Website: www.arttherapy.org
E-mail: info@arttherapy.org

American Association of Acupuncture and Oriental Medicine
P.O. Box 162340
Sacramento, CA 95816
Toll-Free: 866-455-7999
Phone: 916-443-4770
Fax: 916-443-4766
Website: www.aaaomonline.org

American Association of Colleges of Osteopathic Medicine
5550 Friendship Boulevard
Suite 310
Chevy Chase, MD 20815-7231
Phone: 301-968-4100
Fax: 301-968-4101
Website: www.aacom.org

American Association of Integrative Medicine
2750 East Sunshine
Springfield, MO 65804
Toll-Free: 877-718-3053
Phone: 417-881-9995
Fax: 417-823-9959
Website: www.aaimedicine.com

American Association of Naturopathic Physicians
4435 Wisconsin Avenue NW
Suite 403
Washington, DC 20016
Toll-Free: 866-538-2267
Phone: 202-237-8150
Fax: 202-237-8152
Website: www.naturopathic.org
E-mail: member.services@naturopathic.org

American Botanical Council
6200 Manor Road
Austin, TX 78723
Phone: 512-926-4900
Fax: 512-926-2345
Website: abc.herbalgram.org
E-mail: abc@herbalgram.org

American Chiropractic Association
1701 Clarendon Boulevard
Arlington, VA 22209
Phone: 703-276-8800
Fax: 703-243-2593
Website: www.acatoday.org

American Dance Therapy Association
10632 Little Patuxent Parkway
Suite 108
Columbia, MD 21044-3263
Phone: 410-997-4040
Fax: 410-997-4048
Website: www.adta.org
E-mail: info@adta.org

American Feng Shui Institute
111 N. Atlantic Boulevard
Suite 352
Monterey Park, CA 91754
Website: www.amfengshui.com
E-mail: fsinfo@amfengshui.com

American Heart Association
National Center
7272 Greenville Avenue
Dallas, TX 75231
Toll-Free: 800-AHA-USA-1
(242-8721)
Website: www.americanheart.org

American Herbalists Guild
141 Nob Hill Road
Cheshire, CT 06410
Phone: 203-272-6731
Fax: 203-272-8550
Website:
www.americanherbalistsguild.com
E-mail: ahgoffice@earthlink.net

American Holistic Health Association
P.O. Box 17400
Anaheim, CA 92817-7400
Phone: 714-779-6152
Website: www.ahha.org
E-mail: mail@ahha.org

American Holistic Medical Association
23366 Commerce Park
Suite 101B
Beachwood, OH 44122
Phone: 216-292-6644
Fax: 216-292-6688
Website:
www.holisticmedicine.org
E-mail:
info@holisticmedicine.org

American Massage Therapy Association
500 Davis Street, Suite 900
Evanston, IL 60201
Toll-Free: 877-905-2700
Phone: 847-864-0123
Fax: 847-864-5196
Website: www.amtamassage.org
E-mail: info@amtamassage.org

American Music Therapy Association
8455 Colesville Road
Suite 1000
Silver Spring, MD 20910
Phone: 301-589-3300
Fax: 301-589-5175
Website: www.musictherapy.org
E-mail: info@musictherapy.org

American Naturopathic Medical Association
P.O. Box 96273
Las Vegas, NV 89193
Phone: 702-897-7053
Fax: 702-897-7140
Website: www.anma.org

American Oriental Bodywork Therapy Association
1010 Haddonfield-Berlin Road
Suite 408
Voorhees, NJ 08043-3514
Phone: 856-782-1616
Fax: 856-782-1653
Website: www.aobta.org
E-mail: office@aobta.org

American Osteopathic Association
1090 Vermont Avenue NW
Suite 510
Washington, DC 20005
Toll-Free: 800-962-9008
Phone: 202-414-0140
Fax: 202-544-3525
Website: www.osteopathic.org

American Polarity Therapy Association
122 N. Elm Street
Suite 512
Greensboro, NC 27401
Phone: 336-574-1121
Fax: 336-574-1151
Website:
www.polaritytherapy.org
E-mail: APTAoffices@
polaritytherapy.org

American Psychological Association
750 First Street NE
Washington, DC 20002-4242
Toll-Free: 800-374-2721
Phone: 202-336-5500
Website: www.apa.org

American Reflexology Certification Board
P.O. Box 5147
Gulfport, FL 33737
Phone: 303-933-6921
Fax: 303-904-0460
Website: www.arcb.net
E-mail: info@arcb.net

American Society for the Alexander Technique
P.O. Box 2307
Dayton, OH 45401
Toll-Free: 800-473-0620
Phone: 937-586-3732
Fax: 937-586-3699
Website: www.alexandertech.org

American Society of Clinical Hypnosis
140 N. Bloomingdale Road
Bloomingdale, IL 60108
Phone: 630-980-4740
Fax: 630-351-8490
Website: www.asch.net
E-mail: info@asch.net

American Tai Chi and Qigong Association
2465 J-17 Centreville Road, #150
Herndon, VA 20171
Website:
www.americantaichi.org

American Yoga Association
P.O. Box 19986
Sarasota, FL 34276
Website:
www.americanyogaassociation.org
E-mail: info@
americanyogaassociation.org

Arizona Center for Integrative Medicine
P.O. Box 245153
Tucson, AZ 85724-5153
Phone: 520-626-6417
Fax: 520-626-3518
Website: integrativemedicine
.arizona.edu

Associated Bodywork and Massage Professionals
25188 Genesee Trail Road
Golden, CO 80401
Toll-Free: 800-458-2267
Fax: 800-667-8260
Website: www.abmp.com
E-mail: expectmore@abmp.com

Association for Applied Psychophysiology and Biofeedback
10200 West 44th Avenue
Suite 304
Wheat Ridge, CO 80033
Toll-Free: 800-477-8892
Website: www.aapb.org
E-mail: aapb@resourcenter.com

Association of Reflexologists
5 Fore Street
Taunton, Somerset TA1 1HX
United Kingdom
Phone: 011-44-1823-351010
Website: www.aor.org.uk
E-mail: info@aor.org.uk

Atlantic Institute of Aromatherapy
16018 Saddlestring Drive
Tampa, FL 33612
Phone: 813-265-2222
Website:
www.atlanticinstitute.com

Ayurvedic Institute
P.O. Box 23445
Albuquerque, NM 87192-1445
Phone: 505-291-9698
Fax: 505-294-7572
Website: www.ayurveda.com

The Bach Centre
Mount Vernon, Baker's Lane
Brightwell-cum-Sotwell, Oxon
OX10 0PZ
United Kingdom
Phone: 011-44-1491-834678
Website: www.bachcentre.com

Bastyr Center for Natural Health
3670 Stone Way North
Seattle, WA 98103
Phone: 206-834-4100
Website: www.bastyrcenter.org

Benson-Henry Institute for Mind Body Medicine
151 Merrimac Street
Fourth Floor
Boston, MA 02114
Phone: 617-643-6090
Fax: 617-643-6077
Website: www.massgeneral.org/bhi
E-mail: mindbody@partners.org

Biodynamic Craniosacral Therapy Association of North America
150 Cross Creek Court
Chapel Hill, NC 27517
Phone: 734-904-0546
Website: www.craniosacraltherapy.org
E-mail: info@craniosacraltherapy.org

Biofeedback Certification Institute of America
10200 W. 44th Avenue
Suite 310
Wheat Ridge, CO 80033-2840
Toll-Free: 866-908-8713
Phone: 303-420-2902
Fax: 303-422-8894
Website: www.bcia.org
E-mail: info@bcia.org

Buteyko Breathing Association
15 Stanley Place
Chipping Ongar, Essex CM5 9SU
United Kingdom
Phone: 011-44-1277-366906
Website: www.buteykobreathing.org
E-mail: info@buteykobreathing.org

Center for Integrative Health and Healing
388 Kenwood Avenue
Delmar, NY 12054
Phone: 518-689-2244
Fax: 518-689-2081
Website: www.cihh.net

Center for Integrative Medicine
University of Maryland School of Medicine
Kernan Hospital Mansion
2200 Kernan Drive
Baltimore, MD 21207-6697
Phone: 410-448-6871
Fax: 410-448-6875
Website: www.compmed.umm.edu
E-mail: info@compmed.umm.edu

Center for Mindfulness in Medicine, Health Care, and Society
University of Massachusetts
Medical School
55 Lake Avenue North
Worcester, MA 01655
Phone: 508-856-2656
Fax: 508-856-1977
Website: www.umassmed.edu/
Content.aspx?id=41252
E-mail:
mindfulness@umassmed.edu

Chi Energy
Website: chienergy.co.uk

Complementary Healthcare Information Service
Website: www.chisuk.org.uk
E-mail: info@chisuk.org.uk

DrWeil.com
Website: www.drweil.com

Feldenkrais Educational Foundation of North America
5436 N. Albina Avenue
Portland, OR 97217
Toll-Free: 800-775-2118
Phone: 503-221-6612
Fax: 503-221-6616
Website: www.feldenkrais.com

Feldenkrais Resources
3680 6th Avenue
San Diego, CA 92103
Toll-Free: 800-765-1907
Phone: 619-220-8776
Fax: 619-330-4993
Website: www.
feldenkraisresources.com
E-mail: office@
feldenkraisresources.com

Flower Essence Society
P.O. Box 459
Nevada City, CA 95959
Toll-Free: 800-736-9222
Phone: 530-265-9163
Fax: 530-265-0584
Website: www.flowersociety.org
E-mail: info@flowersociety.org

Hellerwork International
P.O. Box 17373
Anaheim, CA 92817
Phone: 714-873-6131
Website: www.hellerwork.com
E-mail: info@hellerwork.com

Holistic Network
Website:
www.holisticnetwork.org

Homeopathic Educational Services
2124B Kittredge Street
Berkeley, CA 94704
Phone: 510-649-0294
Fax: 510-649-1955
Website: www.homeopathic.com

Institute of Traditional Medicine
2017 SE Hawthorne Boulevard
Portland, OR 97214
Phone: 503-233-4907
Website: www.itmonline.org

International Association of Reiki Professionals
Website: www.iarpreiki.org
E-mail: info@iarp.org

International Association of Yoga Therapists
P.O. Box 12890
Prescott, AZ 86304
Phone: 928-541-0004
Website: www.iayt.org

International Center for Reiki Training
21421 Hilltop Street, Unit #28
Southfield, MI 48033
Toll-Free: 800-332-8112
Phone: 248-948-8112
Fax: 248-948-9534
Website: www.reiki.org
E-mail: center@reiki.org

International Chiropractors Association
1110 N. Glebe Road, Suite 650
Arlington, VA 22201
Toll-Free: 800-423-4690
Phone: 703-528-5000
Fax: 703-528-5023
Website: www.chiropractic.org

International College of Applied Kinesiology
Website: www.icak.com

International Feng Shui Guild
705 B SE Melody Lane
Suite 166
Lees Summit, MO 64063
Toll-Free: 888-881-IFSG
(881-4374)
Website: www.ifsguild.org
E-mail: office@ifsguild.org

International Institute of Reflexology
5650 First Avenue North
St. Petersburg, FL 33733-2642
Phone: 727-343-4811
Fax: 727-381-2807
Website:
www.reflexology-usa.net
E-mail: iir@reflexology-usa.net

International Medical and Dental Hypnotherapy Association
P.O. Box 2468
Laceyville, PA 18623
Toll-Free: 800-553-6886
Phone: 570-869-1021
Fax: 570-869-1249
Website: www.imdha.com
E-mail: info@imdha.com

International Thai Therapists Association
4715 Bruton Road
Plant City, FL 33565
Phone: 706-358-8646
Website: www.thaimassage.com
E-mail: itta@core.com

Mayo Clinic
Website: www.mayoclinic.org

Moores Cancer Center
University of California–San
Diego Medical Center
3855 Health Sciences Drive
La Jolla, CA 92093
Phone: 858-822-6146
Website: cancer.ucsd.edu

**National Association for
Drama Therapy**
44365 Premier Plaza, Suite 220
Ashburn, VA 20147
Phone: 571-333-2991
Fax: 571-223-6440
Website: www.nadt.org
E-mail: nadt.office@nadt.org

**National Association for
Holistic Aromatherapy**
P.O. Box 1868
Banner Elk, NC 28604
Phone: 828-898-6161
Fax: 828-898-1965
Website: www.naha.org
E-mail: info@naha.org

**National Association of
Cognitive-Behavioral
Therapists**
P.O. Box 2195
Weirton, WV 26062
Toll-Free: 800-853-1135
Website: www.nacbt.org
E-mail: nacbt@nacbt.org

**National Association of
Nutrition Professionals**
P.O. 2752
Berkeley, CA 94702
Toll-Free: 800-342-8037
Fax: 510-580-9429
Website: www.nanp.org

**National Center for
Homeopathy**
101 S Whiting Street
Suite 16
Alexandria, VA 22304
Phone: 703-548-7790
Fax: 703-548-7792
Website:
www.homeopathic.org

**National Center on
Physical Activity and
Disability**
1640 W. Roosevelt Road
Chicago, IL 60608-6904
Toll-Free: 800-900-8086
Website: www.ncpad.org
E-mail: ncpad@uic.edu

**National Certification
Commission for
Acupuncture and
Oriental Medicine**
76 South Laura Street
Suite 1290
Jacksonville, FL 32202
Phone: 904-598-1005
Fax: 904-598-5001
Website: www.nccaom.org

**National College of
Naturopathic Medicine**
049 SW Porter Street
Portland, OR 97201
Phone: 503-552-1555
Website: www.ncnm.edu
E-mail: reception@ncnm.edu

National Headache Foundation
820 N. Orleans, Suite 217
Chicago, IL 60610
Toll-Free: 888-NHF-5552
(643-5552)
Phone: 312-274-2650
Website: www.headaches.org
E-mail: info@headaches.org

National Institute of Ayurvedic Medicine
584 Milltown Road
Brewster, NY 10509
Phone: 845-278-8700
Fax: 845-278-8215
Website: www.niam.com
E-mail: ayurveda@niam.com

National Qigong Association
P.O. Box 270065
St. Paul, MN 55127
Toll-Free: 888-815-1893
Fax: 888-359-9526
Website: www.nqa.org

Natural Medicines Comprehensive Database
Website:
www.naturaldatabase.com

Nemours Foundation Center for Children's Health Media
1600 Rockland Road
Wilmington, DE 19803
Phone: 302-651-4000
Website: www.kidshealth.org
E-mail: info@kidshealth.org

Physicians Association of Anthroposophic Medicine
1923 Geddes Avenue
Ann Arbor, MI 48104
Website: www.paam.net
E-mail:
paam@anthroposophy.org

Reflexology Association of America
375 North Stephanie Street
Suite 1411
Henderson, NV 89014
Phone: 980-234-0159
Fax: 401-568-6449
Website:
www.reflexology-usa.org
E-mail:
InfoRAA@reflexology-usa.org

Rolf Institute of Structural Integration
5055 Chaparral Court, Suite 103
Boulder, CO 80301
Toll-Free: 800-530-8875
Phone: 303-449-5903
Fax: 303-449-5978
Website: www.rolf.org

Scripps Center for Integrative Medicine
10820 North Torrey Pines Road
La Jolla, CA 92037
Phone: 858-554-3300
Fax: 858-554-2965
Website: www.scripps.org/
services/integrative-medicine

Society for Light Treatment and Biological Rhythms
Website: www.sltbr.org

**Society of Auricular
Acupuncturists**
29 Liverpool Lawn
Ramsgate, Kent CT11 9HJ
United Kingdom
Phone: 011-44-845-0949186
Website: www.
auricularacupuncturecollege.com

**Thai Yoga Center/SomaVeda
Institute**
4715 Bruton Road
Plant City, FL 33565
Phone: 706-358-8646
Website:
www.thaiyogacenter.com

**Therapeutic Touch
International
Association, Inc.**
P.O. Box 419
Craryville, NY 12521
Phone: 518-325-1185
Fax: 509-693-3537
Website:
www.therapeutic-touch.org

Trager International
Website: www.trager.com
E-mail: admin@trager.com

**University of Minnesota
Center for Spirituality
and Healing**
420 Delaware St. SE
Mayo Memorial Building
5th floor, MMC #505, C592
Minneapolis, MN 55455
Phone: 612-624-9459
Fax: 612-626-5280
Website: www.csh.umn.edu
E-mail: mclau033@umn.edu

**University of Texas M.D.
Anderson Cancer Center**
1515 Holcombe Boulevard
Houston, TX 77030
Phone: 877-MDA-6789
(632-6789)
Website:
www.mdanderson.org

**Vegetarian Resource
Group**
P.O. Box 1463
Baltimore, MD 21203
Phone: 410-366-8343
Website: www.vrg.org
E-mail: vrg@vrg.org

WholeHealthMD
46040 Center Oak Plaza
Suite 130
Sterling, VA 20166
Website:
www.wholehealthmd.com

**Zero Balancing Health
Association**
Kings Contrivance Village
Center
8640 Guilford Road
Suite 240
Columbia, MD 21046
Phone: 410-381-8956
Fax: 410-381-9634
Website:
www.zerobalancing.com
E-mail:
zbha@zerobalancing.com

Index

Index

Page numbers followed by 'n' indicate a footnote. Page numbers in *italics* indicate a table or illustration.

A

AAFA *see* Asthma and Allergy Foundation of America
AAFP *see* American Academy of Family Physicians
"About Art Therapy" (American Art Therapy Association) 299n
"About Zero Balancing" (Zero Balancing Association) 487n
Academy for Guided Imagery, contact information 601
Accutane (isotretinoin), acne 134
Acupressure Institute, contact information 601
acupuncture
    allergies 506
    arthritis 498, 500–502
    defined 593
    described 25, 60, 75, 458
    headache 533–34
    mental health care 576
    overview 81–84
    posttraumatic stress disorder 583–84
"Acupuncture" (National Headache Foundation) 533n
"Acupuncture: An Introduction" (NCCAM) 81n
"Acupuncture May Help Symptoms of Posttraumatic Stress Disorder" (NCCAM) 583n
"Acupuncture Relieves Pain and Improves Function in Knee Osteoarthritis" (NCCAM) 491n
"Acupuncture Shows Promise in Improving Rates of Pregnancy Following IVF" (NCCAM) 561n
A.D.A.M., Inc., touch therapy publication 479n
Adequate Intakes (AI), vitamin A 130
adjustments, described 23
adolescents
    detoxification diets 265
    supplements 117–19
    vegetarians 282
adverse events, hyperbaric oxygen therapy 289
African Americans, osteoporosis 149–50
Agency for Healthcare Research and Quality (AHRQ) contact information 599

Agency for Healthcare Research
and Quality (AHRQ), continued
hyperbaric oxygen therapy
publication 285n
Age-Related Eye Disease
Study 157–58, 210–11
age-related macular
degeneration (AMD)
vitamin E 157–58
zinc 210–11
AHRQ *see* Agency for Healthcare
Research and Quality
AI *see* Adequate Intakes
ai chi, described 384, 392–95
ai chi ne, described 385
alcohol addiction,
electroacupuncture 579–80
alcohol use
beta-carotene 134
energy drinks 232
vitamin B6 139
Alexander, F.M. 379, 381–82
Alexander Technique, overview
371–82
Alexander Technique International,
contact information 601
allergies
bee sting 255
bee stings 255
bioresonance therapy 484–85
CAM therapies 503–6
echinacea 207
fish oils 185
alpha-carotene, vitamin A 130
alpha-linolenic acid 176
alpha-lipoic acid, diabetes mellitus
524–25
alpha-tocopherol, vitamin E 153–54
Alpha-Tocopherol Beta-Carotene
Cancer Prevention Study 131
"Alternative Approaches to Mental
Health Care" (SAMHSA) 574n
alternative medicine, described 4, 21
Alternative Medicine Foundation,
contact information 601
"Alternative Therapies" (AAFA) 503n
Alzheimer disease
grape seed extract 517–18
research 27–28

Alzheimer's Disease Cooperative
Study 146
American Academy of Anti-Aging
Medicine, contact information 601
American Academy of Family
Physicians (AAFP), contact
information 602
American Academy of Medical
Acupuncture, contact information
602
American Apitherapy Association,
apitherapy publication 253n
American Apitherapy Society,
contact information 602
American Art Therapy Association
art therapy publication 299n
contact information 602
American Association of Acupuncture
and Oriental Medicine, contact
information 602
American Association of Colleges
of Osteopathic Medicine, contact
information 602
American Association of Integrative
Medicine, contact information 602
American Association of Naturopathic
Physicians, contact information 268,
602
American Board of Psychological
Hypnosis, contact information 326
American Botanical Council,
contact information 603
American Chiropractic Association,
contact information 603
American Dance Therapy Association
contact information 603
dance therapy publication 359n
American Feng Shui Institute,
contact information 603
American Heart Association,
contact information 603
American Herbalists Guild,
contact information 603
American Holistic Health Association,
contact information 603
American Holistic Medical Association,
contact information 603
American Massage Therapy
Association, contact information 603

American Music Therapy Association
contact information 604
music therapy publication 335n
American Naturopathic Medical
Association, contact information
604
American Oriental Bodywork
Therapy Association, contact
information 604
American Osteopathic Association,
contact information 604
American Polarity Therapy
Association
contact information 604
polarity therapy publication 467n
American Pregnancy Association,
infertility treatment publication
560n
American Psychological Association
contact information 604
publications
hypnosis 324n
relaxation training 345n
American Reflexology Certification
Board
contact information 604
reflexology publication 431n
American Society for the Alexander
Technique, contact information 604
American Society of Clinical Hypnosis,
contact information 326, 605
American Tai Chi and Qigong
Association, contact information 605
American Yoga Association, contact
information 605
anaphylaxis, bee stings 255
M.D. Anderson Cancer Center,
contact information 611
androstenedione, described 227
anemia
folic acid 161
vitamin B12 144
angina pectoris, fish oils 178
angioplasty, fish oils 181
animal-assisted therapies,
mental health care 575
antibiotic medications, probiotics 220
anticonvulsant medications, folic acid
163

antioxidants
age-related macular
degeneration 210–11
research 250
vitamin A 130
vitamin E 153–54, 158
anxiety, self-hypnosis 582
apitherapy, overview 253–55
"Applied Kinesiology" (Natural
Medicines Comprehensive
Database) 448n
applied kinesiology, overview 448–49
apricot pits 54
"Aquatic Therapy" (NCPAD) 383n
aquatic therapy, overview 383–98
"Are Detox Diets Safe?" (Nemours
Foundation) 264n
"Are You Considering CAM?"
(NCCAM) 7n
ARIC study *see* Atherosclerosis Risk
in Communities study
Arizona Center for Integrative
Medicine, contact information 605
Arnold, Joan 371n
aromatherapy
defined 593
overview 257–61
"Aromatherapy and Essential
Oils" (NCI) 257n
Artemisia annua 61
artemisinin 61
arthritis
Alexander technique 374
apitherapy 253–54
CAM therapies 491–502
health fraud 46
selenium 195
art therapy
mental health care 575
overview 299–302
Associated Bodywork and
Massage Professionals,
contact information 605
Association for Applied
Psychophysiology and Biofeedback
biofeedback publication 303n
contact information 605
Association of American Indian
Physicians, contact information 80

Association of Reflexologists,
contact information 605
asthma
Alexander technique 374–75
CAM therapies 503–6
fish oils 179
Asthma and Allergy Foundation
of America (AAFA), alternative
therapies publication 503n
atherosclerosis, fish oils 176, 179
Atherosclerosis Risk in Communities
study (ARIC study) 172
athletes
Alexander technique 378
sports supplements 226–30
Atlantic Institute of Aromatherapy,
contact information 605
attention deficit hyperactivity disorder
(ADHD), CAM therapies 580–81
autonomic nervous system,
meditation 331
Awareness Through
Movement 409–10
Ayurveda
defined 593
described 25, 61–62
mental health care 577
overview 65–71
Ayurvedic Institute, contact
information 605
"Ayurvedic Medicine: An
Introduction" (NCCAM) 65n

B

The Bach Centre, contact
information 605
BackHab, described 385, 390
back pain, CAM therapies 563–65
bacteria, probiotics 219–20
Bad Ragaz, described 385
baiguo 214
bai guo ye 214
balance
acupuncture 81–82
Ayurvedic medicine 67–69
Native American medicine 79
naturopathy 91
traditional Chinese medicine 75

barbiturates, folic acid 163
Bastyr Center for Natural Health,
contact information 606
Beal, Flint 520
Beecher, Henry 294
bee stings *see* apitherapy
Bekhterev, Vladimir 431
Benefin 54
Benson, Herbert 345–47
Benson-Henry Institute for
Mind Body Medicine, contact
information 606
Berman, Brian M, 501–2
beta-carotene, vitamin A 130
beta-cryptoxanthin, vitamin A 130
Bifidobacterium bifidus 220
Biodynamic Craniosacral Therapy
Association of North America,
contact information 606
bioelectromagnetic-based
therapies, described 5
biofeedback
allergies 506
defined 593
headache 534–35
mental health care 577
overview 303–9
"Biofeedback" (National
Headache Foundation) 533n
Biofeedback Certification Institute of
America, contact information 606
"Biofeedback: Consumer Questions
Answered" (Moss) 303n
biofield, described 456
biofield therapies, described 5
"Biologically Based Practices: An
Overview" (NCCAM) 243n
biologically based therapies
defined 594
described 4, 22
overview 243–51
bioresonance therapy, overview
484–85
bipolar disorder, fish oils 179
Black Beauties (slang) 53–54
black cohosh, menopause 569
blood pressure levels,
magnesium 169–70
body-based practices, defined 596

Bompey, Nanci 484n
bone health
  calcium 198–200
  vitamin D 147
borage, arthritis 493
Boswellia, arthritis 496
"Botanical Dietary Supplements:
  Background Information" (ODS)
  107n
botanicals
  arthritis 491–97
  Ayurvedic medicine 70
  defined 594
  menopause 569–71
  overview 107–10
"Bowen Technique" (Natural Medicines
  Comprehensive Database) 449n
Bowen technique, overview 449–50
brain injury, hyperbaric oxygen
  therapy 287
breastfeeding
  fish oils 186–87
  probiotics 220
"A Brief History of Foot Reflexology"
  (American Reflexology Certification
  Board) 431n
Briggs, Josephine 201
Brunschwiler, Arjana 387
Burdenko Method, described 385
Buteyko Breathing Association,
  contact information 606

C

caffeine
  energy drinks 231–32
  green tea 237
  sports supplements 228
calcidiol, described 147
calcitriol, described 147
calcium
  bone health 147, 198–200
  vegans 278
  vegetarians 280
"Calcium Supplements: What to
  Look for" (NIAMS) 198n
calorie restriction, described 557–58
CAM *see* complementary and
  alternative medicine

"CAM and Diabetes: A Focus on
  Dietary Supplements" (NCCAM)
  523n
"CAM and Fibromyalgia: At a
  Glance" (NCCAM) 529n
"CAM and Hepatitis C: A Focus on
  Herbal Supplements" (NCCAM)
  541n
Camellia sinensis 236
"Cam Use and Children" (NCCAM) 17n
"Cancer and CAM" (NCCAM) 507n
cancers
  aromatherapy 258
  CAM therapies 507–16
  deep breathing exercises 311–15
  fish oils 179
  folic acid 165
  Gerson therapy 269–72
  health fraud 45–46
  macrobiotics 273–74
  research 26–27
  selenium 193–94
  spiritual distress 342–44
  vitamin A 131
  vitamin D 150–51
  vitamin E 156–57
Cannon, Walter 294
"Can't Sleep? Science Is Seeking
  New Answers" (NIH) 585n
"Can We Prevent Aging?" (NIA) 547n
Caraka Samhita 66
carbohydrate metabolism,
  magnesium 170–71
carbohydrates, energy drinks 233
cardiac arrhythmias, fish oils 179
cardiovascular disease
  fish oils 177–78, 181
  folic acid 164
  magnesium 173–74
  vitamin B12 144–45
Carotene and Retinol Efficiency
  Trial (CARET) 131
carotenoids, overview 129–35
carpal tunnel syndrome
  Alexander technique 375, 377
  vitamin B6 139
cataracts, vitamin E 157–58
CDC *see* Centers for Disease
  Control and Prevention

Cellular Tea 54
Center for Integrative Health
  and Healing
  contact information 606
  publications
     craniosacral therapy 403n
     guided imagery 322n
     lymphatic drainage
      massage 419n
     Shiatsu 475n
     Tui Na 421n
Center for Integrative Medicine,
  contact information 606
Center for Mindfulness in Medicine,
  Health Care, and Society, contact
  information 607
Centers for Disease Control and
  Prevention (CDC), contact
  information 599
cerebral palsy, hyperbaric
  oxygen therapy 287–88
certification
  art therapy 299–300, 302
  Ayurvedic medicine 70
  biofeedback 306
  CAM practitioners 33
  dance therapy 359–60
  homeopathy 88–89
  massage therapy 417
  naturopathy 94
  Reiki 473
  traditional Chinese
    medicine 77
  Trager approach 451
  yoga 355
  see also licensing requirements
chakras
  color therapy 358
  polarity therapy 468
CHD *see* coronary heart
  disease
chelation therapy
  defined 594
  heart disease 537–40
  research 26
chi *see* qi
Chi Energy
  feng shui publication 317n
  website address 607

children
  complementary and alternative
    medicine 16, 17–19
  Rolfing 446
  vegetarians 281–82
Chinese herbal medicine, described 75
Chinese massage, overview 421–22
Chinese Materia Medica, described 61
Chinese tea 236
chiropractic
  allergies 506
  defined 594
  described 23
  headache 535
  overview 399–402
"Chiropractic: An Introduction"
  (NCCAM) 399n
"Chiropractors" (National
  Headache Foundation) 533n
cholecalciferol, described 148
cholesterol levels
  fish oils 177
  selenium 195
  vitamin E 154–55
chondroitin
  arthritis 496–97
  overview 201–4
  research 27
chromium, diabetes mellitus 525
"Chromotherapy" (Natural Medicines
  Comprehensive Database) 358n
Clegg, Daniel O. 201, 203
Cleland, Rich 51–52
clinical trials
  aromatherapy 259
  beta-carotene 134
  CAM practitioners 36
  complementary and alternative
    medicine 11
  defined 594
  dietary supplements 246, 249–51
  Gerson therapy 271–72
  ginkgo biloba 215
  homeopathy 63–64
  magnesium 170, 172
  manipulative and body-based
    practices 364–67
  PC-SPES 510, 512
  selenium 194

clinical trials, continued
  thunder god vine 492
  vitamin D 150–51
  vitamin E 155–59
  zinc 209–11
cod liver oil 176
coenzyme Q10
  Parkinson disease 519–21
  research 250
cognitive function
  vitamin B12 145–46
  vitamin E 158–59
coldwater fish 176
colonic irrigation, detoxification
  diets 264–65
color therapy, overview 358–59
complementary and alternative
  medicine (CAM)
  defined 594
  overview 3–11
"Complementary and Alternative
  Medicine (CAM)" (NIA) 21n
Complementary Healthcare
  Information Service, contact
  information 607
complementary medicine,
  described 3–4, 21
constitution, Ayurvedic medicine 67
conventional medicine, defined 594
Cooke, David A. 78n, 267n, 273n,
  285n, 303n, 322n, 403n, 419n, 450n,
  486n, 491n, 503n, 517n, 537n, 574n
Cornelius, Alfons 431
coronary artery bypass grafting,
  fish oils 181
coronary heart disease (CHD)
  chelation therapy 537–40
  vitamin E 154–56
cranberry juice, research 250–51
"Craniosacral Therapy" (Center for
  Integrative Health and Healing)
  403n
craniosacral therapy, overview 403–5
creatine, described 227–28
Crohn disease, fish oils 179–80
"Crystal and Gem Therapy"
  (University of California) 486n
crystal therapy 486–87
Cuentos, mental health care 577

cupping, described 76
curcumin, arthritis 496
cyclosporine, fish oils 178, 182
cystic fibrosis, fish oils 180

D

Daily Value (DV), defined 594–95
dance therapy
  mental health care 576
  overview 359–60
DASH diet *see* Dietary Approaches
  to Stop Hypertension
decoction, described 108
deep breathing exercises,
  overview 311–15
dehydroepiandrosterone (DHEA)
  described 227, 552–53
  menopause 571
dementia
  CAM therapies 517–19
  fish oils 180
  vitamin B12 145–46
Department of Health and Human
  Services (DHHS) *see* US Department
  of Health and Human Services
depression
  fish oils 180
  St. John's wort 216
detoxification diets, overview 264–66
DHA (docosahexaenoic acid)
  described 55
  fish oils 176
DHEA *see* dehydroepiandrosterone
DHHS *see* US Department of Health
  and Human Services
diabetes mellitus
  CAM therapies 523–27
  fish oils 182
  health fraud 47
  magnesium 170–72
diarrhea, zinc 209
diet and nutrition
  arthritis 497–98
  CAM therapies 264–83
  folic acid 161–62
  Gerson therapy 269–72
  macrobiotics 273–74
  mental health care 575

diet and nutrition, continued
  veganism 275–79
  vegetarianism 279–83
  vitamin A 130–31, 135
  vitamin B6 138, 140–41
Dietary Approaches to Stop
  Hypertension (DASH diet) 170
Dietary Reference Intakes (DRI),
  folic acid 162
Dietary Supplement Health and
  Education Act (DSHEA; 1994)
  biologically based therapies 243–44
  definitions 101, 107–8, 111
  regulations 53
dietary supplements
  adolescents 117–19
  arthritis 491–97
  defined 595
  described 121–22
  diabetes mellitus 525–27
  health fraud 47
  online safety 52–56
  overview 101–5, 111–15
  vitamin B12 144
  vitamin D 148
  see also botanicals
"Dietary Supplements: Background
  Information" (ODS) 101n
"Dietary Supplements Glucosamine
  and/or Chondroitin Fare No Better
  than Placebo in Slowing Structural
  Damage of Knee Osteoarthritis"
  (NIH) 201n
dietary therapy, described 76
"The Differences between Reflexology
  and Massage" (American Reflexology
  Certification Board) 431n
digestive tract, probiotics 220–21
digitalis 491
dilutions principle 86
distant healing, described 460
DNA (deoxyribonucleic acid)
  folic acid 161
  vitamin B12 143
Dodge, Hiroko 518
dong quai, menopause 569–70
doshas
  Ayurvedic medicine 67–68
  described 25

drug interactions
  fish oils 187–88
  St. John's wort 217, 251
  vitamin B6 139
DrWeil.com, website address 607
Dull, Harold 387
DV *see* Daily Value
dysmenorrhea, fish oils 180

E

echinacea
  naturopathy 62
  overview 206–7
  research 251
"Echinacea" (NCCAM) 206n
eczema, fish oils 180
EDTA chelation therapy, heart
  disease 537–40
EGCG (epigallocatechin gallate) 236
"Electroacupuncture May Help
  Alcohol Addiction" (NCCAM) 579n
electromagnetic energy
  arthritis 498–99
  described 460–61
  feng shui 317–19
electronic communications,
  mental health care 578
elements, traditional Chinese
  medicine 75
enemas, Gerson therapy 270–72
  see also detoxification diets
energy drinks, overview 231–33
"Energy Drinks: Power Boosts or
  Empty Boasts?" (SAMHSA) 231n
energy medicine
  defined 595
  described 5, 22–23
  overview 455–61
"Energy Medicine: An Overview"
  (NCCAM) 455n
EPA (eicosapentaenoic acid)
  described 55
  fish oils 176
ephedra
  adolescents 118
  traditional Chinese medicine 77
ephedrine, dietary supplements 53
epigallocatechin gallate (EGCG) 236

epinephrine, bee stings 255
ergocalciferol, described 148
ergogenic aids, described 226
essential oils
  apitherapy 253
  overview 257–61
estrogen, described 554–57
evening primrose oil, arthritis 493
exercises
  relaxation 313–15
  water therapy 389–95
extract, described 108
eye disorders, vitamin E 157–58

F

fasting
  hormone therapy 557–58
  overview 267–68
"Fasting" (University of California)
  267n
fat burners, sports supplements 228
fats, vegans 277
FDA *see* US Food and Drug
  Administration
"FDA 101: Health Fraud
  Awareness" (FDA) 45n
Feldenkrais, Moshe 385, 407, 411–12
Feldenkrais Educational Foundation
  of North America
  Feldenkrais method
    publication 407n
  website address 607
Feldenkrais method
  described 385
  overview 407–12
Feldenkrais Resources, website
  address 607
feng shui, overview 317–19
"Feng Shui Principles" (ChiEnergy)
  317n
feverfew
  arthritis 496
  headache 535–36
"Feverfew (*Tanacetum Parthenium*)"
  (National Headache Foundation)
  533n
fibromyalgia, CAM therapies 529–32
fight or flight, described 294

financial considerations
  acupuncture 84
  biofeedback 308
  CAM therapies 39–40, 44
  dietary supplements 245
  macrobiotics 274
  manipulative and body-based
    practices 368–69
  see also insurance coverage
fish body oil 176
fish extract 176
fish liver oil 176
fish oils
  arthritis 493–94
  overview 176–90
Fitzgerald, William 431
flaxseed, overview 190–91
"Flaxseed and Flaxseed Oils"
  (NCCAM) 190n
flexible spending arrangements
  (FSA), described 42
Flower Essence Society, website
  address 607
"Folate" (ODS) 161n
folic acid (folate), overview 161–67
Food, Drug, and Cosmetic Act (1938)
  86
Food and Drug Administration
  (FDA) *see* US Food and Drug
  Administration
fossil tree 214
fraud
  dietary supplements 124
  overview 45–49
frequency therapy 458
"Frequently Asked Questions"
  (Arnold; Gillerman) 371n
"Frequently Asked Questions"
  (Feldenkrais Educational
  Foundation) 407n
"Frequently Asked Questions"
  (Rolf Institute of Structural
  Integration) 438n
"Frequently Asked Questions
  about Apitherapy" (American
  Apitherapy Association) 253n
"Frequently Asked Questions About
  Music Therapy" (American Music
  Therapy Association) 335n

FSA (flexible spending arrangements), described 42
Functional Integration 410

G

gamma-linolenic acid 493
garlic, research 26
gem therapy 486–87
Gerson, Max B. 269–71
"Gerson Therapy" (NCI) 269n
Gerson therapy, overview 269–72
Gillerman, Hope 371n
ginger, arthritis 495–96
"Ginkgo" (NCCAM) 214n
ginkgo biloba
    dementia 518–19
    overview 214–15
ginseng
    hepatitis C 542
    menopause 570
glucosamine
    arthritis 496–97
    overview 201–4
    research 27
glycyrrhizin, hepatitis C 542
GMP *see* good manufacturing practices
goat weed 216
good manufacturing practices (GMP)
    biologically based therapies 243
    botanicals 110
    dietary supplements 104, 112
    sports supplements 226
grape seed extract, Alzheimer disease 517–18
"Grape Seed Extract May Help Prevent and Treat Alzheimer's" (NCCAM) 517n
Green Hornet 54
"Green Tea" (NCCAM) 236n
green tea, overview 236–37
guarine, energy drinks 232
guided imagery
    defined 595
    mental health care 577
    overview 322–24
    see also imagery

"Guided Imagery" (Center for Integrative Health and Healing) 322n

H

Haas, Richard 520
Hahnemann, Samuel Christian 63, 85
halibut oil 176
Halliwick, described 386
hatha yoga *see* yoga
Hayashi, Chujiro 471
Head, Henry 431
headache, CAM therapies 533–36
healing touch therapy, described 22
health care providers
    CAM discussions 37–38
    dietary supplements 123
    see also practitioners
Healthfinder, contact information 599
health fraud, overview 45–49
health insurance *see* insurance coverage
Health Professionals' Follow-up Study (HFS)
    magnesium 171
    vitamin E 157
health risks
    acupuncture 82
    carotenoids 134–35
    chiropractic 401
    dietary supplements 122–23
    folic acid 166–67
    homeopathy 88
    magnet therapy 466
    manipulative and body-based practices 368
    naturopathy 95–96
    online products 52
    probiotics 222–23
    spinal manipulation 565
    tai chi 351
    vitamin A 133–34
    vitamin B6 140
    yoga 355
health savings account (HSA), described 43

heart disease
  selenium 195
  vitamin B6 140
Heart Outcomes Prevention
  Evaluation (HOPE) 155, 157
Heller, Joseph 436
Hellerwork International
  Hellerwork publication 436n
  website address 607
Hellerwork structural integration,
  overview 436–37
hemoglobin
  described 137
  vitamin B12 143
hemoglobin A1C levels,
  magnesium 172
hepatitic C, CAM therapy 541–45
herbal supplements
  adolescents 117–19
  defined 595
  hepatitis C 542
  see also botanicals
HFS *see* Health Professionals'
  Follow-up Study
HHS *see* US Department of
  Health and Human Services
high blood pressure *see* hypertension
HIV (human immunodeficiency virus)
  health fraud 46
  selenium 195–96
Holistic Network, website address 607
Homeopathic Educational Services,
  contact information 607
homeopathy
  arthritis 500
  defined 595
  described 25, 63–64, 459
  overview 85–89
"Homeopathy: An Introduction"
  (NCCAM) 85n
homocysteine
  Alzheimer disease 28
  vitamin B6 140
"Hoodia" (NCCAM) 238n
hoodia, overview 238–39
hormones, sports supplements 227–28
hormone therapies
  menopause 568
  overview 547–58

HSA (health savings account),
  described 43
Huang Di Nei Jing 75
Hubbard, William 51–52
human growth hormone,
  described 550–51
human pathogenic trial,
  homeopathy 63
hydrotherapy
  arthritis 499–500
  naturopathy 92
  overview 383–98
hyperbaric oxygen therapy,
  overview 285–89
"Hyperbaric Oxygen Therapy for
  Brain Injury, Cerebral Palsy, and
  Stroke" (AHRQ) 285n
hypercholesterolemia, fish oils 182
hyperglycemia, magnesium 171
Hypericum perforatum
  see St. John's wort
hypertension (high blood
  pressure), fish oils 177
hypertriglyceridemia, fish oils 177
hypervitaminosis A, described 133
hypnosis
  allergies 506
  anxiety 582
  defined 595
  described 312
  overview 324–27
"Hypnosis Today: Looking beyond
  the media portrayal" (American
  Psychological Association) 324n
hypomagnesemia,
  magnesium 170–73

I

IgA nephropathy, fish oils 180
imagery, described 24, 296, 312
  see also guided imagery
immune system
  craniosacral therapy 403
  echinacea 206–7
  mind-body medicine 295–96
  probiotics 221
  touch therapy 460
  vitamin B6 137

immune system, continued
vitamin D 147
vitamin E 153–54
zinc 208–11
infants
eye/brain development
and omega 3 fatty acids180
vegetarians 281
infertility
CAM therapies 561–62
herbal remedies 560–61
influenza, health fraud 48
infusion, described 108
Ingham, Eunice D. 431
Inner Canon of the Yellow
Emperor 75
Institute for Traditional Medicine,
contact information 80
Institute of Traditional Medicine,
contact information 608
insurance coverage
alternative medicine 504
apitherapy 254
CAM practitioners 33, 34
CAM therapies 39–44
chiropractic 402
music therapy 338–40
integrative medicine,
described 4, 21
interconnectedness,
Ayurvedic medicine 67
International Association
of Reiki Professionals,
contact information 608
International Association of Yoga
Therapists, contact information 608
International Center for Reiki
Training, contact information 608
International Chiropractors
Association, contact information 608
International College of Applied
Kinesiology, website address 608
International Feng Shui Guild,
contact information 608
International Institute of Reflexology,
contact information 608
International Medical and Dental
Hypnotherapy Association, contact
information 608

International Society of Hypnosis,
contact information 327
International Thai Therapists
Association, contact information 608
"An Introduction to Naturopathy"
(NCCAM) 91n
"An Introduction to Probiotics"
(NCCAM) 219n
iron
vegans 278
vegetarians 281
isoniazid, vitamin B6 139
isotretinoin, acne 134

J

Japanese silver apricot 214
Japanese tea 236
juice therapies, overview 267–68

K

Kalahari cactus 238
Kano, Jigaro 411–12
kapha, Ayurvedic medicine 68
Katz, Stephen I. 203, 501
kava
menopause 570
research 251
kew tree 214
ki *see* qi
kinesiology 448–49
Kirlian photography 317
Klamath weed 216
Kneipp, Sebastian 92
Konno, Jun 384
Krieger, Dolores 479–80
Kunz, Dora 479–80

L

labels, dietary supplements 102–4,
114–15
Lactobacillus acidophilus 220
lactoferrin 544
lacto-ovo vegetarians, defined 279, 597
lacto-vegetarians, defined 280, 597
Laetrile 54
Lane, Andrew J. 54

laser therapy, allergies 506
law of minimum dose 86
licensing requirements
    biofeedback 306
    CAM practitioners 18, 33
    chiropractic 401
    homeopathy 88–89
    massage therapy 417
    naturopathy 94
    Reiki 473
    yoga 355
    see also certification
licorice, hepatitis C 543
life forces, Ayurvedic
    medicine 67–68
light therapy, described 458
like cures like 85
list of medications
    CAM practitioners 35
    health care providers 38
long chain polyunsaturated
    fatty acids 176
Lubar, Joel 306
lupus erythematosus,
    fish oils 180
Lust, Benedict 92
lutein, vitamin A 130
lycopene, vitamin A 130
"Lymphatic Drainage Massage"
    (Center for Integrative Health
    and Healing) 419n
lymphatic drainage massage,
    overview 419–20
Lyu Ki Dou, described 386

M

mackerel oil 176
"Macrobiotics" (University of
    California) 273n
macrobiotics, overview 273–74
"Magnesium" (ODS) 169n
magnesium, overview 169–74
"Magnets for Pain" (NCCAM) 463n
magnet therapy
    arthritis 498–99
    defined 595
    described 22, 457
    overview 463–66

ma huang (ephedra)
    adolescents 118
    described 228
    traditional Chinese
        medicine 77
maidenhair tree 214
Manheimer, Eric 562
manipulation
    defined 595
    described 23
    naturopathy 92
    see also chiropractic; Rolfing
manipulative and body-based
    practices
    described 4, 23
    overview 363–69
"Manipulative and Body-Based
    Practices: An Overview"
    (NCCAM) 363n
manipulative practices,
    defined 596
marine oil 176
massage, defined 596
massage therapy
    described 23, 313–17
    hydrotherapy 386
    mental health care 578
    overview 414–18
"Massage Therapy: An
    Introduction" (NCCAM) 414n
Mayo Clinic, website address 608
medications
    folic acid 163
    online cautions 51–56
    see also drug interactions
meditation
    defined 596
    described 24, 296
    guided imagery 322–23
    mental health care 577
    overview 329–33
"Meditation: An Introduction"
    (NCCAM) 329n
melatonin
    described 551–52
    sleep disorders 588–89
menhaden oil 176
"Menopausal Symptoms and
    CAM" (NCCAM) 567n

menopause, CAM therapies 567–72
mental health care,
   CAM therapies 574–79
Mentastics 451
meridians
   acupuncture 82
   described 60
   traditional Chinese
      medicine 75
metformin, folic acid 163
methionine, described 143
methotrexate, folic acid 163, 165
MGN-3 54
milk thistle
   hepatitis C 542
   research 250
millimeter wave therapy,
   described 457–58
mind-body medicine
   defined 596
   described 4, 23–24
   overview 293–98
"Mind-Body Medicine:
   An Overview" (NCCAM) 293n
mindfulness meditation,
   described 331
mineral, defined 596
Moores Cancer Center,
   contact information 609
Moss, Donald 303n
movement therapy,
   mental health care 576
moxibustion, described 25, 60, 76
multiple sclerosis (MS)
   apitherapy 253–54
   shiatsu 477
music therapy
   described 315
   mental health care 576
   overview 335–40
   sound energy therapy 458

N

National Association for Drama
   Therapy, contact information 609
National Association for Holistic
   Aromatherapy, contact
   information 609
National Association of Cognitive-
   Behavioral Therapists, contact
   information 609
National Association of Nutrition
   Professionals, contact information
   609
National Cancer Institute (NCI)
   contact information 599
   publications
      aromatherapy 257n
      cancer, CAM 507n
      deep breathing exercises 311n
      Gerson therapy 269n
      spirituality 341n
National Center for Complementary
   and Alternative Medicine (NCCAM)
   contact information 600
   publications
      acupuncture 81n
      alcohol addiction 579n
      arthritis 491n
      attention deficit hyperactivity
         disorder 580n
      Ayurvedic medicine 65n
      biologically based practices
         243n
      CAM, children 17n
      CAM, United States 13n
      CAM overview 3n, 7n
      CAM practitioners 32n, 37n
      CAM treatment financial
         considerations 39n
      cancer 507n
      chelation therapy, heart
         disease 537n
      chiropractic 399n
      diabetes mellitus 523n
      dietary supplements 111n
      echinacea 206n
      energy medicine 455n
      fibromyalgia 529n
      flaxseed 190n
      ginkgo biloba 214n
      ginkgo extract 517n
      grape seed extract 517n
      green tea 236n
      hepatitis C 541n
      homeopathy 85n
      hoodia 238n

National Center for Complementary
and Alternative Medicine (NCCAM),
continued
publications, continued
infertility treatment 561n
low back pain 563n
magnet therapy 463n
manipulative and body based
therapies 363n
massage therapy 414n
meditation 329n
menopausal symptoms 567n
mind-body medicine 293n
naturopathy 91n
posttraumatic stress
disorder 583n
probiotics 219n
Reiki 471n
St. John's wort 216n
self-hypnosis 582n
tai chi 349n
traditional Chinese
medicine 74n
whole medical systems 59n
yoga 353n
National Center for Homeopathy,
contact information 609
National Center on Physical Activity
and Disability (NCPAD)
contact information 609
hydrotherapy publication 383n
National Certification Commission for
Acupuncture and Oriental Medicine,
contact information 609
National College of Naturopathic
Medicine, contact information 609
National Headache Foundation
contact information 610
publications
acupuncture 533n
biofeedback 533n
chiropractic 533n
feverfew 533n
National Institute of Arthritis
and Musculoskeletal and Skin
Diseases (NIAMS)
calcium supplements
publication 198n
contact information 600

National Institute of Ayurvedic
Medicine, contact information 610
National Institute of Diabetes and
Digestive and Kidney Diseases
(NIDDK), contact information 600
National Institute of Neurological
Disorders and Stroke (NINDS)
coenzyme Q10 publication 517n
contact information 600
National Institute on Aging (NIA)
contact information 600
publications
aging prevention 547n
CAM use 21n
National Institutes of Health (NIH)
contact information 600
publications
glucosamine/
chondroitin 201n
sleep disorders 585n
National Library of Medicine
(NLM), contact information 601
National Qigong Association
contact information 610
qigong publication 427n
Native American medicine
mental health care 577
overview 78–80
"Native American Medicine"
(University of California) 78n
Natural Medicines Comprehensive
Database, publications
applied kinesiology 448n
Bowen technique 449n
color therapy 358n
Natural Medicines Comprehensive
Database, website address 610
Natural Standard, fish oils
publication 176n
naturopathy
defined 596
described 26, 62–63
overview 91–97
NCCAM *see* National Center for
Complementary and Alternative
Medicine
NCI *see* National Cancer Institute
NCPAD *see* National Center on
Physical Activity and Disability

Nemours Foundation
  contact information 610
  publications
     detoxification diets 264n
     Pilates 423n
     sports supplements 226n
     vegetarianism 279n
Neoral (cyclosporine), fish oils 178,
  182
nephrotic syndrome, fish oils 181
new dietary ingredient,
  described 101, 102–3
NIA *see* National Institute on
  Aging
niacin, vitamin B6 137
NIAMS *see* National Institute of
  Arthritis and Musculoskeletal
  and Skin Diseases
NIDDK *see* National Institute
  of Diabetes and Digestive and
  Kidney Diseases
NIH *see* National Institutes
  of Health
NINDS *see* National Institute of
  Neurological Disorders and Stroke
NLM *see* National Library of
  Medicine
noise, feng shui 319
Nurses' Health Study
  magnesium 171
  vitamin A 132
  vitamin E 157
Nutrition Labeling and Education
  Act (NLEA; 1990) 245

O

Oakes, David 521
ODS *see* Office of Dietary
  Supplements
Office of Dietary Supplements
  (ODS)
  contact information 600
  publications
     botanicals 107n
     dietary supplements 101n
     folate 161n
     magnesium 169n
     selenium 193n

Office of Dietary Supplements
  (ODS), continued
  publications, continued
     vitamin A 129n
     vitamin B6 137n
     vitamin B12 143n
     vitamin D 147n
     vitamin E 153n
     zinc 208n
Ogden, David 387
older adults
  CAM therapies 547–58
  complementary and alternative
    medicine 21–30
  dietary supplements 121–27
  folic acid 166
omega-3 fatty acids
  Alzheimer disease 28
  defined 596
  diabetes mellitus 525–26
  overview 176–91
  regulations 55
  vegans 278
  see also fish oils; flaxseed
  "Omega-3 Fatty Acids, Fish Oil,
    Alpha-Linoleic Acid" (Natural
    Standard) 176n
omega-6 fatty acids 493
omega fatty acids 176
osteoarthritis
  acupuncture 27, 500–502
  shiatsu 476
osteopathic manipulation,
  overview 399–402
osteoporosis
  magnesium 174
  vitamin A 132–33
  vitamin D 149–50
Otikon Otic Solution 62–63
otitis media, naturopathy 62–63
out of pocket expenses,
  CAM therapies 39
  see also financial considerations;
    insurance coverage
ovo-vegetarians, defined 279
oxalic acid, calcium 278
oxygen therapy, overview
  285–89
oxymatrine 544

P

paclitaxel 491
"Pain" (NCI) 311n
pain management
  Alexander technique 373–74
  CAM therapies 563–65
  chiropractic 23
  deep breathing exercises 311–15
  magnet therapy 457
  mind-body medicine 294–95
  therapeutic touch 480
panchakarma, Ayurvedic medicine 69
parasympathetic nervous system,
  meditation 332
pastoral counseling, mental health
  care 575
Pavlov, Ivan 431
"Paying for CAM Treatment"
  (NCCAM) 39n
"PC-SPES" (NCI) 507n
PC-SPES, described 510–13
Pearson, Nancy J. 586, 589
pediatricians, complementary
  and alternative medicine 18–19
pernicious anemia, vitamin B12 144
Physicians Association of
  Anthroposophic Medicine, contact
  information 610
phytoestrogens, menopause 570–71
Pilates
  hydrotherapy 386
  overview 423–25
"Pilates" (Nemours Foundation) 423n
Pilates, Joseph 386
Pilates, Joseph H. 423–24
"Pilot Study Provides New Insight
  on Effect of Ginkgo Extract on
  Dementia in the Elderly" (NCCAM)
  517n
pitta, Ayurvedic medicine 68
placebo effect
  alternative medicine 504–5
  described 294, 296–97
polarity therapy, overview 467–69
polyphenols, diabetes mellitus 526–27
polyunsaturated fatty acids (PUFA) 176
posttraumatic stress disorder (PTSD),
  acupuncture 583–84

potentization, described 86
"The power of the relaxation
  response" (American Psychological
  Association) 345n
practitioners
  acupuncture 83–84
  apitherapy 254
  art therapy 301–2
  Ayurvedic medicine 70
  biofeedback 306–8
  chiropractic 400–401
  complementary and
    alternative medicine 10
  Feldenkrais method 411
  guided imagery 323
  manipulative and body-based
    practices 363–64
  music therapy 336
  naturopathy 93–95
  overview 32–36
  polarity therapy 468–69
  Reiki 473
  tai chi 351
  therapeutic touch 480, 482
  traditional Chinese
    medicine 77–78
  yoga 355
prakriti, Ayurvedic medicine 67
prayer, overview 341–44
prebiotics, described 219
preeclampsia, fish oils 181
preformed vitamin A,
  described 129
pregnancy
  Alexander technique 378
  fish oils 186–87
  magnet therapy 499
premenstrual syndrome,
  vitamin B6 139
principle of dilutions 86
principle of similars 63, 85
probiotics
  defined 596
  overview 219–23
professional organizations,
  CAM practitioners 33
progesterone, described 554–57
proprioceptive neuromuscular
  facilitation, described 386

proteins
  vegans 277
  vegetarians 280
provitamin A carotenoid,
  described 129–30
psoriasis, fish oils 181
purification, detoxification
  diets 265
putative energy fields,
  described 455, 458–61
pyridoxal 137
pyridoxamine 137
pyridoxine 137

Q

qi (chi)
  acupuncture 82
  defined 597
  described 24, 69
  feng shui 317–18
  shiatsu 475
  tai chi 349
  traditional Chinese
    medicine 75
qi gong
  described 24, 76, 458–59
  overview 427–29
"Questions and Answers:
  The NIH Trial of EDTA
  Chelation Therapy for
  Coronary Artery Disease"
  (NCCAM) 537n

R

radio psychiatry, mental health
  care 578–79
RDA *see* Recommended Dietary
  Allowances
reactive oxygen species (ROS),
  vitamin E 153–54
Recommended Dietary
  Allowances (RDA)
  folic acid *162*
  vitamin A 130–31
  vitamin B6 138
red clover, menopause 570
redirected thinking, described 312

reflexology
  defined 597
  described 23
  overview 431–33
Reflexology Association of America,
  contact information 610
regulations
  dietary supplements 53, 102–3,
    112–13
  omega-3 fatty acids 55
Reiki
  defined 597
  described 23
  overview 471–74
"Reiki: An Introduction"
  (NCCAM) 471n
relaxation therapy
  allergies 506
  described 312
  overview 345–47
  sleep disorders 588
religious traditions
  counseling, described 313
  meditation 329
  spirituality 341–44
repetitive strain injury,
  Alexander technique 375, 377
resveratrol, described 557–58
retinal, described 129
retinoic acid, described 129
retinoids, described 134
retinol, described 129–30
rheumatoid arthritis
  CAM therapies 491–502
  fish oils 178
"Rheumatoid Arthritis and
  Complementary and Alternative
  Medicine" (NCCAM) 491n
rickets, vitamin D 148
Riley, Joe Shelby 431
RNA (ribonucleic acid), folic acid 161
Roaccutane (isotretinoin), acne 134
Rolf, Ida 436, 438–40, 445–46
Rolfing, overview 438–46
Rolf Institute of Structural
  Integration
  contact information 610
  Rolfing publication 438n
ROS *see* reactive oxygen species

S

Saccharomyces boulardii 220
safety considerations
aromatherapy 260
Ayurvedic medicine 70–71
botanicals 109–10
CAM therapies 28–30
color therapy 359
complementary and
alternative medicine 8–9, 18
dietary supplements 29, 114–15,
122–23
fish oils 184–85
massage therapy 416–17
online medical products 51–56
Reiki 472–73
supplements 118–19
traditional Chinese
medicine 76–77
see also fraud
St. John's wort
attention deficit hyperactivity
disorder 580–81
overview 216–17
research 251
"St. John's Wort" (NCCAM) 216n
"St. John's Wort Shows No Impact
on the Symptoms of ADHD"
(NCCAM) 580n
salmon oil 176
SAMe (S-adenosyl-L-methionine),
research 250
SAMHSA *see* Substance Abuse
and Mental Health Services
Administration
Sawitzke, Allen D. 201–2
schisandra 544
schizophrenia, fish oils 181
Schroter, Aman 387
Scripps Center for Integrative
Medicine, contact information 610
SeaSilver 54
Selected Vegetables/Sun's Soup
513–16
"Selected Vegetables/Sun's Soup"
(NCI) 507n
"Selecting a CAM Practitioner"
(NCCAM) 32n

selenium
overview 193–96
prostate cancer 156–57
research 27, 194
"Selenium" (ODS) 193n
Selenium and Vitamin C Cancer
Prevention Trial (SELECT) 27, 194
self-hypnosis, anxiety 582
"Self-Hypnosis Beneficial for
Women Undergoing Breast
Biopsy" (NCCAM) 582n
serotonin, vitamin B6 138
sexual enhancement, health
fraud 47
shark liver oil 176
Sherrington, Charles 431
"Shiatsu" (Center for Integrative
Health and Healing) 475n
shiatsu, overview 475–78
Shults, Clifford 519–21
side effects
acupuncture 82
aromatherapy 260
chiropractic 401
detoxification diets 265
echinacea 207
fish oils 185–86
flaxseed 191
Gerson therapy 272
ginkgo biloba 215
green tea 237
homeopathy 88
isotretinoin 134
magnet therapy 466
meditation 332
naturopathy 95–96
probiotics 222–23
spinal manipulation 565
tai chi 351
yoga 355
similars principle 63, 85
SkinAnswer 54
sleep disorders, CAM
therapies 585–90
Society for Clinical and Experimental
Hypnosis, contact information 327
Society for Light Treatment and
Biological Rhythms, website
address 610

Society of Auricular Acupuncturists, contact information 611
sound energy therapy, described 458
Sova, Ruth 395
soy, menopause 570
spinal manipulation
   described 23
   pain management 563–65
   see also chiropractic
"Spinal Manipulation for Low-Back Pain" (NCCAM) 563n
spirituality
   defined 597
   overview 341–44
"Spirituality in Cancer Care" (NCI) 341n
sports supplements
   adolescents 117–19
   overview 226–30
"Sports Supplements" (Nemours Foundation) 226n
statistics
   acupuncture 82
   Ayurvedic medicine 66
   CAM therapies 508
   complementary and alternative medicine 13–16, 17
   dietary supplements 112, 244–45
   homeopathy 86
   manipulative and body-based practices 363
   massage therapy 414
   meditation 330
   naturopathy 92–93
   Reiki 472
   tai chi 350
   traditional Chinese medicine 74
   yoga 354
Stone, Randolph 468
Straus, Stephen E. 501, 585
stress management
   Alexander technique 373
   massage therapy 415–516
   mental health care 577–78
   mind-body medicine 297
   relaxation therapy 347
stroke
   fish oils 182
   hyperbaric oxygen therapy 288

"Study Suggests Coenzyme Q10 Slows Functional Decline in Parkinson Disease" (NINDS) 517n
Substance Abuse and Mental Health Services Administration (SAMHSA)
   contact information 601
   publications
      energy drinks 231n
      mental health care 574n
      supplements 117n
sulfasalazine, folic acid 163
Sun's Soup 513–16
supplements *see* dietary supplements; herbal supplements
"Supplements: Added Risk, Doubtful Benefit" (SAMHSA) 117n
support groups, described 313
surgical preparation, mind-body medicine 297
Sushruta Samhita 66
sympathetic nervous system, meditation 332
synbiotics, described 219

T

tai chi
   defined 597
   described 24, 76
   overview 349–52
   qi gong 429
"Tai Chi: An Introduction" (NCCAM) 349n
Takata, Hawayo 471
TCM *see* traditional Chinese medicine
telemedicine, mental health care 578
telephone counseling, mental health care 578
testosterone, described 553–54
Thai Yoga Center/Soma Veda Institute, contact information 611
therapeutic touch *see* touch therapy
"Therapeutic Touch" (A.D.A.M., Inc.) 479n
Therapeutic Touch International Association, contact information 611
thermogenics, described 228
Thomas, Jennifer 53

thunder god vine
 arthritis 492–93
 described 61
tincture, described 108
"Tips for Older Dietary
 Supplement Users" (FDA) 121n
"Tips for Talking with Your Health
 Care Providers about CAM"
 (NCCAM) 37n
TJ-108 544
Tolerable Upper Intake Levels (UL),
 vitamin A 130–31, 134
touch therapy
 described 313, 459–60
 overview 479–82
toxins, described 264
traditional Chinese medicine (TCM)
 defined 597
 described 24–25, 59–60
 mental health care 576–77
 overview 74–78
"Traditional Chinese Medicine: An
 Introduction" (NCCAM) 74n
Trager approach, overview 450–51
Trager International
 contact information 611
 Trager approach publication 450n
transcendental meditation, described
 331
transplant rejections, fish oils 178, 182
"Treating Infertility with Herbal
 Medications" (American Pregnancy
 Association) 560n
triamterene, folic acid 163
triglyceride levels, fish oils 177
Tripterygium wilfordii Hook F 61
tryptophan, vitamin B6 137
Tui Na, overview 421–22
"Tui Na: Chinese Massage" (Center
 for Integrative Health and Healing)
 421n
tuning fork therapy 458
"Turn off Allergies" (Bompey) 484n

U

UL *see* Tolerable Upper Intake Levels
ulcerative colitis, fish oils 182
ultra-high dilutions, described 87

United States Pharmacopeia (USP),
 described 199
University of California,
 publications
 crystal therapy 486n
 fasting 267n
 macrobiotics 273n
 Native American medicine 78n
University of Minnesota Center for
 Spirituality and Healing, contact
 information 611
unpredictable command
 technique, described 387
urinary tract infections,
 naturopathy 62–63
US Department of Health and
 Human Services (DHHS; HHS),
 contact information 601
"Use Caution Buying Medical
 Products Online" (FDA) 51n
"The Use of Complementary and
 Alternative Medicine in the
 United States" (NCCAM) 13n
US Food and Drug Administration
 (FDA)
 contact information 601
 publications
  dietary supplements 121n
  health fraud awareness 45n
  online medical products 51n
"Using Dietary Supplements Wisely"
 (NCCAM) 111n
USP *see* United States
 Pharmacopeia
Usui, Mikao 471

V

valerian
 arthritis 494–95
 research 251
vata, Ayurvedic medicine 68
"Vegan Diets in a Nutshell"
 (Vegetarian Resource Group) 275n
veganism, overview 275–79
vegans, defined 280, 597
"Vegetarianism" (Nemours
 Foundation) 279n
vegetarianism, overview 279–83

Vegetarian Resource Group
  contact information 611
  veganism publication 275n
vegetarians, defined 597
veritable energy fields,
  described 455, 456–58
vibrational therapy 458
vis medicatrix naturae 91
vitamin A, overview 129–35
"Vitamin A and Carotenoids"
  (ODS) 129n
"Vitamin B6" (ODS) 137n
vitamin B6, overview 137–41
vitamin B12
  overview 143–46
  vegans 278–79
  vegetarians 280
"Vitamin B12" (ODS) 143n
vitamin B17 54
vitamin C, research 250
vitamin D
  overview 147–51
  vegans 277
  vegetarians 280
"Vitamin D" (ODS) 147n
vitamin E
  overview 153–59
  research 27, 250
"Vitamin E Fact Sheet" (ODS) 153n
vitamins, defined 597

W

Wassertanzen, described 387
water Pilates, described 386
Watsu, described 387
weight management
  fish oils 182
  green tea 236–37
  health fraud 47
  hoodia 238–39
  resveratrol 557–58
"What can I expect in a typical
  Polarity Therapy session?"
  (American Polarity Therapy
  Association) 467n
"What Hellerwork Structural
  Integration Is" (Hellerwork
  International) 436n

"What is CAM?" (NCCAM) 3n
"What Is Dance/Movement
  Therapy?" (American Dance
  Therapy Association) 359n
"What is Polarity Therapy?"
  (American Polarity Therapy
  Association) 467n
"What is Qigong?" (National
  Qigong Association) 427n
"What Is the Trager Approach?"
  (Trager International) 450n
WholeHealthMD, contact
  information 611
whole medical systems
  defined 597
  described 4, 24–26
  energy medicine 459
  overview 59–64
"Whole Medical Systems: An
  Overview" (NCCAM) 59n
Wills, Lucy 161
wind chime therapy 458
Women's Angiographic
  Vitamin and Estrogen
  study 155
Women's Antioxidant and
  Folic Acid Cardiovascular
  Study 146
Women's Health Study,
  magnesium 171
wound healing
  hydrotherapy 383
  millimeter wave therapy 457
  mind-body medicine 297
  zinc 208–9
Wykle, Mary 387

X

Xhoba 238

Y

yang *see* yin/yang
Yellow Jackets (slang) 53–54
yinhsing 214
yin/yang
  acupuncture 81
  defined 597–98

yin/yang, continued
  described 24, 69
  macrobiotics 273
  polarity therapy 468
  traditional Chinese medicine 75
yoga
  defined 598
  described 24
  hydrotherapy 387
  mental health care 577
  overview 353–56
"Yoga for Health: An Introduction"
  (NCCAM) 353n
Yogalates, described 387–88, 391–92

Z

zeaxanthin, vitamin A 130
Zen macrobiotic diet 273
zero balancing, overview 487–88
Zero Balancing Health Association
  contact information 611
  zero balancing publication 487n
zinc
  overview 208–11
  research 251
  vegans 278
  vegetarians 281
"Zinc" (ODS) 208n

Health Reference Series
Complete Catalog
List price $93 per volume. School and library price $84 per volume.

Adolescent Health Sourcebook, 3rd Edition

Basic Consumer Health Information about Adolescent Growth and Development, Puberty, Sexuality, Reproductive Health, and Physical, Emotional, Social, and Mental Health Concerns of Teens and Their Parents, Including Facts about Nutrition, Physical Activity, Weight Management, Acne, Allergies, Cancer, Diabetes, Growth Disorders, Juvenile Arthritis, Infections, Substance Abuse, and More

Along with Information about Adolescent Safety Concerns, Youth Violence, a Glossary of Related Terms, and a Directory of Resources

Edited by Amy L. Sutton. 600 pages. 2010. 978-0-7808-1140-9.

Adult Health Concerns Sourcebook

Basic Consumer Health Information about Medical and Mental Concerns of Adults, Including Facts about Choosing Healthcare Providers, Navigating Insurance Options, Maintaining Wellness, Preventing Cancer, Heart Disease, Stroke, Diabetes, and Osteoporosis, and Understanding Aging-Related Health Concerns, Including Menopause, Cognitive Changes, and Changes in the Coronary and Vascular Systems

Along with Tips on Caring for Aging Parents and Dealing with Health-Related Work and Travel Issues, a Glossary, and a Directory of Resources for Additional Help and Information

Edited by Sandra J. Judd. 648 pages. 2008. 978-0-7808-0999-4.

"Provides a thorough list of topics that are important to adult health and for caregivers."
—*CHOICE, Nov '08*

"Written in easy-to-understand language... the content is well-organized and is intended to aid adults in making health care-related decisions."
—*AORN Journal, Dec '08*

AIDS Sourcebook, 4th Edition

Basic Consumer Health Information about Human Immunodeficiency Virus (HIV) and Acquired Immunodeficiency Syndrome (AIDS), Featuring Updated Statistics and Facts about Risks, Prevention, Screening, Diagnosis, Treatments, Side Effects, and Complications, and Including a Section about the Impact of HIV/AIDS on the Health of Women, Children, and Adolescents

Along with Tips on Managing Life with AIDS, Reports on Current Research Initiatives and Clinical Trials, a Glossary of Related Terms, and Resource Directories for Further Help and Information

Edited by Ivy L. Alexander. 680 pages. 2008. 978-0-7808-0997-0.

SEE ALSO *Contagious Diseases Sourcebook, 2nd Edition*

Alcoholism Sourcebook, 3rd Edition

Basic Consumer Health Information about Alcohol Use, Abuse, and Dependence, Featuring Facts about the Physical, Mental, and Social Health Effects of Alcohol Addiction, Including Alcoholic Liver Disease, Pancreatic Disease, Cardiovascular Disease, Neurological Disorders, and the Effects of Drinking during Pregnancy

Along with Information about Alcohol Treatment, Medications, and Recovery Programs, in Addition to Tips for Reducing the Prevalence of Underage Drinking, Statistics about Alcohol Use, a Glossary of Related Terms, and Directories of Resources for More Help and Information

Edited by Joyce Brennfleck Shannon. 600 pages. 2010. 978-0-7808-1141-6.

SEE ALSO *Drug Abuse Sourcebook, 3rd Edition*

Allergies Sourcebook, 3rd Edition

Basic Consumer Health Information about Allergic Disorders, Such as Anaphylaxis, Hives,

Eczema, Rhinitis, Sinusitis, and Conjunctivitis, and Their Triggers, Including Pollen, Mold, Dust Mites, Animal Dander, Insects, Chemicals, Food, Food Additives, and Medications

Along with Advice about the Diagnosis and Treatment of Allergy Symptoms, a Glossary of Related Terms, a Directory of Resources for Help and Information, and Suggestions for Additional Reading

Edited by Amy L. Sutton. 588 pages. 2007. 978-0-7808-0950-5.

SEE ALSO Asthma Sourcebook, 2nd Edition

Alzheimer Disease Sourcebook, 4th Edition

Basic Consumer Health Information about Alzheimer Disease, Other Dementias, and Related Disorders, Including Multi-Infarct Dementia, Dementia with Lewy Bodies, Frontotemporal Dementia (Pick Disease), Wernicke-Korsakoff Syndrome (Alcohol-Related Dementia), AIDS Dementia Complex, Huntington Disease, Creutzfeldt-Jacob Disease, and Delirium

Along with Information about Coping with Memory Loss and Forgetfulness, Maintaining Skills, and Long-Term Planning for People with Dementia, and Suggestions Addressing Common Caregiver Concerns, Updated Information about Current Research Efforts, a Glossary of Related Terms, and Directories of Sources for Additional Help and Information

Edited by Karen Bellenir. 603 pages. 2008. 978-0-7808-1001-3.

"An invaluable resource for persons who have received a diagnosis, for caregivers, and for family members dealing with this insidious disease. It is recommended for public, community college, and ready-reference sections in academic libraries."
—American Reference Books Annual, 2009

SEE ALSO Brain Disorders Sourcebook, 3rd Edition

Arthritis Sourcebook, 3rd Edition

Basic Consumer Health Information about the Risk Factors, Symptoms, Diagnosis, and Treatment of Osteoarthritis, Rheumatoid Arthritis, Juvenile Arthritis, Gout, Infectious Arthritis, and Autoimmune Disorders Associated with Arthritis

Along with Facts about Medications, Surgeries, and Self-Care Techniques to Manage Pain and Disability, Tips on Living with Arthritis, a Glossary of Related Terms, and Resources for Additional Help and Information

Edited by Amy L. Sutton. 600 pages. 2010. 978-0-7808-1077-8.

Asthma Sourcebook, 2nd Edition

Basic Consumer Health Information about the Causes, Symptoms, Diagnosis, and Treatment of Asthma in Infants, Children, Teenagers, and Adults, Including Facts about Different Types of Asthma, Common Co-Occurring Conditions, Asthma Management Plans, Triggers, Medications, and Medication Delivery Devices

Along with Asthma Statistics, Research Updates, a Glossary, a Directory of Asthma-Related Resources, and More

Edited by Karen Bellenir. 581 pages. 2006. 978-0-7808-0866-9.

SEE ALSO Lung Disorders Sourcebook; Respiratory Disorders Sourcebook, 2nd Edition

Attention Deficit Disorder Sourcebook

Basic Consumer Health Information about Attention Deficit/Hyperactivity Disorder in Children and Adults, Including Facts about Causes, Symptoms, Diagnostic Criteria, and Treatment Options Such as Medications, Behavior Therapy, Coaching, and Homeopathy

Along with Reports on Current Research Initiatives, Legal Issues, and Government Regulations, and Featuring a Glossary of Related Terms, Internet Resources, and a List of Additional Reading Material

Edited by Dawn D. Matthews. 447 pages. 2002. 978-0-7808-0624-5.

"Recommended reference source."
—Booklist, Jan '03

SEE ALSO Learning Disabilities Sourcebook, 3rd Edition

Autism and Pervasive Developmental Disorders Sourcebook

Basic Consumer Health Information about Autism Spectrum and Pervasive Developmental Disorders, Such as Classical Autism, Asperger Syndrome, Rett Syndrome, and Childhood Disintegrative Disorder, Including Information about Related Genetic Disorders and Medical Problems and Facts about Causes, Screening Methods, Diagnostic Criteria, Treatments and Interventions, and Family and Education Issues

Along with a Glossary of Related Terms, Tips for Evaluating the Validity of Health Claims, and a Directory of Resources for Additional Help and Information

Edited by Sandra J. Judd. 603 pages. 2007. 978-0-7808-0953-6.

"This book provides a current overview of disorders on the autism spectrum and information about various therapies, educational resources, and help for families with practical issues such as workplace adjustments, living arrangements, and estate planning. It is a useful resource for public and consumer health libraries."
—*American Reference Books Annual, 2009*

SEE ALSO Learning Disabilities Sourcebook, 3rd Edition

Back and Neck Disorders Sourcebook, 2nd Edition

Basic Consumer Health Information about Spinal Pain, Spinal Cord Injuries, and Related Disorders, Such as Degenerative Disk Disease, Osteoarthritis, Scoliosis, Sciatica, Spina Bifida, and Spinal Stenosis, and Featuring Facts about Maintaining Spinal Health, Self-Care, Pain Management, Rehabilitative Care, Chiropractic Care, Spinal Surgeries, and Complementary Therapies

Along with Suggestions for Preventing Back and Neck Pain, a Glossary of Related Terms, and a Directory of Resources

Edited by Amy L. Sutton. 607 pages. 2004. 978-0-7808-0738-9.

"Recommended... An easy to use, comprehensive medical reference book."
—*E-Streams, Sep '05*

"For anyone who has back or neck problems, this book is ideal. Its easy-to-understand language and variety of topics makes this sourcebook a worthwhile read. The price... is reasonable for the amount of information contained in the book"
—*Occupational Therapy in Health Care, 2007*

Blood & Circulatory Disorders Sourcebook, 3rd Edition

Basic Consumer Health Information about Blood and Circulatory System Disorders, Such as Anemia, Leukemia, Lymphoma, Rh Disease, Hemophilia, Thrombophilia, Other Bleeding and Clotting Deficiencies, and Artery, Vascular, and Venous Diseases, Including Facts about Blood Types, Blood Donation, Bone Marrow and Stem Cell Transplants, Tests and Medications, and Tips for Maintaining Circulatory Health

Along with a Glossary of Related Terms and a List of Resources for Additional Help and Information

Edited by Sandra J. Judd. 600 pages. 2010. 978-0-7808-1081-5.

SEE ALSO Leukemia Sourcebook

Brain Disorders Sourcebook, 3rd Edition

Basic Consumer Health Information about Acquired and Traumatic Brain Injuries, Brain Tumors, Cerebral Palsy and Other Genetic and Congenital Brain Disorders, Infections of the Brain, Epilepsy, and Degenerative Neurological Disorders Such as Dementia, Huntington Disease, and Amyotrophic Lateral Sclerosis (ALS)

Along with Information on Brain Structure and Function, Treatment and Rehabilitation Options, a Glossary of Terms Related to Brain Disorders, and a Directory of Resources for More Information

Edited by Joyce Brennfleck Shannon. 600 pages. 2010. 978-0-7808-1083-9.

SEE ALSO Alzheimer Disease Sourcebook, 4th Edition

Breast Cancer Sourcebook, 3rd Edition

Basic Consumer Health Information about Breast Health and Breast Cancer, Including Facts about Environmental, Genetic, and Other Risk Factors, Prevention Efforts, Screening and Diagnostic Methods, Surgical Treatment Options and Other Care Choices, Complementary and Alternative Therapies, and Post-Treatment Concerns

Along with Statistical Data, News about Research Advances, a Glossary of Related Terms, and Directories of Resources for Additional Information and Support

Edited by Karen Bellenir. 606 pages. 2009. 978-0-7808-1030-3.

"A very useful reference for people wanting to learn more about breast cancer and how to negotiate their care or the care of a loved one. The third edition is necessary as information/treatment options continue to evolve."
—Doody's Review Service, 2009

SEE ALSO *Cancer Sourcebook for Women, 3rd Edition, Women's Health Concerns Sourcebook, 3rd Edition*

Breastfeeding Sourcebook

Basic Consumer Health Information about the Benefits of Breastmilk, Preparing to Breastfeed, Breastfeeding as a Baby Grows, Nutrition, and More, Including Information on Special Situations and Concerns Such as Mastitis, Illness, Medications, Allergies, Multiple Births, Prematurity, Special Needs, and Adoption

Along with a Glossary and Resources for Additional Help and Information

Edited by Jenni Lynn Colson. 367 pages. 2002. 978-0-7808-0332-9.

SEE ALSO *Pregnancy and Birth Sourcebook, 3rd Edition*

Burns Sourcebook

Basic Consumer Health Information about Various Types of Burns and Scalds, Including Flame, Heat, Cold, Electrical, Chemical, and Sun Burns

Along with Information on Short-Term and Long-Term Treatments, Tissue Reconstruction, Plastic Surgery, Prevention Suggestions, and First Aid

Edited by Allan R. Cook. 604 pages. 1999. 978-0-7808-0204-9.

"This is an exceptional addition to the series and is highly recommended for all consumer health collections, hospital libraries, and academic medical centers."
—E-Streams, Mar '00

"This key reference guide is an invaluable addition to all health care and public libraries in confronting this ongoing health issue."
—American Reference Books Annual, 2000

SEE ALSO *Dermatological Disorders Sourcebook, 2nd Edition*

Cancer Sourcebook, 5th Edition

Basic Consumer Health Information about Major Forms and Stages of Cancer, Featuring Facts about Head and Neck Cancers, Lung Cancers, Gastrointestinal Cancers, Genitourinary Cancers, Lymphomas, Blood Cell Cancers, Endocrine Cancers, Skin Cancers, Bone Cancers, Metastatic Cancers, and More

Along with Facts about Cancer Treatments, Cancer Risks and Prevention, a Glossary of Related Terms, Statistical Data, and a Directory of Resources for Additional Information

Edited by Karen Bellenir. 1105 pages. 2007. 978-0-7808-0947-5.

"The 5th, updated edition of Cancer Sourcebook should be in every public and health lending library collection... An unparalleled discussion essential for any health collections considering an all-in-one basic general reference."
—California Bookwatch, Aug '07

SEE ALSO *Breast Cancer Sourcebook, 3rd Edition, Cancer Survivorship Sourcebook, Leukemia Sourcebook*

Cancer Sourcebook for Women, 4th Edition

Basic Consumer Health Information about Gynecologic Cancers and Other Cancers of Special Concern to Women, Including Cancers of the Breast, Cervix, Colon, Lung, Ovaries, Thyroid, and Uterus

Along with Facts about Benign Conditions of the Female Reproductive System, Cancer Risk

642

Factors, Diagnostic and Treatment Procedures, Side Effects of Cancer and Cancer Treatments, Women's Issues in Cancer Survivorship, a Glossary of Related Terms, and a Directory of Resources for Additional Help and Information

Edited by Karen Bellenir. 600 pages. 2010. 978-0-7808-1139-3.

SEE ALSO Breast Cancer Sourcebook, 3rd Edition, Women's Health Concerns Sourcebook, 3rd Edition

Cancer Survivorship Sourcebook

Basic Consumer Health Information about the Physical, Educational, Emotional, Social, and Financial Needs of Cancer Patients from Diagnosis, through Cancer Treatment, and Beyond, Including Facts about Researching Specific Types of Cancer and Learning about Clinical Trials and Treatment Options, and Featuring Tips for Coping with the Side Effects of Cancer Treatments and Adjusting to Life after Cancer Treatment Concludes

Along with Suggestions for Caregivers, Friends, and Family Members of Cancer Patients, a Glossary of Cancer Care Terms, and Directories of Related Resources

Edited by Karen Bellenir. 633 pages. 2007. 978-0-7808-0985-7.

"Well organized and comprehensive in coverage, the book speaks to issues encountered both during and after cancer treatment. Recommended for consumer health and public libraries."
—*Library Journal, Aug 1 '07*

"Cancer Survivorship Sourcebook will be useful to anyone who has a friend or loved one with a cancer diagnosis."
—*American Reference Books Annual, 2008*

SEE ALSO *Cancer Sourcebook, 5th Edition, Disease Management Sourcebook*

Cardiovascular Disorders Sourcebook, 4th Edition

Basic Consumer Health Information about Heart and Blood Vessel Diseases and Disorders, Such as Angina, Heart Attack, Heart Failure, Cardiomyopathy, Arrhythmias, Valve Disease, Atherosclerosis, Aneurysms, and

Congenital Heart Defects, Including Information about Cardiovascular Disease in Women, Men, Children, Adolescents, and Minorities

Along with Facts about Diagnosing, Managing, and Preventing Cardiovascular Disease, a Glossary of Related Medical Terms, and a Directory of Resources for Additional Information

Edited by Amy L. Sutton. 600 pages. 2010. 978-0-7808-1080-8.

Caregiving Sourcebook

Basic Consumer Health Information for Caregivers, Including a Profile of Caregivers, Caregiving Responsibilities and Concerns, Tips for Specific Conditions, Care Environments, and the Effects of Caregiving

Along with Facts about Legal Issues, Financial Information, and Future Planning, a Glossary, and a Listing of Additional Resources

Edited by Joyce Brennfleck Shannon. 583 pages. 2001. 978-0-7808-0331-2.

"Essential for most collections."
—*Library Journal, Apr 1 '02*

"An ideal addition to the reference collection of any public library. Health sciences information professionals may also want to acquire the Caregiving Sourcebook for their hospital or academic library for use as a ready reference tool by health care workers interested in aging and caregiving."
—*E-Streams, Jan '02*

Child Abuse Sourcebook, 2nd Edition

Basic Consumer Health Information about the Physical, Sexual, and Emotional Abuse of Children, Neglect, Münchhausen Syndrome by Proxy (MSBP), and Shaken Baby Syndrome, and Featuring Facts about Withholding Medical Care, Corporal Punishment, Child Maltreatment in Youth Sports, and Parental Substance Abuse

Along with Information about Child Protective Services, Foster Care, Adoption, Parenting Challenges, Abuse Prevention Programs, and Intervention, Treatment, and Recovery Guidelines, a Glossary of Related Terms, and Resources for Additional Help and Information

Edited by Joyce Brennfleck Shannon. 600 pages. 2009. 978-0-7808-1037-2.

SEE ALSO *Domestic Violence Sourcebook, 3rd Edition*

Childhood Diseases and Disorders Sourcebook, 2nd Edition

Basic Consumer Health Information about the Physical, Mental, and Developmental Health of Pre-Adolescent Children, Including Facts about Infectious Diseases, Asthma, Allergies, Diabetes, and Other Acute and Chronic Conditions Affecting the Gastrointestinal Tract, Ears, Nose, Throat, Liver, Kidneys, Heart, Blood, Brain, Muscles, Bones, and Skin

Along with Reports on Recommended Childhood Vaccinations, Wellness Guidelines, a Glossary of Related Medical Terms, and a List of Resources for Parents

Edited by Sandra J. Judd. 694 pages. 2009. 978-0-7808-1031-0.

"The strength of this source is the wide range of information given about childhood health issues... It is most appropriate for public libraries and academic libraries that field medical questions."
—*American Reference Books Annual, 2009*

SEE ALSO *Healthy Children Sourcebook*

Colds, Flu and Other Common Ailments Sourcebook

Basic Consumer Health Information about Common Ailments and Injuries, Including Colds, Coughs, the Flu, Sinus Problems, Headaches, Fever, Nausea and Vomiting, Menstrual Cramps, Diarrhea, Constipation, Hemorrhoids, Back Pain, Dandruff, Dry and Itchy Skin, Cuts, Scrapes, Sprains, Bruises, and More

Along with Information about Prevention, Self-Care, Choosing a Doctor, Over-the-Counter Medications, Folk Remedies, and Alternative Therapies, and Including a Glossary of Important Terms and a Directory of Resources for Further Help and Information

Edited by Chad T. Kimball. 622 pages. 2001. 978-0-7808-0435-7.

"A good starting point for research on common illnesses. It will be a useful addition to public and consumer health library collections."
—*American Reference Books Annual, 2002*

"Will prove valuable to any library seeking to maintain a current, comprehensive reference collection of health resources... Excellent reference."
—*The Bookwatch, Aug '01*

SEE ALSO *Contagious Diseases Sourcebook, 2nd Edition*

Communication Disorders Sourcebook

Basic Information about Deafness and Hearing Loss, Speech and Language Disorders, Voice Disorders, Balance and Vestibular Disorders, and Disorders of Smell, Taste, and Touch

Edited by Linda M. Ross. 533 pages. 1996. 978-0-7808-0077-9.

"This is skillfully edited and is a welcome resource for the layperson. It should be found in every public and medical library."
—*Booklist Health Sciences Supplement, Oct '97*

Complementary & Alternative Medicine Sourcebook, 4th Edition

Basic Consumer Health Information about Ayurveda, Acupuncture, Aromatherapy, Chiropractic Care, Diet-Based Therapies, Guided Imagery, Herbal and Vitamin Supplements, Homeopathy, Hypnosis, Massage, Meditation, Naturopathy, Pilates, Reflexology, Reiki, Shiatsu, Tai Chi, Traditional Chinese Medicine, Yoga, and Other Complementary and Alternative Medical Therapies

Along with Statistics, Tips for Selecting a Practitioner, Treatments for Specific Health Conditions, a Glossary of Related Terms, and a Directory of Resources for Additional Help and Information

Edited by Amy L. Sutton. 600 pages. 2010. 978-0-7808-1082-2.

Congenital Disorders Sourcebook, 2nd Edition

Basic Consumer Health Information about Nonhereditary Birth Defects and Disorders

Related to Prematurity, Gestational Injuries, Congenital Infections, and Birth Complications, Including Heart Defects, Hydrocephalus, Spina Bifida, Cleft Lip and Palate, Cerebral Palsy, and More

Along with Facts about the Prevention of Birth Defects, Fetal Surgery and Other Treatment Options, Research Initiatives, a Glossary of Related Terms, and Resources for Additional Information and Support

Edited by Sandra J. Judd. 619 pages. 2007. 978-0-7808-0945-1.

"Congenital Disorders Sourcebook provides an excellent, non-technical overview of many aspects of pregnancy with the focus on congenital disorders."
—American Reference Books Annual, 2008

"An excellent readable reference aimed at the lay public for difficult to understand medical problems. An excellent starting point for the interested parent or family member who may then be motivated to seek more information."
—Doody's Review Service, 2007

SEE ALSO Pregnancy and Birth Sourcebook, 3rd Edition

Contagious Diseases Sourcebook, 2nd Edition

Basic Consumer Health Information about Diseases Spread from Person to Person through Direct Physical Contact, Airborne Transmissions, Sexual Contact, or Contact with Blood or Other Body Fluids, Including Pneumococcal, Staphylococcal, and Streptococcal Diseases, Colds, Influenza, Lice, Measles, Mumps, Tuberculosis, and Others

Along with Facts about Self-Care and Over-the-Counter Medications, Antibiotics and Drug Resistance, Disease Prevention, Vaccines, and Bioterrorism, a Glossary, and a Directory of Resources for More Information

Edited by Joyce Brennfleck Shannon. 600 pages. 2010. 978-0-7808-1075-4.

SEE ALSO AIDS Sourcebook, 4th Edition, Hepatitis Sourcebook

Cosmetic and Reconstructive Surgery Sourcebook, 2nd Edition

Basic Consumer Information about Plastic Surgery and Non-Surgical Appearance-Enhancing Procedures, Including Facts about Botulinum Toxin, Collagen Replacement, Dermabrasion, Chemical Peels, Eyelid Surgery, Nose Reshaping, Lip Augmentation, Liposuction, Breast Enlargement and Reduction, Tummy Tucking, and Other Skin, Hair, Facial, and Body Shaping Procedures

Along with Information about Reconstructive Procedures for Congenital Disorders, Disfiguring Diseases, Burns, and Traumatic Injuries, a Glossary of Related Terms, and a Directory of Additional Resources

Edited by Karen Bellenir. 483 pages. 2007. 978-0-7808-0951-2.

"A comprehensive source for people considering cosmetic surgery... also recommended for medical students who will perform these procedures later in their careers; and public librarians and academic medical librarians who may assist patrons interested in this information."
—Medical Reference Services Quarterly, Fall '08

"A practical guide for health care consumers and health care workers... This easy-to-read reference guide would be useful for novice and veteran health care consumers, surgical technology students, nursing students, and perioperative nurses new to plastic and reconstructive surgery. It also may be helpful for medical-surgical nurses as a guide for patient teaching in their practices."
—AORN Journal, Aug '08

SEE ALSO Surgery Sourcebook, 2nd Edition

Death and Dying Sourcebook, 2nd Edition

Basic Consumer Health Information about End-of-Life Care and Related Perspectives and Ethical Issues, Including End-of-Life Symptoms and Treatments, Pain Management, Quality-of-Life Concerns, the Use of Life Support, Patients' Rights and Privacy Issues, Advance Directives, Physician-Assisted Suicide, Caregiving, Organ and Tissue Donation, Autopsies, Funeral Arrangements, and Grief

Along with Statistical Data, Information about the Leading Causes of Death, a Glossary, and Directories of Support Groups and Other Resources

Edited by Joyce Brennfleck Shannon. 626 pages. 2006. 978-0-7808-0871-3.

Dental Care and Oral Health Sourcebook, 3rd Edition

Basic Consumer Health Information about Dental Care and Oral Health Throughout the Lifespan, Including Facts about Cavities, Bad Breath, Cold and Canker Sores, Dry Mouth, Toothaches, Gum Disease, Malocclusion, Temporomandibular Joint and Muscle Disorders, Oral Cancers, and Dental Emergencies

Along with Information about Mouth Hygiene, Crowns, Bridges, Implants, and Fillings, Surgical, Orthodontic, and Cosmetic Dental Procedures, Pain Management, Health Conditions that Impact Oral Care, a Glossary of Related Terms, and a Directory of Additional Resources

Edited by Amy L. Sutton. 619 pages. 2008. 978-0-7808-1032-7.

"Could serve as turning point in the battle to educate consumers in issues concerning oral health. Tightly written in terms the average person can understand, yet comprehensive in scope and authoritative in tone, it is another excellent sourcebook in the Health Reference Series... Should be in the reference department of all public libraries, and in academic libraries that have a public constituency."
—American Reference Books Annual, 2009

Depression Sourcebook, 2nd Edition

Basic Consumer Health Information about Unipolar Depression, Bipolar Disorder, Dysthymia, Seasonal Affective Disorder, Postpartum Depression, and Other Depressive Disorders, Including Facts about Populations at Special Risk, Coexisting Medical Conditions, Symptoms, Treatment Options, and Suicide Prevention

Along with Statistical Data, a Glossary of Related Terms, and a Directory of Resources for Additional Help and Information

Edited by Sandra J. Judd. 646 pages. 2008. 978-0-7808-1003-7.

"Recommended for public libraries."
—American Reference Books Annual, 2009

SEE ALSO Mental Health Disorders Sourcebook, 4th Edition

Dermatological Disorders Sourcebook, 2nd Edition

Basic Consumer Health Information about Conditions and Disorders Affecting the Skin, Hair, and Nails, Such as Acne, Rosacea, Rashes, Dermatitis, Pigmentation Disorders, Birthmarks, Skin Cancer, Skin Injuries, Psoriasis, Scleroderma, and Hair Loss, Including Facts about Medications and Treatments for Dermatological Disorders and Tips for Maintaining Healthy Skin, Hair, and Nails

Along with Information about How Aging Affects the Skin, a Glossary of Related Terms, and a Directory of Resources for Additional Help and Information

Edited by Amy L. Sutton. 617 pages. 2006. 978-0-7808-0795-2.

"Well organized... presents a plethora of information in a manner that is appropriate in style and readability for the intended audience."
—Physical Therapy, Nov '06

"Helpfully brings together... sources in one convenient place, saving the user hours of research time."
—American Reference Books Annual, 2006

SEE ALSO Burns Sourcebook

Diabetes Sourcebook, 4th Edition

Basic Consumer Health Information about Type 1 and Type 2 Diabetes Mellitus, Gestational Diabetes, Monogenic Forms of Diabetes, and Insulin Resistance, with Guidelines for Lifestyle Modifications and the Medical Management of Diabetes, Including Facts about Insulin, Insulin Delivery Devices, Oral Diabetes Medications, Self-Monitoring of Blood Glucose, Meal Planning, Physical Activity Recommendations, Foot Care, and Treatment Options for People with Kidney Failure

Along with a Section about Diabetes Complications and Co-Occurring Conditions, a Glossary of Related Terms, and Directories of Resources for Additional Help and Information

Edited by Karen Bellenir. 627 pages. 2008. 978-0-7808-1005-1.

"Completely and comprehensively covering almost everything a student or physician would need to know... well worth the investment."
—*Internet Bookwatch, Dec '08*

SEE ALSO *Endocrine and Metabolic Disorders Sourcebook, 2nd Edition*

Diet and Nutrition Sourcebook, 3rd Edition

Basic Consumer Health Information about Dietary Guidelines and the Food Guidance System, Recommended Daily Nutrient Intakes, Serving Proportions, Weight Control, Vitamins and Supplements, Nutrition Issues for Different Life Stages and Lifestyles, and the Needs of People with Specific Medical Concerns, Including Cancer, Celiac Disease, Diabetes, Eating Disorders, Food Allergies, and Cardiovascular Disease

Along with Facts about Federal Nutrition Support Programs, a Glossary of Nutrition and Dietary Terms, and Directories of Additional Resources for More Information about Nutrition

Edited by Joyce Brennfleck Shannon. 605 pages. 2006. 978-0-7808-0800-3.

"A valuable resource tool for any individual."
—*Journal of Dental Hygiene, Apr '07*

"From different recommended eating habits to reduce disease and common ailments to nutrition advice for those with specific conditions, Diet and Nutrition Sourcebook is especially important because so much is changing in this area, and so rapidly."
—*California Bookwatch, Jun '06*

SEE ALSO *Eating Disorders Sourcebook, 2nd Edition, Vegetarian Sourcebook*

Digestive Diseases and Disorders Sourcebook

Basic Consumer Health Information about Diseases and Disorders that Impact the Upper and Lower Digestive System, Including Celiac Disease, Constipation, Crohn's Disease, Cyclic Vomiting Syndrome, Diarrhea, Diverticulosis and Diverticulitis, Gallstones, Heartburn, Hemorrhoids, Hernias, Indigestion (Dyspepsia), Irritable Bowel Syndrome, Lactose Intolerance, Ulcers, and More

Along with Information about Medications and Other Treatments, Tips for Maintaining a Healthy Digestive Tract, a Glossary, and Directory of Digestive Diseases Organizations

Edited by Karen Bellenir. 323 pages. 2000. 978-0-7808-0327-5.

"An excellent addition to all public or patient-research libraries."
—*American Reference Books Annual, 2001*

"Recommended reference source."
—*Booklist, May '00*

SEE ALSO *Gastrointestinal Diseases and Disorders Sourcebook, 2nd Edition*

Disabilities Sourcebook

Basic Consumer Health Information about Physical and Psychiatric Disabilities, Including Descriptions of Major Causes of Disability, Assistive and Adaptive Aids, Workplace Issues, and Accessibility Concerns

Along with Information about the Americans with Disabilities Act, a Glossary, and Resources for Additional Help and Information

Edited by Dawn D. Matthews. 602 pages. 2000. 978-0-7808-0389-3.

"A must for libraries with a consumer health section."
—*American Reference Books Annual, 2002*

"A much needed addition to the Omnigraphics Health Reference Series. A current reference work to provide people with disabilities, their families, caregivers or those who work with them, a broad range of information in one volume, has not been available until now... It is recommended for all public and academic library reference collections."
—*E-Streams, May '01*

"An excellent source book in easy-to-read format covering many current topics; highly recommended for all libraries."
—*CHOICE, Jan '01*

Disease Management Sourcebook

Basic Consumer Health Information about Coping with Chronic and Serious Illnesses, Navigating the Health Care System, Communicating with Health Care Providers, Assessing Health Care Quality, and Making Informed Health Care Decisions, Including Facts about Second Opinions, Hospitalization, Surgery, and Medications

Along with a Section about Children with Chronic Conditions, Information about Legal, Financial, and Insurance Issues, a Glossary of Related Terms, and Directories of Additional Resources

Edited by Joyce Brennfleck Shannon. 621 pages. 2008. 978-0-7808-1002-0.

"Consumers need to know how to manage their health care the same way they manage anything else in their lives. The text is very readable and is written for the layperson and consumer. The cost is not prohibitive. This book should be in all collections of health care libraries and public libraries."
— American Reference Books Annual, 2009

"The information is very current, and the selection of font and layout make the book easy to read. A hardback that will stand up to much usage, this is an excellent resource for consumers... Recommended. General readers."
—CHOICE, Nov '08

"Intended for lay readers, this resource clarifies the many confusing and overwhelming details associated with chronic disease care. Meticulous and clearly explained, the book even includes diagrams intended to ease comprehension of over-the-counter medication labels. An essential guide to navigating the health-care rapids."
—Library Journal, Aug '08

Domestic Violence Sourcebook, 3rd Edition

Basic Consumer Health Information about Warning Signs, Risk Factors, and Health Consequences of Intimate Partner Violence, Sexual Violence and Rape, Stalking, Human Trafficking, Child Maltreatment, Teen Dating Violence, and Elder Abuse

Along with Facts about Victims and Perpetrators, Strategies for Violence Prevention, and Emergency Interventions, Safety Plans, and Financial and Legal Tips for Victims, a Glossary of Related Terms, and Directories of Resources for Additional Information and Support

Edited by Joyce Brennfleck Shannon. 634 pages. 2009. 978-0-7808-1038-9.

"A recommended pick for any library interested in consumer health and social issues... A 'must' for any serious health collection."
—California Bookwatch, Jul '09

SEE ALSO Child Abuse Sourcebook, 2nd Edition

Drug Abuse Sourcebook, 3rd Edition

Basic Consumer Health Information about the Abuse of Cocaine, Club Drugs, Hallucinogens, Heroin, Inhalants, Marijuana, and Other Illicit Substances, Prescription Medications, and Over-the-Counter Medicines

Along with Facts about Addiction and Related Health Effects, Drug Abuse Treatment and Recovery, Drug Testing, Prevention Programs, Glossaries of Drug-Related Terms, and Directories of Resources for More Information

Edited by Joyce Brennfleck Shannon. 600 pages. 2010. 978-0-7808-1079-2.

SEE ALSO Alcoholism Sourcebook, 3rd Edition

Ear, Nose, and Throat Disorders Sourcebook, 2nd Edition

Basic Consumer Health Information about Disorders of the Ears, Hearing Loss, Vestibular Disorders, Nasal and Sinus Problems, Throat and Vocal Cord Disorders, and Otolaryngologic Cancers, Including Facts about Ear Infections and Injuries, Genetic and Congenital Deafness, Sensorineural Hearing Disorders, Tinnitus, Vertigo, Ménière Disease, Rhinitis, Sinusitis, Snoring, Sore Throats, Hoarseness, and More

Along with Reports on Current Research Initiatives, a Glossary of Related Medical Terms, and a Directory of Sources for Further Help and Information

Edited by Sandra J. Judd. 631 pages. 2007. 978-0-7808-0872-0.

"A resource book for the general public that provides comprehensive coverage of basic up-to-date medical information about the causes, symptoms, diagnosis, and treatment of diseases and disorders that affect the ears, nose, sinuses, throat, and voice... The majority of information is presented in question and answer format, much like questions a patient might ask of a health care provider. An extensive index facilitates the reader's ability to easily access information on any specific topic."

—*Journal of Dental Hygiene, Oct '07*

"A handy compilation of information on common and some not so common ailments of the ears, nose, and throat."

—*Doody's Review Service, 2007*

▓

Eating Disorders Sourcebook, 2nd Edition

Basic Consumer Health Information about Anorexia Nervosa, Bulimia, Binge Eating, Compulsive Exercise, Female Athlete Triad, and Other Eating Disorders, Including Facts about Body Image and Other Cultural and Age-Related Risk Factors, Prevention Efforts, Adverse Health Effects, Treatment Options, and the Recovery Process

Along with Guidelines for Healthy Weight Control, a Glossary, and Directories of Additional Resources

Edited by Joyce Brennfleck Shannon. 557 pages. 2007. 978-0-7808-0948-2.

"Recommended for the reference collection of large public libraries."

—*American Reference Books Annual, 2008*

"A basic health reference any health or general library needs."

—*Internet Bookwatch, Jun '07*

SEE ALSO Diet and Nutrition Sourcebook, 3rd Edition, Mental Health Disorders Sourcebook, 4th Edition

▓

Emergency Medical Services Sourcebook

Basic Consumer Health Information about Preventing, Preparing for, and Managing Emergency Situations, When and Who to Call for Help, What to Expect in the Emergency Room, the Emergency Medical Team,

Patient Issues, and Current Topics in Emergency Medicine

Along with Statistical Data, a Glossary, and Sources of Additional Help and Information

Edited by Jenni Lynn Colson. 472 pages. 2002. 978-0-7808-0420-3.

"Handy and convenient for home, public, school, and college libraries. Recommended."

—*CHOICE, Apr '03*

"This reference can provide the consumer with answers to most questions about emergency care in the United States, or it will direct them to a resource where the answer can be found."

—*American Reference Books Annual, 2003*

SEE ALSO Injury and Trauma Sourcebook

▓

Endocrine and Metabolic Disorders Sourcebook, 2nd Edition

Basic Consumer Health Information about Hormonal and Metabolic Disorders that Affect the Body's Growth, Development, and Functioning, Including Disorders of the Pancreas, Ovaries and Testes, and Pituitary, Thyroid, Parathyroid, and Adrenal Glands, with Facts about Growth Disorders, Addison Disease, Cushing Syndrome, Conn Syndrome, Diabetic Disorders, Multiple Endocrine Neoplasia, Inborn Errors of Metabolism, and More

Along with Information about Endocrine Functioning, Diagnostic and Screening Tests, a Glossary of Related Terms, and Directories of Additional Resources

Edited by Joyce Brennfleck Shannon. 597 pages. 2007. 978-0-7808-0952-9.

SEE ALSO Diabetes Sourcebook, 4th Edition

▓

Environmental Health Sourcebook, 3rd Edition

Basic Consumer Health Information about the Environment and Its Effects on Human Health, Including Facts about Air, Water, and Soil Contamination, Hazardous Chemicals, Foodborne Hazards and Illnesses, Household Hazards Such as Radon, Mold, and Carbon Monoxide, Consumer Hazards from Toxic Products and Imported Goods, and Disorders

Linked to Environmental Causes, Including Chemical Sensitivity, Cancer, Allergies, and Asthma

Along with Information about the Impact of Environmental Hazards on Specific Populations, a Glossary of Related Terms, and Resources for Additional Help and Information.

Edited by Laura Larsen. 600 pages. 2010. 978-0-7808-1078-5

Ethnic Diseases Sourcebook

Basic Consumer Health Information for Ethnic and Racial Minority Groups in the United States, Including General Health Indicators and Behaviors, Ethnic Diseases, Genetic Testing, the Impact of Chronic Diseases, Women's Health, Mental Health Issues, and Preventive Health Care Services

Along with a Glossary and a Listing of Additional Resources

Edited by Joyce Brennfleck Shannon. 648 pages. 2001. 978-0-7808-0336-7.

"Not many books have been written on this topic to date, and the Ethnic Diseases Sourcebook is a strong addition to the list. It will be an important introductory resource for health consumers, students, health care personnel, and social scientists. It is recommended for public, academic, and large hospital libraries."
— American Reference Books Annual, 2002

"Will prove valuable to any library seeking to maintain a current, comprehensive reference collection of health resources... An excellent source of health information about genetic disorders which affect particular ethnic and racial minorities in the U.S."
—The Bookwatch, Aug '01

Eye Care Sourcebook, 3rd Edition

Basic Consumer Health Information about Eye Care and Eye Disorders, Including Facts about the Diagnosis, Prevention, and Treatment of Refractive Disorders, Cataracts, Glaucoma, Macular Degeneration, and Problems Affecting the Cornea, Retina, and Lacrimal Glands

Along with Advice about Preventing Eye Injuries and Tips for Living with Low Vision or Blindness, a Glossary of Related Terms, and Directories of Resources for More Help and Information

Edited by Amy L. Sutton. 646 pages. 2008. 978-0-7808-1000-6.

"A solid reference tool for eye care and a valuable addition to a collection."
—American Reference Books Annual, 2009

Family Planning Sourcebook

Basic Consumer Health Information about Planning for Pregnancy and Contraception, Including Traditional Methods, Barrier Methods, Hormonal Methods, Permanent Methods, Future Methods, Emergency Contraception, and Birth Control Choices for Women at Each Stage of Life

Along with Statistics, a Glossary, and Sources of Additional Information

Edited by Amy Marcaccio Keyzer. 503 pages. 2001. 978-0-7808-0379-4.

"Recommended for public, health, and undergraduate libraries as part of the circulating collection."
—E-Streams, Mar '02

"Will prove valuable to any library seeking to maintain a current, comprehensive reference collection of health resources... Excellent reference."
—The Bookwatch, Aug '01

SEE ALSO Pregnancy and Birth Sourcebook, 3rd Edition

Fitness and Exercise Sourcebook, 3rd Edition

Basic Consumer Health Information about the Physical and Mental Benefits of Fitness, Including Cardiorespiratory Endurance, Muscular Strength, Muscular Endurance, and Flexibility, with Facts about Sports Nutrition and Exercise-Related Injuries and Tips about Physical Activity and Exercises for People of All Ages and for People with Health Concerns

Along with Advice on Selecting and Using Exercise Equipment, Maintaining Exercise Motivation, a Glossary of Related Terms, and a Directory of Resources for More Help and Information

Edited by Amy L. Sutton. 635 pages. 2007. 978-0-7808-0946-8.

"Updates the consumer information on the physical and mental benefits of physical activity throughout the lifespan offered in earlier editions... Recommended. All readers; all levels."

—CHOICE, Oct '07

"An exceptionally well-rounded coverage perfect for any concerned about developing and understanding a fitness program."

—California Bookwatch, Jun '07

SEE ALSO Sports Injuries Sourcebook, 3rd Edition

Food Safety Sourcebook

Basic Consumer Health Information about the Safe Handling of Meat, Poultry, Seafood, Eggs, Fruit Juices, and Other Food Items, and Facts about Pesticides, Drinking Water, Food Safety Overseas, and the Onset, Duration, and Symptoms of Foodborne Illnesses, Including Types of Pathogenic Bacteria, Parasitic Protozoa, Worms, Viruses, and Natural Toxins

Along with the Role of the Consumer, the Food Handler, and the Government in Food Safety, a Glossary, and Resources for Additional Help and Information

Edited by Dawn D. Matthews. 327 pages. 1999. 978-0-7808-0326-8.

"Recommended reference source."

—Booklist, May '00

"This book takes the complex issues of food safety and foodborne pathogens and presents them in an easily understood manner. [It does] an excellent job of covering a large and often confusing topic."

— American Reference Books Annual, 2000

Forensic Medicine Sourcebook

Basic Consumer Information for the Layperson about Forensic Medicine, Including Crime Scene Investigation, Evidence Collection and Analysis, Expert Testimony, Computer-Aided Criminal Identification, Digital Imaging in the Courtroom, DNA Profiling, Accident Reconstruction, Autopsies, Ballistics, Drugs and Explosives Detection, Latent Fingerprints, Product Tampering, and Questioned Document Examination

Along with Statistical Data, a Glossary of Forensics Terminology, and Listings of Sources for Further Help and Information

Edited by Annemarie S. Muth. 574 pages. 1999. 978-0-7808-0232-2.

"Given the expected widespread interest in its content and its easy to read style, this book is recommended for most public and all college and university libraries."

—E-Streams, Feb '01

"A wealth of information, useful statistics, references are up-to-date and extremely complete. This wonderful collection of data will help students who are interested in a career in any type of forensic field. It is a great resource for attorneys who need information about types of expert witnesses needed in a particular case. It also offers useful information for fiction and nonfiction writers whose work involves a crime. A fascinating compilation. All levels."

—CHOICE, Jan '00

"There are several items that make this book attractive to consumers who are seeking certain forensic data... This is a useful current source for those seeking general forensic medical answers."

—American Reference Books Annual, 2000

Gastrointestinal Diseases and Disorders Sourcebook, 2nd Edition

Basic Consumer Health Information about the Upper and Lower Gastrointestinal (GI) Tract, Including the Esophagus, Stomach, Intestines, Rectum, Liver, and Pancreas, with Facts about Gastroesophageal Reflux Disease, Gastritis, Hernias, Ulcers, Celiac Disease, Diverticulitis, Irritable Bowel Syndrome, Hemorrhoids, Gastrointestinal Cancers, and Other Diseases and Disorders Related to the Digestive Process

Along with Information about Commonly Used Diagnostic and Surgical Procedures, Statistics, Reports on Current Research Initiatives and Clinical Trials, a Glossary, and Resources for Additional Help and Information

Edited by Sandra J. Judd. 654 pages. 2006. 978-0-7808-0798-3.

"The text is designed for the general reader seeking information on prevention, disease warning signs, diagnostic and therapeutic questions... It is an excellent resource for the general reader to conveniently locate credible, coordinated and indexed information... The sourcebook will prove very helpful for patients, caregivers and should be available in every physician waiting room."

—*Doody's Review Service, 2006*

SEE ALSO *Diet and Nutrition Sourcebook, 3rd Edition, Digestive Diseases and Disorders Sourcebook*

Genetic Disorders Sourcebook, 4th Edition

Basic Consumer Health Information about Hereditary Diseases and Disorders, Including Facts about the Human Genome, Genetic Inheritance Patterns, Disorders Associated with Specific Genes, Such as Sickle Cell Disease, Hemophilia, and Cystic Fibrosis, Chromosome Disorders, Such as Down Syndrome, Fragile X Syndrome, and Turner Syndrome, and Complex Diseases and Disorders Resulting from the Interaction of Environmental and Genetic Factors, Such as Allergies, Cancer, and Obesity

Along with Facts about Genetic Testing, Suggestions for Parents of Children with Special Needs, Reports on Current Research Initiatives, a Glossary of Genetic Terminology, and Resources for Additional Help and Information

Edited by Sandra J. Judd. 600 pages. 2010. 978-0-7808-1076-1.

Head Trauma Sourcebook

Basic Information for the Layperson about Open-Head and Closed-Head Injuries, Treatment Advances, Recovery, and Rehabilitation

Along with Reports on Current Research Initiatives

Edited by Karen Bellenir. 414 pages. 1997. 978-0-7808-0208-7.

Headache Sourcebook

Basic Consumer Health Information about Migraine, Tension, Cluster, Rebound and Other Types of Headaches, with Facts about

the Cause and Prevention of Headaches, the Effects of Stress and the Environment, Headaches during Pregnancy and Menopause, and Childhood Headaches

Along with a Glossary and Other Resources for Additional Help and Information

Edited by Dawn D. Matthews. 342 pages. 2002. 978-0-7808-0337-4.

"Highly recommended for academic and medical reference collections."

—*Library Bookwatch, Sep '02*

SEE ALSO *Pain Sourcebook, 3rd Edition*

Healthy Aging Sourcebook

Basic Consumer Health Information about Maintaining Health through the Aging Process, Including Advice on Nutrition, Exercise, and Sleep, Help in Making Decisions about Midlife Issues and Retirement, and Guidance Concerning Practical and Informed Choices in Health Consumerism

Along with Data Concerning the Theories of Aging, Different Experiences in Aging by Minority Groups, and Facts about Aging Now and Aging in the Future; and Featuring a Glossary, a Guide to Consumer Help, Additional Suggested Reading, and Practical Resource Directory

Edited by Jenifer Swanson. 537 pages. 1999. 978-0-7808-0390-9.

"Recommended reference source."

—*Booklist, Feb '00*

SEE ALSO *Adult Health Sourcebook, Physical and Mental Issues in Aging Sourcebook*

Healthy Children Sourcebook

Basic Consumer Health Information about the Physical and Mental Development of Children between the Ages of 3 and 12, Including Routine Health Care, Preventative Health Services, Safety and First Aid, Healthy Sleep, Dental Care, Nutrition, and Fitness, and Featuring Parenting Tips on Such Topics as Bedwetting, Choosing Day Care, Monitoring TV and Other Media, and Establishing a Foundation for Substance Abuse Prevention

Along with a Glossary of Commonly Used Pediatric Terms and Resources for Additional Help and Information.

Edited by Chad T. Kimball. 624 pages. 2003. 978-0-7808-0247-6.

"**Should be required reading for parents and teachers.**"
— *E-Streams, Jun '04*

"**It is hard to imagine that any other single resource exists that would provide such a comprehensive guide of timely information on health promotion and disease prevention for children aged 3 to 12.**"
— *American Reference Books Annual, 2004*

"**This easy-to-read volume is a tremendous resource.**"
— *AORN Journal, May '05*

SEE ALSO *Childhood Diseases and Disorders Sourcebook, 2nd Edition*

Healthy Heart Sourcebook for Women

Basic Consumer Health Information about Cardiac Issues Specific to Women, Including Facts about Major Risk Factors and Prevention, Treatment and Control Strategies, and Important Dietary Issues

Along with a Special Section Regarding the Pros and Cons of Hormone Replacement Therapy and Its Impact on Heart Health, and Additional Help, Including Recipes, a Glossary, and a Directory of Resources

Edited by Dawn D. Matthews. 321 pages. 2000. 978-0-7808-0329-9.

"**A good reference source and recommended for all public, academic, medical, and hospital libraries.**"
— *Medical Reference Services Quarterly, Summer '01*

"**Contains very important information about coronary artery disease that all women should know. The information is current and presented in an easy-to-read format. The book will make a good addition to any library.**"
— *American Medical Writers Association Journal, Summer '00*

SEE ALSO *Cardiovascular Diseases and Disorders Sourcebook, 4th Edition, Women's Health Concerns Sourcebook, 3rd Edition*

Hepatitis Sourcebook

Basic Consumer Health Information about Hepatitis A, Hepatitis B, Hepatitis C, and Other Forms of Hepatitis, Including Autoimmune Hepatitis, Alcoholic Hepatitis, Nonalcoholic Steatohepatitis, and Toxic Hepatitis, with Facts about Risk Factors, Screening Methods, Diagnostic Tests, and Treatment Options

Along with Information on Liver Health, Tips for People Living with Chronic Hepatitis, Reports on Current Research Initiatives, a Glossary of Terms Related to Hepatitis, and a Directory of Sources for Further Help and Information

Edited by Sandra J. Judd. 570 pages. 2006. 978-0-7808-0749-5.

"**The breadth of information found in this one book would not be readily found in another source. Highly recommended.**"
— *American Reference Books Annual, 2006*

SEE ALSO *Contagious Diseases Sourcebook, 2nd Edition*

Household Safety Sourcebook

Basic Consumer Health Information about Household Safety, Including Information about Poisons, Chemicals, Fire, and Water Hazards in the Home

Along with Advice about the Safe Use of Home Maintenance Equipment, Choosing Toys and Nursery Furniture, Holiday and Recreation Safety, a Glossary, and Resources for Further Help and Information

Edited by Dawn D. Matthews. 587 pages. 2002. 978-0-7808-0338-1.

"**As a sourcebook on household safety this book meets its mark. It is encyclopedic in scope and covers a wide range of safety issues that are commonly seen in the home.**"
— *E-Streams, Jul '02*

Hypertension Sourcebook

Basic Consumer Health Information about the Causes, Diagnosis, and Treatment of High Blood Pressure, with Facts about Consequences, Complications, and Co-Occurring Disorders, Such as Coronary Heart Disease, Diabetes, Stroke, Kidney Disease, and Hypertensive Retinopathy, and Issues in Blood Pressure

Control, Including Dietary Choices, Stress Management, and Medications

Along with Reports on Current Research Initiatives and Clinical Trials, a Glossary, and Resources for Additional Help and Information

Edited by Dawn D. Matthews and Karen Bellenir. 588 pages. 2004. 978-0-7808-0674-0.

"Academic, public, and medical libraries will want to add the Hypertension Sourcebook to their collections."
—*E-Streams, Aug '05*

"The strength of this source is the wide range of information given about hypertension."
—*American Reference Books Annual, 2005*

SEE ALSO *Stroke Sourcebook, 2nd Edition*

Immune System Disorders Sourcebook, 2nd Edition

Basic Consumer Health Information about Disorders of the Immune System, Including Immune System Function and Response, Diagnosis of Immune Disorders, Information about Inherited Immune Disease, Acquired Immune Disease, and Autoimmune Diseases, Including Primary Immune Deficiency, Acquired Immunodeficiency Syndrome (AIDS), Lupus, Multiple Sclerosis, Type 1 Diabetes, Rheumatoid Arthritis, and Graves' Disease

Along with Treatments, Tips for Coping with Immune Disorders, a Glossary, and a Directory of Additional Resources

Edited by Joyce Brennfleck Shannon. 643 pages. 2005. 978-0-7808-0748-8.

"Highly recommended for academic and public libraries."
—*American Reference Books Annual, 2006*

"The updated second edition is a 'must' for any consumer health library seeking a solid resource covering the treatments, symptoms, and options for immune disorder sufferers... An excellent guide."
—*MBR Bookwatch, Jan '06*

SEE ALSO *AIDS Sourcebook, 4th Edition, Arthritis Sourcebook, 3rd Edition*

Infant and Toddler Health Sourcebook

Basic Consumer Health Information about the Physical and Mental Development of Newborns, Infants, and Toddlers, Including Neonatal Concerns, Nutrition Recommendations, Immunization Schedules, Common Pediatric Disorders, Assessments and Milestones, Safety Tips, and Advice for Parents and Other Caregivers

Along with a Glossary of Terms and Resource Listings for Additional Help

Edited by Jenifer Swanson. 570 pages. 2000. 978-0-7808-0246-9.

"As a reference for the general public, this would be useful in any library."
—*E-Streams, May '01*

"Recommended reference source."
—*Booklist, Feb '01*

Infectious Diseases Sourcebook

Basic Consumer Health Information about Non-Contagious Bacterial, Viral, Prion, Fungal, and Parasitic Diseases Spread by Food and Water, Insects and Animals, or Environmental Contact, Including Botulism, E. Coli, Encephalitis, Legionnaires' Disease, Lyme Disease, Malaria, Plague, Rabies, Salmonella, Tetanus, and Others, and Facts about Newly Emerging Diseases, Such as Hantavirus, Mad Cow Disease, Monkeypox, and West Nile Virus

Along with Information about Preventing Disease Transmission, the Threat of Bioterrorism, and Current Research Initiatives, with a Glossary and Directory of Resources for More Information

Edited by Karen Bellenir. 610 pages. 2004. 978-0-7808-0675-7.

"This reference continues the excellent tradition of the Health Reference Series in consolidating a wealth of information on a selected topic into a format that is easy to use and accessible to the general public."
—*American Reference Books Annual, 2005*

"Recommended for public and academic libraries."
—*E-Streams, Jan '05*

SEE ALSO *Environmental Health Sourcebook, 3rd Edition*

Injury and Trauma Sourcebook

Basic Consumer Health Information about the Impact of Injury, the Diagnosis and Treatment of Common and Traumatic Injuries, Emergency Care, and Specific Injuries Related to Home, Community, Workplace, Transportation, and Recreation

Along with Guidelines for Injury Prevention, a Glossary, and a Directory of Additional Resources

Edited by Joyce Brennfleck Shannon. 675 pages. 2002. 978-0-7808-0421-0.

"Practitioners should be aware of guides such as this in order to facilitate their use by patients and their families."
—*Doody's Health Sciences Book Review Journal, Sep-Oct '02*

"Recommended reference source."
—*Booklist, Sep '02*

"Highly recommended for academic and medical reference collections."
—*Library Bookwatch, Sep '02*

SEE ALSO *Emergency Medical Services Sourcebook, Sports Injuries Sourcebook, 3rd Edition*

Learning Disabilities Sourcebook, 3rd Edition

Basic Consumer Health Information about Dyslexia, Auditory and Visual Processing Disorders, Communication Disorders, Dyscalculia, Dysgraphia, and Other Conditions That Impede Learning, Including Attention Deficit/Hyperactivity Disorder, Autism Spectrum Disorders, Hearing and Visual Impairments, Chromosome-Based Disorders, and Brain Injury

Along with Facts about Brain Function, Assessment, Therapy and Remediation, Accommodations, Assistive Technology, Legal Protections, and Tips about Family Life, School Transitions, and Employment Strategies, a Glossary of Related Terms, and Directories of Additional Resources

Edited by Joyce Brennfleck Shannon. 613 pages. 2009. 978-0-7808-1039-6.

"Intended to be a starting point for people who need to know about learning disabilities. Each chapter on a specific disability includes readable, well-organized descriptions... The book is well indexed and a glossary is included. Chapters on organizations and helpful websites will aid the reader who needs more information."
—*American Reference Books Annual, 2009*

"This book provides the necessary information to better understand learning disabilities and work with children who have them... It would be difficult to find another book that so comprehensively explains learning disabilities without becoming incomprehensible to the average parent who needs this information."
—*Doody's Review Service, 2009*

SEE ALSO *Attention Deficit Disorder Sourcebook, Autism and Pervasive Developmental Disorders Sourcebook*

Leukemia Sourcebook

Basic Consumer Health Information about Adult and Childhood Leukemias, Including Acute Lymphocytic Leukemia (ALL), Chronic Lymphocytic Leukemia (CLL), Acute Myelogenous Leukemia (AML), Chronic Myelogenous Leukemia (CML), and Hairy Cell Leukemia, and Treatments Such as Chemotherapy, Radiation Therapy, Peripheral Blood Stem Cell and Marrow Transplantation, and Immunotherapy

Along with Tips for Life During and After Treatment, a Glossary, and Directories of Additional Resources

Edited by Joyce Brennfleck Shannon. 564 pages. 2003. 978-0-7808-0627-6.

"Unlike other medical books for the layperson... the language does not talk down to the reader... This volume is highly recommended for all libraries."
—*American Reference Books Annual, 2004*

"A fine title which ranges from diagnosis to alternative treatments, staging, and tips for life during and after diagnosis."
—*The Bookwatch, Dec '03*

SEE ALSO *Blood & Circulatory Disorders Sourcebook, 3rd Edition, Cancer Sourcebook, 5th Edition*

Liver Disorders Sourcebook

Basic Consumer Health Information about the Liver and How It Works; Liver Diseases, Including Cancer, Cirrhosis, Hepatitis, and

Toxic and Drug Related Diseases; Tips for Maintaining a Healthy Liver; Laboratory Tests, Radiology Tests, and Facts about Liver Transplantation

Along with a Section on Support Groups, a Glossary, and Resource Listings

Edited by Joyce Brennfleck Shannon. 580 pages. 2000. 978-0-7808-0383-1.

"This title is recommended for health sciences and public libraries with consumer health collections."
—E-Streams, Oct '00

"Recommended reference source."
—Booklist, Jun '00

SEE ALSO Gastrointestinal Diseases and Disorders Sourcebook, 2nd Edition, Hepatitis Sourcebook

Lung Disorders Sourcebook

Basic Consumer Health Information about Emphysema, Pneumonia, Tuberculosis, Asthma, Cystic Fibrosis, and Other Lung Disorders, Including Facts about Diagnostic Procedures, Treatment Strategies, Disease Prevention Efforts, and Such Risk Factors as Smoking, Air Pollution, and Exposure to Asbestos, Radon, and Other Agents

Along with a Glossary and Resources for Additional Help and Information

Edited by Dawn D. Matthews. 657 pages. 2002. 978-0-7808-0339-8.

"Highly recommended for academic and medical reference collections."
—Library Bookwatch, Sep '02

SEE ALSO Asthma Sourcebook, 2nd Edition, Respiratory Disorders Sourcebook, 2nd Edition

Medical Tests Sourcebook, 3rd Edition

Basic Consumer Health Information about X-Rays, Blood Tests, Stool and Urine Tests, Biopsies, Mammography, Endoscopic Procedures, Ultrasound Exams, Computed Tomography, Magnetic Resonance Imaging (MRI), Nuclear Medicine, Genetic Testing, Home-Use Tests, and More

Along with Facts about Preventive Care and Screening Test Guidelines, Screening and

Assessment Tests Associated with Such Specific Concerns as Cancer, Heart Disease, Allergies, Diabetes, Thyroid Disfunction, and Infertility, a Glossary of Related Terms, and a Directory of Resources for Additional Help and Information

Edited by Karen Bellenir. 627 pages. 2008. 978-0-7808-1040-2

"This volume has a wide scope that makes it useful... Can be a valuable reference guide."
—American Reference Books Annual, 2009

"Would be a valuable contribution to any consumer health or public library."
—Doody's Book Review Service, 2009

Men's Health Concerns Sourcebook, 3rd Edition

Basic Consumer Health Information about Wellness in Men and Gender-Related Differences in Health, With Facts about Heart Disease, Cancer, Traumatic Injury, and Other Leading Causes of Death in Men, Reproductive Concerns, Sexual Dysfunction, Disorders of the Prostate, Penis, and Testes, Sex-Linked Genetic Disorders, and Other Medical and Mental Concerns of Men

Along with Statistical Data, a Glossary of Related Terms, and a Directory of Resources for Additional Information

Edited by Sandra J. Judd. 632 pages. 2009. 978-0-7808-1033-4.

"A good addition to any reference shelf in academic, consumer health, or hospital libraries."
—ARBAOnline, Oct '09

SEE ALSO Prostate and Urological Disorders Sourcebook

Mental Health Disorders Sourcebook, 4th Edition

Basic Consumer Health Information about the Causes and Symptoms of Mental Health Problems, Including Depression, Bipolar Disorder, Anxiety Disorders, Posttraumatic Stress Disorder, Obsessive-Compulsive Disorder, Eating Disorders, Addictions, and Personality and Psychotic Disorders

Along with Information about Medications and Treatments, Mental Health Concerns in

Children, Adolescents, and Adults, Tips on Living with Mental Health Disorders, a Glossary of Related Terms, and a Directory of Resources for Additional Help and Information

Edited by Amy L. Sutton. 680 pages. 2009. 978-0-7808-1041-9.

"Mental health concerns are presented in everyday language and intended for patients and their families as well as the general public... This resource is comprehensive and up to date... The easy-to-understand writing style helps to facilitate assimilation of needed facts and specifics on often challenging topics."
—*ARBAOnline, Oct '09*

"No health collection should be without this resource, which will reach into many a general lending library as well."
—*Internet Bookwatch, Oct '09*

SEE ALSO *Depression Sourcebook, 2nd Edition, Stress-Related Disorders Sourcebook, 2nd Edition*

Mental Retardation Sourcebook

Basic Consumer Health Information about Mental Retardation and Its Causes, Including Down Syndrome, Fetal Alcohol Syndrome, Fragile X Syndrome, Genetic Conditions, Injury, and Environmental Sources

Along with Preventive Strategies, Parenting Issues, Educational Implications, Health Care Needs, Employment and Economic Matters, Legal Issues, a Glossary, and a Resource Listing for Additional Help and Information

Edited by Joyce Brennfleck Shannon. 627 pages. 2000. 978-0-7808-0377-0.

"Public libraries will find the book useful for reference and as a beginning research point for students, parents, and caregivers."
—*American Reference Books Annual, 2001*

"The strength of this work is that it compiles many basic fact sheets and addresses for further information in one volume. It is intended and suitable for the general public."
—*E-Streams, Nov '00*

"An invaluable overview."
—*Reviewer's Bookwatch, Jul '00*

Movement Disorders Sourcebook, 2nd Edition

Basic Consumer Health Information about the Symptoms and Causes of Movement Disorders, Including Parkinson Disease, Amyotrophic Lateral Sclerosis, Cerebral Palsy, Muscular Dystrophy, Multiple Sclerosis, Myasthenia, Myoclonus, Spina Bifida, Dystonia, Essential Tremor, Choreatic Disorders, Huntington Disease, Tourette Syndrome, and Other Disorders That Cause Slowed, Absent, or Excessive Movements

Along with Information about Surgical and Nonsurgical Interventions, Physical Therapies, Strategies for Independent Living, a Glossary of Related Terms, and a Directory of Resources for Additional Help and Information

Edited by Amy L. Sutton. 618 pages. 2009. 978-0-7808-1034-1.

"The second updated edition of Movement Disorders Sourcebook is a winner, providing the latest research and health findings on all kinds of movement disorders in children and adults... a top pick for any health or general lending library's health reference collection."
—*California Bookwatch, Aug '09*

SEE ALSO *Muscular Dystrophy Sourcebook*

Multiple Sclerosis Sourcebook

Basic Consumer Health Information about Multiple Sclerosis (MS) and Its Effects on Mobility, Vision, Bladder Function, Speech, Swallowing, and Cognition, Including Facts about Risk Factors, Causes, Diagnostic Procedures, Pain Management, Drug Treatments, and Physical and Occupational Therapies

Along with Guidelines for Nutrition and Exercise, Tips on Choosing Assistive Equipment, Information about Disability, Work, Financial, and Legal Issues, a Glossary of Related Terms, and a Directory of Additional Resources

Edited by Joyce Brennfleck Shannon. 553 pages. 2007. 978-0-7808-0998-7.

Muscular Dystrophy Sourcebook

Basic Consumer Health Information about Congenital, Childhood-Onset, and Adult-Onset

Forms of Muscular Dystrophy, Such as Duchenne, Becker, Emery-Dreifuss, Distal, Limb-Girdle, Facioscapulohumeral (FSHD), Myotonic, and Ophthalmoplegic Muscular Dystrophies, Including Facts about Diagnostic Tests, Medical and Physical Therapies, Management of Co-Occurring Conditions, and Parenting Guidelines

Along with Practical Tips for Home Care, a Glossary, and Directories of Additional Resources

Edited by Joyce Brennfleck Shannon. 552 pages. 2004. 978-0-7808-0676-4.

"This book is highly recommended for public and academic libraries as well as health care offices that support the information needs of patients and their families."
—*E-Streams, Apr '05*

"Excellent reference."
—*The Bookwatch, Jan '05*

SEE ALSO *Movement Disorders Sourcebook, 2nd Edition*

■

Obesity Sourcebook
Basic Consumer Health Information about Diseases and Other Problems Associated with Obesity, and Including Facts about Risk Factors, Prevention Issues, and Management Approaches

Along with Statistical and Demographic Data, Information about Special Populations, Research Updates, a Glossary, and Source Listings for Further Help and Information

Edited by Wilma Caldwell and Chad T. Kimball. 360 pages. 2001. 978-0-7808-0333-6.

"The book synthesizes the reliable medical literature on obesity into one easy-to-read and useful resource for the general public."
—*American Reference Books Annual, 2002*

"Well suited for the health reference collection of a public library or an academic health science library that serves the general population."
—*E-Streams, Sep '01*

■

Osteoporosis Sourcebook
Basic Consumer Health Information about Primary and Secondary Osteoporosis and Juvenile Osteoporosis and Related Conditions, Including Fibrous Dysplasia, Gaucher Disease, Hyperthyroidism, Hypophosphatasia,

Myeloma, Osteopetrosis, Osteogenesis Imperfecta, and Paget's Disease

Along with Information about Risk Factors, Treatments, Traditional and Non-Traditional Pain Management, a Glossary of Related Terms, and a Directory of Resources

Edited by Allan R. Cook. 568 pages. 2001. 978-0-7808-0239-1.

"This resource is recommended as a great reference source for public, health, and academic libraries, and is another triumph for the editors of Omnigraphics."
—*American Reference Books Annual, 2002*

"Will prove valuable to any library seeking to maintain a current, comprehensive reference collection of health resources... From prevention to treatment and associated conditions, this provides an excellent survey."
—*The Bookwatch, Aug '01*

SEE ALSO *Healthy Aging Sourcebook, Women's Health Concerns Sourcebook, 3rd Edition*

■

Pain Sourcebook, 3rd Edition
Basic Consumer Health Information about Acute and Chronic Pain, Including Nerve Pain, Bone Pain, Muscle Pain, Cancer Pain, and Disorders Characterized by Pain, Such as Arthritis, Temporomandibular Muscle and Joint (TMJ) Disorder, Carpal Tunnel Syndrome, Headaches, Heartburn, Sciatica, and Shingles, and Facts about Diagnostic Tests and Treatment Options for Pain, Including Over-the-Counter and Prescription Drugs, Physical Rehabilitation, Injection and Infusion Therapies, Implantable Technologies, and Complementary Medicine

Along with Tips for Living with Pain, a Glossary of Related Terms, and a Directory of Additional Resources

Edited by Joyce Brennfleck Shannon. 644 pages. 2008. 978-0-7808-1006-8.

"Excellent for ready-reference users and can be used for beginning students in health fields... appropriate for the consumer health collection in both public and academic libraries."
—*American Reference Books Annual, 2009*

SEE ALSO Arthritis Sourcebook, 3rd Edition; Back and Neck Sourcebook, 2nd Edition;

Pediatric Cancer Sourcebook

Basic Consumer Health Information about Leukemias, Brain Tumors, Sarcomas, Lymphomas, and Other Cancers in Infants, Children, and Adolescents, Including Descriptions of Cancers, Treatments, and Coping Strategies

Along with Suggestions for Parents, Caregivers, and Concerned Relatives, a Glossary of Cancer Terms, and Resource Listings

Edited by Edward J. Prucha. 575 pages. 1999. 978-0-7808-0245-2.

"An excellent source of information. Recommended for public, hospital, and health science libraries with consumer health collections."
—E-Streams, Jun '00

"A valuable addition to all libraries specializing in health services and many public libraries."
—American Reference Books Annual, 2000

SEE ALSO *Childhood Diseases and Disorders Sourcebook, 2nd Edition, Healthy Children Sourcebook*

Physical and Mental Issues in Aging Sourcebook

Basic Consumer Health Information on Physical and Mental Disorders Associated with the Aging Process, Including Concerns about Cardiovascular Disease, Pulmonary Disease, Oral Health, Digestive Disorders, Musculoskeletal and Skin Disorders, Metabolic Changes, Sexual and Reproductive Issues, and Changes in Vision, Hearing, and Other Senses

Along with Data about Longevity and Causes of Death, Information on Acute and Chronic Pain, Descriptions of Mental Concerns, a Glossary of Terms, and Resource Listings for Additional Help

Edited by Jenifer Swanson. 660 pages. 1999. 978-0-7808-0233-9.

"This is a treasure of health information for the layperson."
—CHOICE Health Sciences Supplement, May '00

"Recommended for public libraries."
—American Reference Books Annual, 2000

SEE ALSO *Healthy Aging Sourcebook*

Podiatry Sourcebook, 2nd Edition

Basic Consumer Health Information about Disorders, Diseases, and Deformities that Affect the Foot and Ankle, Including Sprains, Corns, Calluses, Bunions, Plantar Warts, Plantar Fasciitis, Neuromas, Clubfoot, Flat Feet, Achilles Tendonitis, and Much More

Along with Information about Selecting a Foot Care Specialist, Foot Fitness, Shoes and Socks, Diagnostic Tests and Corrective Procedures, Financial Assistance for Corrective Devices, a Glossary of Related Terms, and a Directory of Resources for Additional Help and Information

Edited by Ivy L. Alexander. 516 pages. 2007. 978-0-7808-0944-4.

"An excellent resource... Although there have been various types of 'foot books' published in the past, none are as comprehensive as this one. 5 Stars (out of 5)!"
—Doody's Review Service, 2007

"Perfect for both health libraries and general-interest lending collections."
—Internet Bookwatch, Jul '07

Pregnancy and Birth Sourcebook, 3rd Edition

Basic Consumer Health Information about Pregnancy and Fetal Development, Including Facts about Fertility and Conception, Physical and Emotional Changes during Pregnancy, Prenatal Care and Diagnostic Tests, High-Risk Pregnancies and Complications, Labor, Delivery, and the Postpartum Period

Along with Tips on Maintaining Health and Wellness during Pregnancy and Caring for Newborn Infants, a Glossary of Related Terms, and Directories of Resources for Additional Help and Information

Edited by Amy L. Sutton. 645 pages. 2009. 978-0-7808-1074-7.

SEE ALSO *Breastfeeding Sourcebook, Congenital Disorders Sourcebook, 2nd Edition, Family Planning Sourcebook, Women's Health Concerns Sourcebook, 3rd Edition*

Prostate and Urological Disorders Sourcebook

Basic Consumer Health Information about Urogenital and Sexual Disorders in Men, Including Prostate and Other Andrological Cancers, Prostatitis, Benign Prostatic Hyperplasia, Testicular and Penile Trauma, Cryptorchidism, Peyronie Disease, Erectile Dysfunction, and Male Factor Infertility, and Facts about Commonly Used Tests and Procedures, Such as Prostatectomy, Vasectomy, Vasectomy Reversal, Penile Implants, and Semen Analysis

Along with a Glossary of Andrological Terms and a Directory of Resources for Additional Information

Edited by Karen Bellenir. 604 pages. 2006. 978-0-7808-0797-6.

"Certain to be a popular pick among library reference holdings... No prior knowledge is assumed for any of the conditions or terms herein, making it a most accessible general-interest reference."
—*California Bookwatch, Apr '06*

SEE ALSO *Men's Health Concerns Sourcebook, 3rd Edition, Urinary Tract and Kidney Diseases and Disorders Sourcebook, 2nd Edition*

Prostate Cancer Sourcebook

Basic Consumer Health Information about Prostate Cancer, Including Information about the Associated Risk Factors, Detection, Diagnosis, and Treatment of Prostate Cancer

Along with Information on Non-Malignant Prostate Conditions, and Featuring a Section Listing Support and Treatment Centers and a Glossary of Related Terms

Edited by Dawn D. Matthews. 340 pages. 2001. 978-0-7808-0324-4.

"Recommended reference source."
—*Booklist, Jan '02*

"A valuable resource for health care consumers seeking information on the subject... All text is written in a clear, easy-to-understand language that avoids technical jargon. Any library that collects consumer health resources would strengthen their collection with the addition of the Prostate Cancer Sourcebook."
—*American Reference Books Annual, 2002*

SEE ALSO *Cancer Sourcebook, 5th Edition, Men's Health Concerns Sourcebook, 3rd Edition*

Rehabilitation Sourcebook

Basic Consumer Health Information about Rehabilitation for People Recovering from Heart Surgery, Spinal Cord Injury, Stroke, Orthopedic Impairments, Amputation, Pulmonary Impairments, Traumatic Injury, and More, Including Physical Therapy, Occupational Therapy, Speech/Language Therapy, Massage Therapy, Dance Therapy, Art Therapy, and Recreational Therapy

Along with Information on Assistive and Adaptive Devices, a Glossary, and Resources for Additional Help and Information

Edited by Dawn D. Matthews. 519 pages. 2000. 978-0-7808-0236-0.

"This is an excellent resource for public library reference and health collections."
—*American Reference Books Annual, 2001*

"Recommended reference source."
—*Booklist, May '00*

Respiratory Disorders Sourcebook, 2nd Edition

Basic Consumer Health Information about Infectious, Inflammatory, and Chronic Conditions Affecting the Lungs and Respiratory System, Including Pneumonia, Bronchitis, Influenza, Tuberculosis, Sarcoidosis, Asthma, Cystic Fibrosis, Chronic Obstructive Pulmonary Disease, Lung Abscesses, Pulmonary Embolism, Occupational Lung Diseases, and Other Bacterial, Viral, and Fungal Infections

Along with Facts about the Structure and Function of the Lungs and Airways, Methods of Diagnosing Respiratory Disorders, and Treatment and Rehabilitation Options, a Glossary of Related Terms, and a Directory of Resources for Additional Help and Information

Edited by Sandra L. Judd. 638 pages. 2008. 978-0-7808-1007-5.

"An excellent book for patients, their families, or for those who are just curious about respiratory disease. Public libraries and physician offices would find this a valuable resource as well. 4 Stars! (out of 5)"
—*Doody's Review Service, 2009*

"A great addition for public and school libraries because it provides concise health information... readers can start with this reference source and get satisfactory answers before proceeding to other medical reference tools for

more in depth information... A good guide for health education on lung disorders."
—*American Reference Books Annual, 2009*

SEE ALSO *Asthma Sourcebook, 2nd Edition, Lung Disorders Sourcebook*

Sexually Transmitted Diseases Sourcebook, 4th Edition

Basic Consumer Health Information about Chlamydial Infections, Gonorrhea, Hepatitis, Herpes, HIV/AIDS, Human Papillomavirus, Pubic Lice, Scabies, Syphilis, Trichomoniasis, Vaginal Infections, and Other Sexually Transmitted Diseases, Including Facts about Risk Factors, Symptoms, Diagnosis, Treatment, and the Prevention of Sexually Transmitted Infections

Along with Updates on Current Research Initiatives, a Glossary of Related Terms, and Resources for Additional Help and Information

Edited by Laura Larsen. 623 pages. 2009. 978-0-7808-1073-0.

"Extremely beneficial... The question-and-answer format along with the index and table of contents make this well-organized resource extremely easy to reference, read, and comprehend... an invaluable medical reference source for lay readers, and a highly appropriate addition for public library collections, health clinics, and any library with a consumer health collection"
—*ARBAOnline, Oct '09*

SEE ALSO *AIDS Sourcebook, 4th Edition, Contagious Diseases Sourcebook, 2nd Edition, Men's Health Concerns Sourcebook, 3rd Edition, Women's Health Concerns Sourcebook, 3rd Edition*

Sleep Disorders Sourcebook, 3rd Edition

Basic Consumer Health Information about Sleep Disorders, Including Insomnia, Sleep Apnea and Snoring, Jet Lag and Other Circadian Rhythm Disorders, Narcolepsy, and Parasomnias, Such as Sleep Walking and Sleep Talking, and Featuring Facts about Other Health Problems that Affect Sleep, Why Sleep Is Necessary, How Much Sleep Is Needed, the Physical and Mental Effects of Sleep Deprivation, and Pediatric Sleep Issues

Along with Tips for Diagnosing and Treating Sleep Disorders, a Glossary of Related Terms, and a List of Resources for Additional Help and Information

Edited by Sandra J. Judd. 600 pages. 2010. 978-0-7808-1084-6.

Smoking Concerns Sourcebook

Basic Consumer Health Information about Nicotine Addiction and Smoking Cessation, Featuring Facts about the Health Effects of Tobacco Use, Including Lung and Other Cancers, Heart Disease, Stroke, and Respiratory Disorders, Such as Emphysema and Chronic Bronchitis

Along with Information about Smoking Prevention Programs, Suggestions for Achieving and Maintaining a Smoke-Free Lifestyle, Statistics about Tobacco Use, Reports on Current Research Initiatives, a Glossary of Related Terms, and Directories of Resources for Additional Help and Information

Edited by Karen Bellenir. 595 pages. 2004. 978-0-7808-0323-7.

"Provides everything needed for the student or general reader seeking practical details on the effects of tobacco use."
—*The Bookwatch, Mar '05*

"Public libraries and consumer health care libraries will find this work useful."
—*American Reference Books Annual, 2005*

SEE ALSO *Respiratory Disorders Sourcebook, 2nd Edition*

Sports Injuries Sourcebook, 3rd Edition

Basic Consumer Health Information about Sprains and Strains, Fractures, Growth Plate Injuries, Overtraining Injuries, and Injuries to the Head, Face, Shoulders, Elbows, Hands, Spinal Column, Knees, Ankles, and Feet, and with Facts about Heat-Related Illness, Steroids and Sport Supplements, Protective Equipment, Diagnostic Procedures, Treatment Options, and Rehabilitation

Along with a Glossary of Related Terms and a Directory of Resources for Additional Help and Information

Edited by Sandra J. Judd. 623 pages. 2007. 978-0-7808-0949-9.

SEE ALSO *Fitness and Exercise Sourcebook, 3rd Edition, Podiatry Sourcebook, 2nd Edition*

Stress-Related Disorders Sourcebook, 2nd Edition

Basic Consumer Health Information about Stress and Stress-Related Disorders, Including Types of Stress, Sources of Acute and Chronic Stress, the Impact of Stress on the Body's Systems, and Mental and Emotional Health Problems Associated with Stress, Such as Depression, Anxiety Disorders, Substance Abuse, Posttraumatic Stress Disorder, and Suicide

Along with Advice about Getting Help for Stress-Related Disorders, Information about Stress Management Techniques, a Glossary of Stress-Related Terms, and a Directory of Resources for Additional Help and Information

Edited by Amy L. Sutton. 608 pages. 2007. 978-0-7808-0996-3.

"Accessible to the lay reader. Highly recommended for medical and psychiatric collections."
—*Library Journal, Mar '08*

"Well-written for a general readership, the 2nd Edition of Stress-Related Disorders Sourcebook is a useful addition to the health reference literature."
—*American Reference Books Annual, 2008*

SEE ALSO *Mental Health Disorders Sourcebook, 4th Edition*

Stroke Sourcebook, 2nd Edition

Basic Consumer Health Information about Stroke, Including Ischemic, Hemorrhagic, and Mini Strokes, as Well as Risk Factors, Prevention Guidelines, Diagnostic Tests, Medications and Surgical Treatments, and Complications of Stroke

Along with Rehabilitation Techniques and Innovations, Tips on Staying Healthy and Maintaining Independence after Stroke, a Glossary of Related Terms, and a Directory of Resources for Stroke Survivors and Their Families

Edited by Amy L. Sutton. 626 pages. 2008. 978-0-7808-1035-8.

"An encyclopedic handbook on stroke that is written in a language the layperson can understand... This is one of the most helpful, readable books on stroke. This volume is highly recommended and should be in every medical, hospital and public library; in addition, every family practitioner should have a copy in his or her office."
—*American Reference Books Annual, 2009*

SEE ALSO *Brain Disorders Sourcebook, 3rd Edition, Hypertension Sourcebook*

Surgery Sourcebook, 2nd Edition

Basic Consumer Health Information about Common Inpatient and Outpatient Surgeries, Including Critical Care and Trauma, Gastrointestinal, Gynecologic and Obstetric, Cardiac and Vascular, Neurologic, Ophthalmologic, Orthopedic, Reconstructive and Cosmetic, and Other Major and Minor Surgeries

Along with Information about Anesthesia and Pain Relief Options, Risks and Complications, Postoperative Recovery Concerns, and Innovative Surgical Techniques and Tools, a Glossary of Related Terms, and a Directory of Additional Resources

Edited by Amy L. Sutton. 645 pages. 2008. 978-0-7808-1004-4.

"Large public libraries and medical libraries would benefit from this material in their reference collections."
—*American Reference Books Annual, 2009*

SEE ALSO *Cosmetic and Reconstructive Surgery Sourcebook, 2nd Edition*

Thyroid Disorders Sourcebook

Basic Consumer Health Information about Disorders of the Thyroid and Parathyroid Glands, Including Hypothyroidism, Hyperthyroidism, Graves Disease, Hashimoto Thyroiditis, Thyroid Cancer, and Parathyroid Disorders, Featuring Facts about Symptoms, Risk Factors, Tests, and Treatments

Along with Information about the Effects of Thyroid Imbalance on Other Body Systems, Environmental Factors That Affect the Thyroid Gland, a Glossary, and a Directory of Additional Resources

Edited by Joyce Brennfleck Shannon. 573 pages. 2005. 978-0-7808-0745-7.

"Recommended for consumer health collections."
—American Reference Books Annual, 2006

"Highly recommended pick for Basic Consumer health reference holdings at all levels."
—The Bookwatch, Aug '05

SEE ALSO Endocrine and Metabolic Disorders Sourcebook, 2nd Edition

Transplantation Sourcebook

Basic Consumer Health Information about Organ and Tissue Transplantation, Including Physical and Financial Preparations, Procedures and Issues Relating to Specific Solid Organ and Tissue Transplants, Rehabilitation, Pediatric Transplant Information, the Future of Transplantation, and Organ and Tissue Donation

Along with a Glossary and Listings of Additional Resources

Edited by Joyce Brennfleck Shannon. 610 pages. 2002. 978-0-7808-0322-0.

"Recommended for libraries with an interest in offering consumer health information."
—E-Streams, Jul '02

"This is a unique and valuable resource for patients facing transplantation and their families."
—Doody's Review Service, Jun '02

Traveler's Health Sourcebook

Basic Consumer Health Information for Travelers, Including Physical and Medical Preparations, Transportation Health and Safety, Essential Information about Food and Water, Sun Exposure, Insect and Snake Bites, Camping and Wilderness Medicine, and Travel with Physical or Medical Disabilities

Along with International Travel Tips, Vaccination Recommendations, Geographical Health Issues, Disease Risks, a Glossary, and a Listing of Additional Resources

Edited by Joyce Brennfleck Shannon. 619 pages. 2000. 978-0-7808-0384-8.

"Recommended reference source."
—Booklist, Feb '01

"This book is recommended for any public library, any travel collection, and especially any collection for the physically disabled."
—American Reference Books Annual, 2001

SEE ALSO Worldwide Health Sourcebook

Urinary Tract and Kidney Diseases and Disorders Sourcebook, 2nd Edition

Basic Consumer Health Information about the Urinary System, Including the Bladder, Urethra, Ureters, and Kidneys, with Facts about Urinary Tract Infections, Incontinence, Congenital Disorders, Kidney Stones, Cancers of the Urinary Tract and Kidneys, Kidney Failure, Dialysis, and Kidney Transplantation

Along with Statistical and Demographic Information, Reports on Current Research in Kidney and Urologic Health, a Summary of Commonly Used Diagnostic Tests, a Glossary of Related Terms, and a Directory of Resources for Additional Help and Information

Edited by Ivy L. Alexander. 621 pages. 2005. 978-0-7808-0750-1.

"A good choice for a consumer health information library or for a medical library needing information to refer to their patients."
—American Reference Books Annual, 2006

SEE ALSO Prostate and Urological Disorders Sourcebook

Vegetarian Sourcebook

Basic Consumer Health Information about Vegetarian Diets, Lifestyle, and Philosophy, Including Definitions of Vegetarianism and Veganism, Tips about Adopting Vegetarianism, Creating a Vegetarian Pantry, and Meeting Nutritional Needs of Vegetarians, with Facts Regarding Vegetarianism's Effect on Pregnant and Lactating Women, Children, Athletes, and Senior Citizens

Along with a Glossary of Commonly Used Vegetarian Terms and Resources for Additional Help and Information

Edited by Chad T. Kimball. 337 pages. 2002. 978-0-7808-0439-5.

"Organizes into one concise volume the answers to the most common questions concerning vegetarian diets and lifestyles. This title is recommended for public and secondary school libraries."

—E-Streams, Apr '03

"**Invaluable reference for public and school library collections alike.**"
—Library Bookwatch, Apr '03

"**The articles in this volume are easy to read and come from authoritative sources. The book does not necessarily support the vegetarian diet but instead provides the pros and cons of this important decision... Recommended for public libraries and consumer health libraries.**"
—American Reference Books Annual, 2003

SEE ALSO *Diet and Nutrition Sourcebook, 3rd Edition*

Women's Health Concerns Sourcebook, 3rd Edition

Basic Consumer Health Information about Issues and Trends in Women's Health and Health Conditions of Special Concern to Women, Including Endometriosis, Uterine Fibroids, Menstrual Irregularities, Menopause, Sexual Dysfunction, Infertility, Cancer in Women, and Other Such Chronic Disorders as Lupus, Fibromyalgia, and Thyroid Disease

Along with Statistical Data, Tips for Maintaining Wellness, a Glossary, and a Directory of Resources for Further Help and Information

Edited by Sandra J. Judd. 679 pages. 2009. 978-0-7808-1036-5.

"**This useful resource provides information about a wide range of topics that will help women understand their bodies, prevent or treat disease, and maintain health... A detailed index helps readers locate information. This is a useful addition to public and consumer health library collections**"
—ARBAOnline, Jun '09

SEE ALSO *Breast Cancer Sourcebook, 3rd Edition, Cancer Sourcebook for Women, 4th Edition, Healthy Heart Sourcebook for Women*

Workplace Health and Safety Sourcebook

Basic Consumer Health Information about Workplace Health and Safety, Including the Effect of Workplace Hazards on the Lungs,

Skin, Heart, Ears, Eyes, Brain, Reproductive Organs, Musculoskeletal System, and Other Organs and Body Parts

Along with Information about Occupational Cancer, Personal Protective Equipment, Toxic and Hazardous Chemicals, Child Labor, Stress, and Workplace Violence

Edited by Chad T. Kimball. 610 pages. 2000. 978-0-7808-0231-5.

"**As a reference for the general public, this would be useful in any library.**"
—E-Streams, Jun '01

"**Provides helpful information for primary care physicians and other caregivers interested in occupational medicine... General readers; professionals.**"
—CHOICE, May '01

Worldwide Health Sourcebook

Basic Information about Global Health Issues, Including Malnutrition, Reproductive Health, Disease Dispersion and Prevention, Emerging Diseases, Risky Health Behaviors, and the Leading Causes of Death

Along with Global Health Concerns for Children, Women, and the Elderly, Mental Health Issues, Research and Technology Advancements, and Economic, Environmental, and Political Health Implications, a Glossary, and a Resource Listing for Additional Help and Information

Edited by Joyce Brennfleck Shannon. 597 pages. 2001. 978-0-7808-0330-5.

"**Named an Outstanding Academic Title.**"
—CHOICE, Jan '02

"**Yet another handy but also unique compilation in the extensive Health Reference Series, this is a useful work because many of the international publications reprinted or excerpted are not readily available. Highly recommended.**"
—CHOICE, Nov '01

SEE ALSO *Traveler's Health Sourcebook*

Teen Health Series
Complete Catalog
List price $69 per volume. School and library price $62 per volume.

Abuse and Violence Information for Teens
Health Tips about the Causes and Consequences of Abusive and Violent Behavior
Including Facts about the Types of Abuse and Violence, the Warning Signs of Abusive and Violent Behavior, Health Concerns of Victims, and Getting Help and Staying Safe

Edited by Sandra Augustyn Lawton. 411 pages. 2008. 978-0-7808-1008-2.

"A useful resource for schools and organizations providing services to teens and may also be a starting point in research projects."
—*Reference and Research Book News, Aug '08*

"Violence is a serious problem for teens... This resource gives teens the information they need to face potential threats and get help—either for themselves or for their friends."
—*American Reference Books Annual, 2009*

Accident and Safety Information for Teens
Health Tips about Medical Emergencies, Traumatic Injuries, and Disaster Preparedness
Including Facts about Motor Vehicle Accidents, Burns, Poisoning, Firearms, Natural Disasters, National Security Threats, and More

Edited by Karen Bellenir. 420 pages. 2008. 978-0-7808-1046-4.

"Aimed at teenage audiences, this guide provides practical information for handling a comprehensive list of emergencies, from sport injuries and auto accidents to alcohol poisoning and natural disasters."
—*Library Journal, Apr 1, '09*

"Useful in the young adult collections of public libraries as well as high school libraries."
—*American Reference Books Annual, 2009*

SEE ALSO *Sports Injuries Information for Teens, 2nd Edition*

Alcohol Information for Teens, 2nd Edition
Health Tips about Alcohol and Alcoholism
Including Facts about Alcohol's Effects on the Body, Brain, and Behavior, the Consequences of Underage Drinking, Alcohol Abuse Prevention and Treatment, and Coping with Alcoholic Parents

Edited by Lisa Bakewell. 410 pages. 2009. 978-0-7808-1043-3.

"This handbook, written for a teenage audience, provides information on the causes, effects, and preventive measures related to alcohol abuse among teens... The chapters are quick to make a connection to their teenage reading audience. The prose is straightforward and the book lends itself to spot reading. It should be useful both for practical information and for research, and it is suitable for public and school libraries."
—*ARBAOnline, Jun '09*

SEE ALSO *Drug Information for Teens, 2nd Edition*

Allergy Information for Teens
Health Tips about Allergic Reactions Such as Anaphylaxis, Respiratory Problems, and Rashes
Including Facts about Identifying and Managing Allergies to Food, Pollen, Mold, Animals, Chemicals, Drugs, and Other Substances

Edited by Karen Bellenir. 410 pages. 2006. 978-0-7808-0799-0.

"This is a comprehensive, readable text on the subject of allergic diseases in teenagers. 5 Stars (out of 5)!"
—*Doody's Review Service, Jun '06*

"This authoritative and useful self-help title is a solid addition to YA collections, whether for personal interest or reports."
—*School Library Journal, Jul '06*

Asthma Information for Teens, 2nd Ed.
Health Tips about Managing Asthma and Related Concerns

Including Facts about Asthma Causes, Triggers and Symptoms, Diagnosis, and Treatment

Edited by Kim Wohlenhaus. 400 pages. 2010. 978-0-7808-1086-0.

Body Information for Teens
Health Tips about Maintaining Well-Being for a Lifetime
Including Facts about the Development and Functioning of the Body's Systems, Organs, and Structures and the Health Impact of Lifestyle Choices

Edited by Sandra Augustyn Lawton. 458 pages. 2007. 978-0-7808-0443-2.

Cancer Information for Teens, 2nd Edition
Health Tips about Cancer Awareness, Symptoms, Prevention, Diagnosis, and Treatment
Including Facts about Common Cancers Affecting Teens, Causes, Detection, Coping Strategies, Clinical Trials, Nutrition and Exercise, Cancer in Friends or Family, and More

Edited by Karen Bellenir and Lisa Bakewell. 445 pages. 2010. 978-0-7808-1085-3.

Complementary and Alternative Medicine Information for Teens
Health Tips about Non-Traditional and Non-Western Medical Practices
Including Information about Acupuncture, Chiropractic Medicine, Dietary and Herbal Supplements, Hypnosis, Massage Therapy, Prayer and Spirituality, Reflexology, Yoga, and More

Edited by Sandra Augustyn Lawton. 407 pages. 2007. 978-0-7808-0966-6.

"This volume covers CAM specifically for teenagers but of general use also. It should be a welcome addition to both public and academic libraries."
—*American Reference Books Annual, 2008*

"This volume provides a solid foundation for further investigation of the subject, making it useful for both public and high school libraries."
—*VOYA: Voice of Youth Advocates, Jun '07*

Diabetes Information for Teens
Health Tips about Managing Diabetes and Preventing Related Complications
Including Information about Insulin, Glucose Control, Healthy Eating, Physical Activity, and Learning to Live with Diabetes

Edited by Sandra Augustyn Lawton. 410 pages. 2006. 978-0-7808-0811-9.

"A comprehensive instructional guide for teens... some of the material may also be directed towards parents or teachers. 5 stars (out of 5)!"
—*Doody's Review Service, 2006*

"Students dealing with their own diabetes or that of a friend or family member or those writing reports on the topic will find this a valuable resource."
—*School Library Journal, Aug '06*

"This text is directed to the teen population and would be an excellent library resource for a health class or for the teacher as a reference for class preparation. It can, however, serve a much wider audience. The clinical educator on diabetes may find it valuable to educate the newly diagnosed client regardless of age. It also would be an excellent reference and education tool for a preventive medicine seminar on diabetes."
—*Physical Therapy, Mar '07*

Diet Information for Teens, 2nd Edition
Health Tips about Diet and Nutrition
Including Facts about Dietary Guidelines, Food Groups, Nutrients, Healthy Meals, Snacks, Weight Control, Medical Concerns Related to Diet, and More

Edited by Karen Bellenir. 432 pages. 2006. 978-0-7808-0820-1.

"A very quick and pleasant read in spite of the fact that it is very detailed in the information it gives... A book for anyone concerned about diet and nutrition."
—*American Reference Books Annual, 2007*

SEE ALSO Eating Disorders Information for Teens, 2nd Edition

Drug Information for Teens, 2nd Edition
Health Tips about the Physical and Mental Effects of Substance Abuse
Including Information about Marijuana, Inhalants, Club Drugs, Stimulants, Hallucinogens, Opiates, Prescription and Over-the-Counter Drugs, Herbal Products, Tobacco, Alcohol, and More

Edited by Sandra Augustyn Lawton. 468 pages. 2006. 978-0-7808-0862-1.

"As with earlier installments in Omnigraphics' Teen Health Series, Drug Information for Teens is designed specifically to meet the needs and interests of middle and high school students... Strongly recommended for both academic and public libraries."
—*American Reference Books Annual, 2007*

"Solid thoughtful advice is given about how to handle peer pressure, drug-related health concerns, and treatment strategies."
—*School Library Journal, Dec '06*

SEE ALSO *Alcohol Information for Teens, 2nd Edition, Tobacco Information for Teens, 2nd Edition*

Eating Disorders Information for Teens, 2nd Edition
Health Tips about Anorexia, Bulimia, Binge Eating, And Other Eating Disorders
Including Information about Risk Factors, Diagnosis and Treatment, Prevention, Related Health Concerns, and Other Issues

Edited by Sandra Augustyn Lawton. 377 pages. 2009. 978-0-7808-1044-0.

"This handy reference offers basic information and addresses specific disorders, consequences, prevention, diagnosis and treatment, healthy eating, and more. It is written in a conversational style that is easy to understand... Will provide plenty of facts for reports as well as browsing potential for students with an interest in the topic.
—*School Library Journal, Jun '09*

"Written in a straightforward style that will appeal to its teenage audience. The author does not play down the danger of living with an eating disorder and urges those struggling with this problem to seek professional help.

This work, as well as others in this series, will be a welcome addition to high school and undergraduate libraries."
—*American Reference Books Annual, 2009*

SEE ALSO *Diet Information for Teens, 2nd Edition*

Fitness Information for Teens, 2nd Edition
Health Tips about Exercise, Physical Well-Being, and Health Maintenance
Including Facts about Conditioning, Stretching, Strength Training, Body Shape and Body Image, Sports Nutrition, and Specific Activities for Athletes and Non-Athletes

Edited by Lisa Bakewell. 432 pages. 2009. 978-0-7808-1045-7.

"This no-nonsense guide packs a great deal into its pages... This is a helpful reference for basic diet and exercise information for health reports or personal use."
—*School Library Journal, April 2009*

"An excellent source for general information on why teens should be active, making time to exercise, the equipment people might need, various types of activities to try, how to maintain health and wellness, and how to avoid barriers to becoming healthier... This would still be an excellent addition to a public library ready-reference collection or a high school health library collection."
—*American Reference Books Annual, 2009*

"This easy to read, well-written, up-to-date overview of fitness for teenagers provides excellent wellness and exercise tips, information, and directions... It is a useful tool for them to obtain a base knowledge in fitness topics and different sports."
—*Doody's Review Service, 2009*

SEE ALSO *Diet Information for Teens, 2nd Edition, Sports Injuries Information for Teens, 2nd Edition*

Learning Disabilities Information for Teens
Health Tips about Academic Skills Disorders and Other Disabilities That Affect Learning

Including Information about Common Signs of Learning Disabilities, School Issues, Learning to Live with a Learning Disability, and Other Related Issues

Edited by Sandra Augustyn Lawton. 400 pages. 2006. 978-0-7808-0796-9.

"This book provides a wealth of information for any reader interested in the signs, causes, and consequences of learning disabilities, as well as related legal rights and educational interventions... Public and academic libraries should want this title for both students and general readers."
—American Reference Books Annual, 2006

Mental Health Information for Teens, 3rd Edition
Health Tips about Mental Wellness and Mental Illness
Including Facts about Mental and Emotional Health, Depression and Other Mood Disorders, Anxiety Disorders, Behavior Disorders, Self-Injury, Psychosis, Schizophrenia, and More

Edited by Karen Bellenir. 400 pages. 2010. 978-0-7808-1087-7.

SEE ALSO Stress Information for Teens, Suicide Information for Teens, 2nd Edition

Pregnancy Information for Teens
Health Tips about Teen Pregnancy and Teen Parenting
Including Facts about Prenatal Care, Pregnancy Complications, Labor and Delivery, Postpartum Care, Pregnancy-Related Lifestyle Concerns, and More

Edited by Sandra Augustyn Lawton. 434 pages. 2007. 978-0-7808-0984-0.

Sexual Health Information for Teens, 2nd Edition
Health Tips about Sexual Development, Reproduction, Contraception, and Sexually Transmitted Infections
Including Facts about Puberty, Sexuality, Birth Control, Chlamydia, Gonorrhea, Herpes, Human Papillomavirus, Syphilis, and More

Edited by Sandra Augustyn Lawton. 430 pages. 2008. 978-0-7808-1010-5.

"This offering represents the most up-to-date information available on an array of topics including abstinence-only sexual education and pregnancy-prevention methods... The range of coverage—from puberty and anatomy to sexually transmitted diseases—is thorough and extensive. Each chapter includes a bibliographic citation, and the three back sections containing additional resources, further reading, and the index are all first-rate... This volume will be well used by students in need of the facts, whether for educational or personal reasons."
—School Library Journal, Nov '08

"Presents information related to the emotional, physical, and biological development of both males and females that occurs during puberty. It also strives to address some of the issues and questions that may arise... The text is easy to read and understand for young readers, with satisfactory definitions within the text to explain new terms."
—American Reference Books Annual, 2009

Skin Health Information for Teens, 2nd Edition
Health Tips about Dermatological Concerns and Skin Cancer Risks
Including Facts about Acne, Warts, Hives, and Other Conditions and Lifestyle Choices, Such as Tanning, Tattooing, and Piercing, That Affect the Skin, Nails, Scalp, and Hair

Edited by Edited by Kim Wohlenhaus. 418 pages. 2009. 978-0-7808-1042-6.

"The material in this work will be easily understood by teenagers and young adults. The publisher has liberally used bulleted lists and sidebars to keep the reader's attention... A useful addition to school and public library collections."
—ARBAOnline, Oct '09

Sleep Information for Teens
Health Tips about Adolescent Sleep Requirements, Sleep Disorders, and the Effects of Sleep Deprivation
Including Facts about Why People Need Sleep, Sleep Patterns, Circadian Rhythms, Dreaming, Insomnia, Sleep Apnea, Narcolepsy, and More

Edited by Karen Bellenir. 355 pages. 2008. 978-0-7808-1009-9.

"Clear, concise, and very readable and would be a good source of sleep information for anyone—not just teenagers. This work is highly recommended for medical libraries, public school libraries, and public libraries."
—*American Reference Books Annual, 2009*

SEE ALSO Body Information for Teens

Sports Injuries Information for Teens, 2nd Edition
Health Tips about Acute, Traumatic, and Chronic Injuries in Adolescent Athletes
Including Facts about Sprains, Fractures, and Overuse Injuries, Treatment, Rehabilitation, Sport-Specific Safety Guidelines, Fitness Suggestions, and More

Edited by Karen Bellenir. 429 pages. 2008. 978-0-7808-1011-2.

"An engaging selection of informative articles about the prevention and treatment of sports injuries... The value of this book is that the articles have been vetted and are often augmented with inserts of useful facts, definitions of technical terms, and quick tips. Sensitive topics like injuries to genitalia are discussed openly and responsibly. This revised edition contains updated articles and defines sport more broadly than the first edition."
—*School Library Journal, Nov '08*

"This work will be useful in the young adult collections of public libraries as well as high school libraries... A useful resource for student research."
—*American Reference Books Annual, 2009*

SEE ALSO Accident and Safety Information for Teens

Stress Information for Teens
Health Tips about the Mental and Physical Consequences of Stress
Including Information about the Different Kinds of Stress, Symptoms of Stress, Frequent Causes of Stress, Stress Management Techniques, and More

Edited by Sandra Augustyn Lawton. 392 pages. 2008. 978-0-7808-1012-9.

"Understanding what stress is, what causes it, how the body and the mind are impacted by it, and what teens can do are the general categories addressed here... The chapters are brief but informative, and the list of community-help organizations is exhaustive. Report writers will find information quickly and easily, as will those who have personal concerns. The print is clear and the format is readable, making this an accessible resource for struggling readers and researchers."
—*School Library Journal, Dec '08*

"The articles selected will specifically appeal to young adults and are designed to answer their most common questions."
— *American Reference Books Annual, 2009*

SEE ALSO Mental Health Information for Teens, 3rd Edition

Suicide Information for Teens, 2nd Edition
Health Tips about Suicide Causes and Prevention
Including Facts about Depression, Risk Factors, Getting Help, Survivor Support, and More

Edited by Kim Wohlenhaus. 400 pages. 2010. 978-0-7808-1088-4.

SEE ALSO Mental Health Information for Teens, 3rd Edition

Tobacco Information for Teens, 2nd Edition
Health Tips about the Hazards of Using Cigarettes, Smokeless Tobacco, and Other Nicotine Products
Including Facts about Nicotine Addiction, Nicotine Delivery Systems, Secondhand Smoke, Health Consequences of Tobacco Use, Related Cancers, Smoking Cessation, and Tobacco Use Statistics

Edited by Karen Bellenir. 400 pages. 2010. 978-0-7808-1153-9.

SEE ALSO Drug Information for Teens, 2nd Edition

Health Reference Series

Adolescent Health Sourcebook, 3rd Edition

Adult Health Concerns Sourcebook

AIDS Sourcebook, 4th Edition

Alcoholism Sourcebook, 3rd Edition

Allergies Sourcebook, 3rd Edition

Alzheimer Disease Sourcebook, 4th Edition

Arthritis Sourcebook, 3rd Edition

Asthma Sourcebook, 2nd Edition

Attention Deficit Disorder Sourcebook

Autism & Pervasive Developmental Disorders Sourcebook

Back & Neck Sourcebook, 2nd Edition

Blood & Circulatory Disorders Sourcebook, 3rd Edition

Brain Disorders Sourcebook, 3rd Edition

Breast Cancer Sourcebook, 3rd Edition

Breastfeeding Sourcebook

Burns Sourcebook

Cancer Sourcebook for Women, 4th Edition

Cancer Sourcebook, 5th Edition

Cancer Survivorship Sourcebook

Cardiovascular Disorders Sourcebook, 4th Edition

Caregiving Sourcebook

Child Abuse Sourcebook

Childhood Diseases & Disorders Sourcebook, 2nd Edition

Colds, Flu & Other Common Ailments Sourcebook

Communication Disorders Sourcebook

Complementary & Alternative Medicine Sourcebook, 4th Edition

Congenital Disorders Sourcebook, 2nd Edition

Contagious Diseases Sourcebook

Cosmetic & Reconstructive Surgery Sourcebook, 2nd Edition

Death & Dying Sourcebook, 2nd Edition

Dental Care & Oral Health Sourcebook, 3rd Edition

Depression Sourcebook, 2nd Edition

Dermatological Disorders Sourcebook, 2nd Edition

Diabetes Sourcebook, 4th Edition

Diet & Nutrition Sourcebook, 3rd Edition

Digestive Diseases & Disorder Sourcebook

Disabilities Sourcebook

Disease Management Sourcebook

Domestic Violence Sourcebook, 3rd Edition

Drug Abuse Sourcebook, 3rd Edition

Ear, Nose & Throat Disorders Sourcebook, 2nd Edition

Eating Disorders Sourcebook, 3rd Edition

Emergency Medical Services Sourcebook

Endocrine & Metabolic Disorders Sourcebook, 2nd Edition

Environmental Health Sourcebook, 3rd Edition

Ethnic Diseases Sourcebook

Eye Care Sourcebook, 3rd Edition

Family Planning Sourcebook

Fitness & Exercise Sourcebook, 4th Edition

Food Safety Sourcebook

Forensic Medicine Sourcebook

Gastrointestinal Diseases & Disorders Sourcebook, 2nd Edition

Genetic Disorders Sourcebook, 3rd Edition

Head Trauma Sourcebook

Headache Sourcebook

Health Insurance Sourcebook

Healthy Aging Sourcebook

Healthy Children Sourcebook

Healthy Heart Sourcebook for Women

Hepatitis Sourcebook

Household Safety Sourcebook

Hypertension Sourcebook

Immune System Disorders Sourcebook, 2nd Edition

Infant & Toddler Health Sourcebook

Infectious Diseases Sourcebook

Injury & Trauma Sourcebook